Non-Small Cell Lung Cancer

Non-Small Cell Lung Cancer

Editor: Jute Cassie

FOSTER ACADEMICS

www.fosteracademics.com

www.fosteracademics.com

FOSTER ACADEMICS

Cataloging-in-Publication Data

Non-small cell lung cancer / edited by Jute Cassie.
p. cm.
Includes bibliographical references and index.
ISBN 978-1-64646-627-6
1. Lungs--Cancer. 2. Small cell lung cancer. 3. Lungs--Cancer--Diagnosis.
4. Lungs--Cancer--Treatment. 5. Lungs--Diseases. I. Cassie, Jute.
RC280.L8 N66 2023
616.994 24--dc23

Foster Academics,
118-35 Queens Blvd., Suite 400,
Forest Hills, NY 11375, USA

ISBN 978-1-64646-627-6 (Hardback)

Contents

Preface

The purpose of the book is to provide a glimpse into the dynamics and to present opinions and studies of some of the scientists engaged in the development of new ideas in the field from very different standpoints. This book will prove useful to students and researchers owing to its high content quality.

Non-small cell lung cancer (NSCLC) refers to a type of disease in which malignant cells develop in lung tissues. The symptoms of NSCLC are shortness of breath and a persistent cough. NSCLC is primarily divided into three types, including adenocarcinoma, squamous cell carcinoma and large cell carcinoma. Smoking is the leading risk factor of NSCLC. Other risk factors include exposure to radiation, family history and exposure to second hand smoke. Chest X-ray, thoracentesis, CT scan, physical exam and health history, sputum cytology and laboratory tests are used to diagnose NSCLC. Patients with NSCLC can receive a variety of treatments, including laser therapy, surgery, chemotherapy, electrocautery, radiation therapy, targeted therapy and cryosurgery. This book provides significant information to help develop a good understanding of non-small cell lung cancer. Those with an interest in the study of this disease would find this book helpful.

At the end, I would like to appreciate all the efforts made by the authors in completing their chapters professionally. I express my deepest gratitude to all of them for contributing to this book by sharing their valuable works. A special thanks to my family and friends for their constant support in this journey.

Editor

1

Exploiting ING2 Epigenetic Modulation as a Therapeutic Opportunity for Non-Small Cell Lung Cancer

Alice Blondel [1], Amine Benberghout [1], Rémy Pedeux [1] and Charles Ricordel [1,2,*]

[1] INSERM U1242, Chemistry Oncogenesis Stress and Signaling, CLCC Eugène Marquis, 35033 Rennes, France; alice.blondel@univ-rennes1.fr (A.B.); benberghout.amine@gmail.com (A.B.); remy.pedeux@univ-rennes1.fr (R.P.)

[2] CHU Rennes, Service de Pneumologie, Université de Rennes 1, 35033 Rennes, France

* Correspondence: charles.ricordel@chu-rennes.fr

Abstract: Non-small cell lung cancer (NSCLC) has been the leading cause of cancer-related death worldwide, over the last few decades. Survival remains extremely poor in the metastatic setting and, consequently, innovative therapeutic strategies are urgently needed. Inhibitor of Growth Gene 2 (ING2) is a core component of the mSin3A/Histone deacetylases complex (HDAC), which controls the chromatin acetylation status and modulates gene transcription. This gene has been characterized as a tumor suppressor gene and its status in cancer has been scarcely explored. In this review, we focused on ING2 and other mSin3A/HDAC member statuses in NSCLC. Taking advantage of existing public databases and known pharmacological properties of HDAC inhibitors, finally, we proposed a therapeutic model based on an ING2 biomarker-guided strategy.

Keywords: ING2; ING1; ING3; ING4; ING5; non-small cell lung cancer; NSCLC; mSin3A/HDAC complex; chromatin remodeling; HDAC inhibitors; therapeutic approach

1. Introduction

Lung cancer is the leading cause of cancer-related death worldwide. Among the different subtypes of lung cancer, non-small cell lung cancer (NSCLC) is the prevailing subtype, accounting for about 80% to 85% of cases. The prognosis of NSCLC is poor with a 5-year survival rate of 15% [1]. Although great therapeutic advances have been made during the last decades, patients are often diagnosed with advanced stage disease, where only palliative chemotherapy or immunotherapy is recommended. In this context, deciphering biological relevance of tumor suppressor genes in cancer, such as the inhibitor of growth gene (*ING*) family, is an attractive approach to develop new therapeutic breakthrough. Among this protein family of chromatin readers, ING2 and ING1 allow the recruitment of mSin3A/HDAC chromatin remodeling complex on Histone H3 trimethylated on lysine 4 marks (H3K4me3) [2–4]. Histone deacetylases enzymes could promote adjacent histones deacetylation that would in turn result in chromatin remodeling and regulation of gene transcription, mainly inducing transcription repression [5]. In addition, as part of the p53 pathway, ING2 is involved in diverse cellular processes that are recognized as hallmarks of cancer [6–8] and its deletion in mice led to spontaneous soft tissue sarcomas formation [9]. ING2 is now characterized as a tumor suppressor gene and as such, its expression is frequently altered in human tumors. In this review, we assess literature and public databases to evaluate ING2 and other mSin3A/HDAC member statuses in NSCLC, in an effort to uncover new therapeutic opportunities.

2. ING2 Modulates Transcriptional Activity Through Chromatin Remodeling

The first member of the inhibitor of growth gene (*ING*) family, ING1, was initially discovered through an in vivo screen based on subtractive hybridization that aimed to identify tumor suppressor genes [10]. Subsequently, an in silico sequence homology search with ING1 allowed the identification of four other members of the ING family—ING2 [11,12], ING3 [13], ING4 and ING5 [14].

ING genes are made up of multiple exons, resulting in numerous transcribed variants, thanks to alternative mRNA splicing. The *ING2* gene is composed of three exons (1a, 1b, and 2) that can be alternatively spliced, thus, leading to two isoforms—ING2a and ING2b [15]. Using quantitative polymerase chain reaction (qPCR) to examine *ING2a* and *ING2b* expression level in different tissues, Unoki and colleagues found that both isoforms were ubiquitously expressed, albeit ING2a isoform expression was predominant. Moreover, as *ING2b* expression has only been detected at the RNA level and was never detected at the protein level, we focused this review on ING2a, which is thereafter referred to as ING2.

The nucleosome, which is the fundamental chromatin subunit, consists of two pairs of each histones H2A, H2B, H3, and H4 with DNA wrapped around this octamer. The N-terminal tail of each histones, which emerges between the gyres of the DNA superhelix [16], contains highly conserved lysine residues that are the sites for various covalent modifications, including methylation [17]. These lysine methylations form binding sites for transcriptional regulator proteins [18]. More specifically, histone H3 trimethylated on lysine 4 (H3K4me3) has been reported to be exclusively associated with active transcription, while H3K4 dimethylated (H3K4me2) occurs at both inactive and active genes [19,20]. ING2 is able to bind to these marks of active transcription, with more affinity for H3K4me3 than for H3K4me2 [2].

The biological roles of ING2 are related to its various domains (Figure 1, panel A) and more particularly, to its plant homeodomain (PHD), which is characterized by a Cys^4-His-Cys^3 zinc-binding motif that allows ING2 stabilization at active chromatin, through the binding to H3K4me3 [2,3]. The PHD motif of ING2 acts as a dual-specificity module that binds to phosphatidylinositol 5-phosphate (PI(5)P) [21], in addition to H3K4me3. PI(5)P also requires the polybasic region (PBR) that is located immediately after the PHD domain (Figure 1, panel A) to bind efficiently to ING2 [22] and this binding is suggested to change the ING2 sub-nuclear distribution, in order to localize it at target gene promoters [23]. This targeting is crucial for recruiting ING2-associated HDAC activity to target gene promoters. Indeed, ING2 is part of the mSin3A-HDAC complex [4], thanks to its interaction with SAP30, mSin3A, and HDAC1 [24]. This interaction is due to its 40–140 N-terminal motif [25], which is involved in chromatin remodeling. Depicting all the mSin3A/HDAC complex members illustrates this mechanism (Figure 1, panel B). Indeed, this multiprotein complex with mSin3A being its core component, is associated with HDAC 1 and 2 [26], that constitutes the major catalytic subunits. An additional core mSin3A/HDAC protein, AT-rich interactive domain-containing protein 4B (ARID4B), is believed to function as a linker between the mSin3A/HDAC complex and the nucleosome, thus, stabilizing their interaction [27]. Some other members of the complex are involved in the recruitment of the HDAC activity, such as BRMS1/L or SAP30/L [28,29], whereas factors as SIN3A Corepressor Complex Component (SUDS3) [30] and O-linked N-acetylglucosamine transferase (OGT) [31] specifically stabilizes HDAC within the complex, while Sin3A Associated Protein 18 (SAP18) [26] and SIN3-HDAC Complex Associated Factor (SINHCAF) [32] help tethering the complex to the target gene promoter, thereby allowing HDAC to regulate gene transcription (Figure 1, panel C). Finally, SAP130 enables the modulation of mSin3A/HDAC transcriptional repression activity by binding a coactivator [33]. Of note, it has been shown that the sumoylation of ING2 at Lysine 195 enhances ING2 association with the mSin3A/HDAC complex [25]. As this lysine residue belongs to a phosphorylation-dependent SUMO modification (PDSM) consensus sequence, some authors suggest phosphorylation could modulate this interaction [25], but it remains to be demonstrated experimentally.

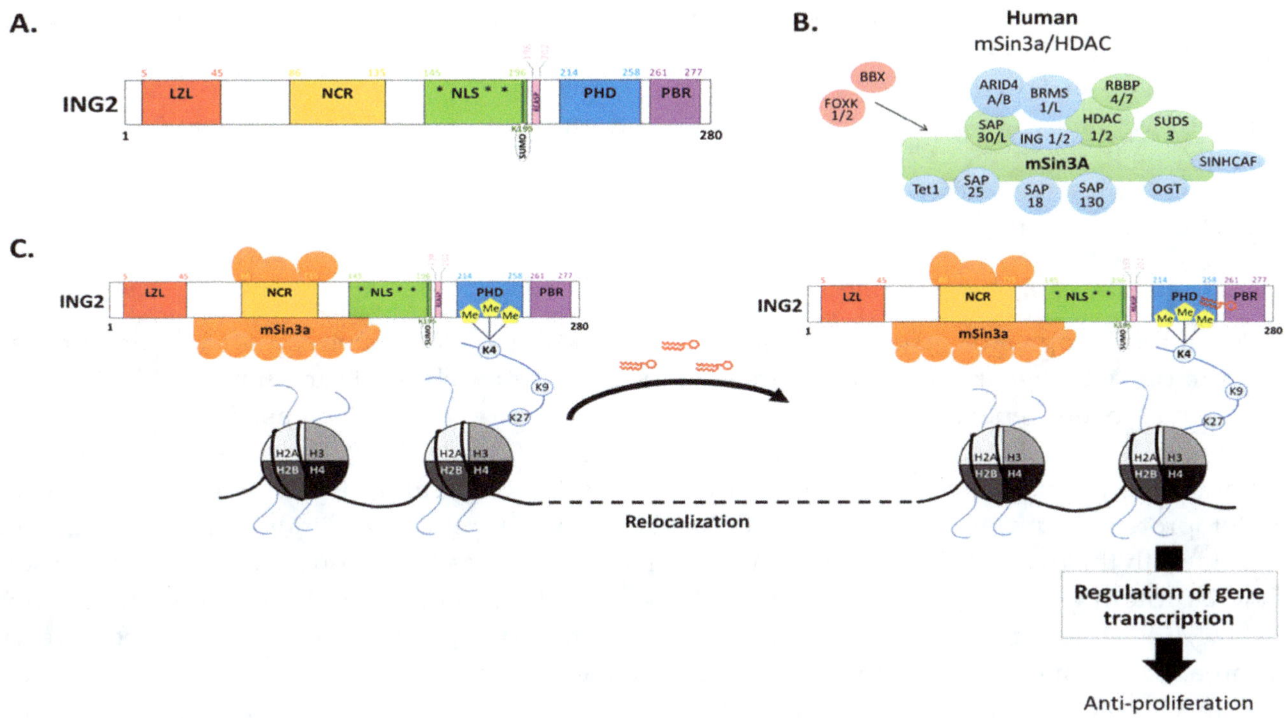

Figure 1. ING2 regulation of gene transcription through its interaction with H3K4me3 and the transcriptional regulator complex mSin3A/HDAC. (**A**) Protein structure of Human ING2. LZL—leucine zipper-like region; NCR—novel conserved region; NLS—nuclear localization signal, *within the NLS three short regions act as a nucleolar targeting signal (NTS); REASP—binding motif; PHD—plant homeodomain; PBR—polybasic region. ING2 structure was built according to UniProtKB ING2_Human (Q9H160). (**B**) Mammalian Sin3A/HDAC complex members. The core Sin3A subunits are depicted in green, the Sin3A associated proteins are depicted in blue, and the transcription factors are depicted in red. The names given for each complex member is the one approved by the HUGO Gene Nomenclature Committee (HGNC). (**C**) Schematic representation of ING2/H3K4me3/Sin3A formation regulating gene transcription. ING2 PHD domain recognizes trimethylated H3K4 (H3K4me3) as well as phosphatidylinositol 5-phosphate (PI(5)P) while the ING2 N-terminal part is detected by the transcriptional regulator complex mSin3-histone deacetylase. The ING2 sumoylation at Lysine 195 increases its association with this complex. An elevation in PI(5)P nuclear level triggers ING2/mSin3A complex relocalization to novel chromatin sites to regulate the transcription of target genes.

Altogether, mSin3A/HDAC chromatin remodeling complex has been originally reported to massively repress the transcription of a number of genes [5,24,34,35]. Nevertheless, the same complex was recently shown to activate some genes [5,24,36], although this capacity seems limited to a small number of genes. Indeed, in a study based on the comparison of gene expression levels in wild-type versus SIN3-deficient cells in *Drosophila* using full-genome oligonucleotide microarrays, a 10-fold difference was found between the number of activated and repressed genes [5]. Hence, ING2 functions as a bridge to link mSin3A/HDAC complex to H3K4me3, thereby, promoting the deacetylation of adjacent acetylated histone residues, which in turn allows chromatin remodeling and regulation of gene transcription (Figure 1, panel C). Of note, ING1 and ING2 are mutually exclusive in the mSin3A/HDAC complex [37] and the binding affinity for H3K4me3 is greater for ING2 compared to the one of ING1 [3].

Another key role for ING2 involves the p53 pathway as ING2 promoter contains two p53 binding sites [38]. Furthermore, the expression of ING2 results in p53 acetylation at Lysine 382 through the histone acetyltransferase p300 [12]. This enhanced acetylation led to p53 activation, ultimately preventing cell proliferation through induction of either senescence [39], apoptosis [40,41], or cell-cycle arrest in G1 [42]. Hence, ING2 is involved in multiple cellular processes, most of which are recognized hallmarks of tumorigenesis (cell-cycle regulation, replicative senescence [7], DNA repair [8], and DNA replication [6]). Moreover, a study conducted on *ING2* knockout mice indicates that ING2 deficiency spontaneously increases soft tissue sarcoma formation [9].

All of these facts highlight *ING2* as a tumor suppressor gene, playing a critical role against tumor development and cancer, notably through the regulation of mSin3A/HDAC-mediated epigenetic functions.

3. ING2 Status in Human Tumors

3.1. ING2 Alterations in Human Tumors

As a tumor suppressor gene, several studies have explored *ING2* gene status in different types of human tumors, whether at the genomic, transcriptomic or protein level. Using immunohistochemistry assay, it has been reported that ING2 protein expression was decreased in patients with, melanoma, breast cancer, hepatocellular carcinoma (16/29 and 44/84) and osteosarcoma [43–45]. This downregulation was correlated with tumor size, histological and pathological classification, alpha-fetoprotein serum level, and the overall survival in hepatocellular carcinoma [44], whereas it only correlated with the overall survival in patients with osteosarcoma [46]. Conversely, overexpression of the ING2 protein was found in patients with endometrial carcinoma and hepatocellular carcinoma (40/84) [44,45]. Moreover, studies on tumor cell lines also found that ING2 was overexpressed in cervical carcinoma, colon cancer, and acute lymphoblastic leukemia (ALL) cell lines [36,45,47]. However, the precise mechanism by which *ING2* expression is altered was not fully elucidated in most studies. Nevertheless, some authors found that miR-153-3p represses *ING2* expression in ALL cells by binding to the 3′-UTR site, and that miR-153-3p is downregulated in ALL cells [47], leading to *ING2* overexpression. Additionally, NF-kB can bind to the *ING2* promoter region and activate *ING2* transcription in colon cancer. Finally, other authors have suggested that activation of NF-kB lead to the upregulation of ING2 [36].

At the transcriptomic level, studies found that ING2 mRNA was downregulated in several tumor types including basal cell carcinoma (75/75), hepatocellular carcinoma and osteosarcoma [44,46,48]. *ING2* downregulation has also been reported in breast, lung, ovarian, pancreatic, and prostate cancer cell lines [49,50]. On one hand, *ING2* upregulation at the mRNA level was reported in patients with colon cancer (18/34) [36], even if the underlying mechanism was not investigated in this study. On the other hand, one publication suggested that the *ING2* gene could be targeted on its 3′-UTR site by miR-8084, which showed tumor-promoting properties in breast cancer [51]. This post-translational regulation of the *ING2* gene expression might explain the discrepancies observed in many publications between *ING2* mRNA level and ING2 protein expression [52].

Finally, at the genomic level, loss of heterozygosity (LOH) of the ING2 chromosomal region has been reported in ameloblastoma (14/28), head and neck squamous cell carcinoma (HNSCC) (30/55) (4q35.1), hepatocellular carcinoma (41.2%) (4q34–35.2), and basal cell carcinoma (3/11) (4q32-35) [53–57]. Moreover, LOH of the 4q35.1 region in HNSCC was correlated with tumor stage and disease-free survival but not with node status or overall survival [54], whereas no correlation has been found in hepatocellular carcinoma [55]. Additionally, deletion of the chromosomic region 4q34–35.2 containing the *ING2* gene has also been reported in uterine leiomyosarcoma (3/6) [58], and hypermethylation of the seven CpG sites in multiple intronic regions of the *ING2* gene has been shown in patients with esophageal squamous cell carcinoma. This was also observed in matched plasma cell-free DNA samples [59], even if the biological consequence of this intronic methylation on *ING2* expression remains unknown.

To explore further *ING2* status in cancer, we used The Cancer Genome Atlas database [60,61] to analyze alterations of the *ING2* gene and the members of the mSin3A/HDAC complex. This analysis revealed that 221 out of 9,892 (2.23%) human cancer samples included in the TCGA Pancancer study presented an alteration of *ING2* gene and 161 of these 221 (73%) alterations were deletions. Moreover, 2,384 out of 9,892 (24.1%) tumor samples presented an alteration in in at least one member of the Sin3a

HDAC complex. Interestingly, one of the tumor types with the most frequent alteration in ING2 was the lung squamous cell carcinoma, comprising 5.54% of the tumors involved (Figure 2, panel A).

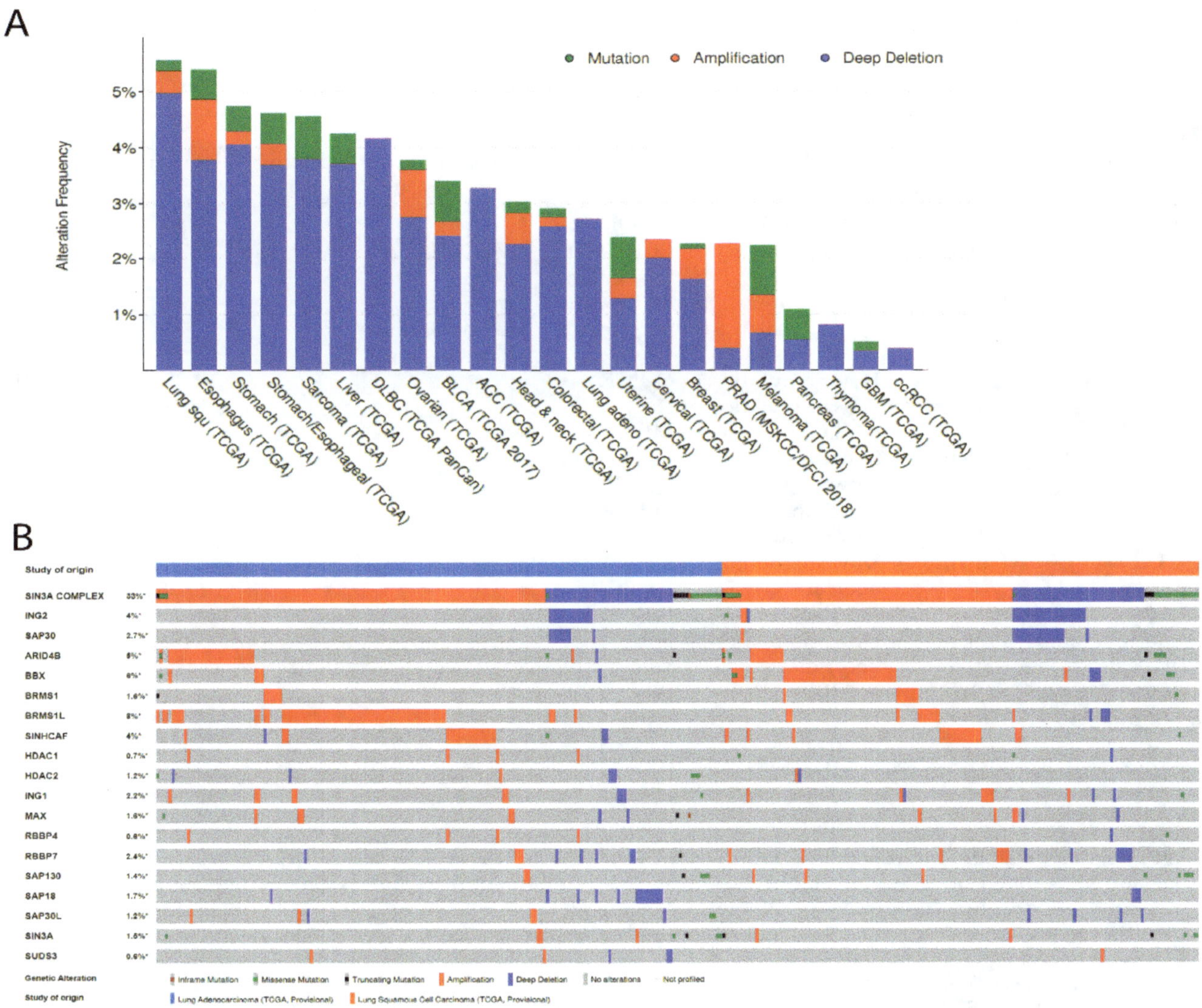

Figure 2. Despite *ING2* being rarely altered at the genomic level in cancers, genomic alteration of at least one member of the mSin3A/HDAC complex is frequent. (**A**) Bar graph showing the alteration frequency according to pathology (from the TCGA database). Blue represents gene deletion, red represents gene amplification, and green represents gene mutation. (**B**) Heatmap representing genomic alterations of mSin3A/HDAC members, according to NSCLC subtype (adenocarcinoma or squamous cell carcinoma) (from the TCGA database). First line is a pool of all mSin3A/HDAC member genomic alterations. Of note, specimens without any genomic alteration concerning the mSin3A/HDAC members are not depicted in the figure.

3.2. ING2 Alterations in Non-Small Cell Lung Cancer

ING2 has also been reported to be altered in NSCLC at the protein, transcriptomic, and genomic level. Indeed, two independent studies showed that ING2 expression levels were decreased at the protein level (independent of the p53 status). A study observed the loss of *ING2* expression in 70 out of 120 (58.3%) NSCLC [62] (Table 1), and was more frequent in adenocarcinoma than in squamous cell carcinoma (68% and 45%, respectively). However, no correlation was observed between ING2 expression in NSCLC and age, gender, disease stage, or patient survival [62]. Another study, conducted on Chinese patient specimens, showed that the ING2 expression was lost in 21 of 64 (32.8%) NSCLC and more frequently in ADK than in SCC (45.8% and 26.3%, respectively) (Table 1). ING2 loss was correlated with lymph node metastasis status and TNM stage in squamous cell carcinoma, but not in adenocarcinome [63]. Whether these discrepancies between these two studies are due to antibody specificity or ethnic disparities (notably, oncogenic driver mutational status was unknown in both studies), remains to be elucidated.

Table 1. ING2a status in human lung cancer.

Tissue Type	Origin	Mutation Type/Expression Change	Methods	Position	Coding	Frequency	Ref.
Lung cancer	Cell lines	Downregulation	RT-QPCR			7/8	[49]
	Patient	Substitution	PCR-SSCP, Sequencing	LZL (13)	Ala -> Ala	6/31	
	Patient	Substitution	PCR-SSCP, Sequencing	6bp downstream exon 1		6/31	
Lung cancer	Cell lines	Downregulation	Q-PCR			2/2	[50]
Lung cancer	Patient	Downregulation	IHC			70/120	[62]
	Patient	No LOH	MM			0/12	
	Patient	Substitution	Sequencing	39	Ala -> Ala	21/22	
	Patient	Downregulation	Q-PCR			15/22	
		No change	Q-PCR			6/22	
		Upregulation	Q-PCR			1/22	
NSCLC	Patient	Downregulation, aberrantly localization	IHC, RT-PCR, WB			21/64 (32.8%)	[63]
Adenocarcinoma	Patient	Downregulation, aberrantly localization	IHC, RT-PCR, WB			11/24 (45.8%)	
Squamous cell carcinoma	Patient	Downregulation, aberrantly localization	IHC, RT-PCR, WB			10/38 (26.3%)	
NSCLC	Patient	Chromosomal deletion	cDNA Microarray	4q34.2–q35.1		2/10 (20%)	[64]

Abbreviations: IHC—Immunohistochemistry; LOH—Loss of Heterozygosity; LZL—Leucine Zipper Like domain; MM—Microsatellite Marker; NSCLC—Non Small Cell Lung Carcinoma; PCR-SSCP—Polymerase Chain Reaction–Single Strand Conformation Polymorphism; RT-PCR—Retro transcription–Polymerase Chain Reaction; Q-PCR—Quantitative-Polymerase Chain Reaction; and WB—Western Blot.

Moreover, some study supports a transcriptional control of *ING2* expression in NSCLC showing a correlation with *ING2* mRNA decrease and low protein expression [62]. Consistently, studies also reported that ING2 was downregulated at the mRNA level in lung cancer cell lines [49,50]. Nevertheless, contradictory results have been found when analyzing TCGA and The Human Protein Atlas (THPA) databases, as the authors did not find any correlation between INGs mRNA and protein expression [52]. It is worth noticing that ING2 degradation has been shown to be mediated by Smad 1 ubiquitination regulatory factor 1 (Smurf 1) [65], a protein highly expressed in lung cancer [66]. Therefore, this mechanism could participate to the contradictory observation made between ING2 mRNA level and protein expression in lung cancer.

Another alteration frequently occurring in NSCLC is the chromosomal deletion of the 4q35.1 region, which includes *ING2* gene. Indeed, it has been reported that the chromosomal region 4q34.2–35.1 was deleted in 2 out of 10 patients with NSCLC [64] (Table 1). However, further investigations on larger samples of patients need to be performed to confirm this observation. Additionally, this chromosomal region contains not only *ING2* gene but also many other genes such as *SAP30* and micro-RNAs (miR-6082; miR-548T; miR-4276; miR-1305; miR-3945; and miR-4455). Therefore, it is still unclear if the deletion of *ING2* alone or the whole chromosomic region is implicated in promoting tumorigenesis. Concerning *ING2* mutations, only silent ones have been found in NSCLC. As an example, a study reported a substitution (C to T) in exon 1 at codon 13 in 6 out of 31 lung cancer (without any change of the encoded amino acid (Alanine) [49]) was likely to be a polymorphism (Table 1).

Interestingly, the analysis of the mSin3A/HDAC complex member alterations in NSCLC via the TCGA database revealed that *ING2* was altered in 20 out of 408 (4.9%) NSCLC and was found to be higher in squamous cell carcinoma than in adenocarcinoma (6.7% and 2.6%, respectively) (Figure 2, panel A). Moreover, the *ING2* gene deep deletion was the most frequent alteration with 17 out of 408 (3.54%) NSCLC and was found to be higher in squamous cell carcinoma than in adenocarcinoma (6.18% and 2.61%, respectively). Only one missense mutation (E204Q) of *ING2* of unknown significance was reported out of the 408 NSCLC samples. Focusing on all members of the mSin3A/HDAC complex, data revealed that 152 of the 408 (37.3%) NSCLC presented an alteration in at least one member of the mSin3A/HDAC complex, occurring in 38.8% of squamous cell carcinoma specimens and 36.1% of adenocarcinoma specimens (Figure 2, panel B). Notably, we found that patients presenting an alteration in at least one member of the mSin3A/HDAC complex had a higher probability of prolonged overall survival, in comparison with patients without any alteration of the complex in lung squamous cell carcinoma ($p = 0.0451$) (data not shown).

In summary, the tumor suppressor protein ING2 was found to be altered in human tumors, especially in NSCLC, mainly at the protein level (varying from 32.8% to 58.3% according to different studies). *ING2* gene alterations in NSCLC are predominantly deletion, but still remain a rare event (less than 3%). Strikingly, genomic alteration of at least one component of the mSin3A/HDAC complex appears to be relatively common in human cancers and NSCLC (24.1% and 33%, respectively) (Figure 2, panel B).

4. Potential Role of the ING2 Epigenetic Modulation in Lung Cancer Treatment

NSCLC is a deadly disease and the leading cause of cancer-related death worldwide. Even if great advances in the field have been made during the last decade, notably thanks to the emergence of targeted therapies and immunotherapies, survival remains poor in the metastatic setting. In this context, developing new therapeutic approaches based on predictive biomarkers is still an active area of research [67]. As discussed above, ING2 genomic alterations are rare in non-small cell lung cancer, and loss at the protein level has been reported within a large proportion range. Even though the number of studies that investigate the expression of ING2 protein are limited in lung cancer, its potential use as a diagnosis biomarker has been suggested by some authors [68].

4.1. Exploring ING2 Dependencies in Cancer Cells

Recently, lot of great efforts have been made to uncover genetic vulnerabilities in cancer, notably taking advantage of the emergent CrispR-screening methods. The Cancer Dependency Map project, led by the Broad Institute, is a systematic high-throughput screening of genotype-specific cancer vulnerabilities in tumor cell lines [69]. According to the latest dataset (CrispR AVANA public 19Q2), many mSin3A/HDAC members are found among the top *ING2* gene co-dependencies in cancer cell lines (Figure 3, panel A). These results suggest that many tumor cells lines are dependent on a functionally active mSin3A/HDAC complex for proliferation. Consequently, we speculate that it could be utilized as an "Achilles' heel", potentially leading to a biomarker-guided therapeutic model (Figure 3, panel B).

Moreover, multiple studies support the important biological role of the mSin3A-HDAC complex in tumors. Of note, it was originally shown that mSin3A/B recruitment was necessary to antagonize c-MYC induced transcriptional activation [70]. *SIN3A*-knockout studies using multiples physiological models demonstrate that a reduction of the mSin3A levels correlates with a loss of proliferative abilities [71,72]. Interestingly, *mSin3A* loss of expression in mouse foregut endoderm lead to severe defect in lung morphogenesis and development [73], underlying its biological role in lung epithelial cells. In cancer cells, whether the mSin3A/HDAC complex as a whole show more tumor suppressive or oncogenic properties, is still under debate [74]. However, the relative high frequencies of genomic alteration concerning at least one member of the mSin3A/HDAC complex in NSCLC TCGA samples, notably gene amplification (23.6% of adenocarcinoma and 17.53% of squamous cell carcinoma) (Figure 2, Panel B), clearly pledges for a "gain-of-function" phenotype predisposing tumors cells to a selective advantage.

Additionally, small molecule inhibitors targeting Paired Amphipathic Helix 2 (PAH2) domain of mSin3A was shown to induce transcriptional reprogramming, impairment of clonogenic abilities, inhibition of proliferation, and metastasis in triple negative breast cancer models [75]. Coherently, the Cancer Dependency Map project database characterizes *SIN3A* gene as a "common essential" gene in a vast majority of cancer cell lines. It is of note that *SIN3A*-knockout mice embryos stop developing after 6.5 weeks [76]. Consequently, targeting mSin3A itself, or specific partners of the complex, appears to be an attractive therapeutic strategy in cancer. Conversely, it is hard to conciliate the fact that ING2 is a recognized tumor suppressor protein belonging to a multi-protein complex that tends to proffer oncogenic properties in cancer cells. However, some could argue that many non-epigenetic functions of ING2 favor its tumor suppressive activity (DNA repair, DNA replication, cell cycle progression, etc.) but it still remains an unresolved issue to date.

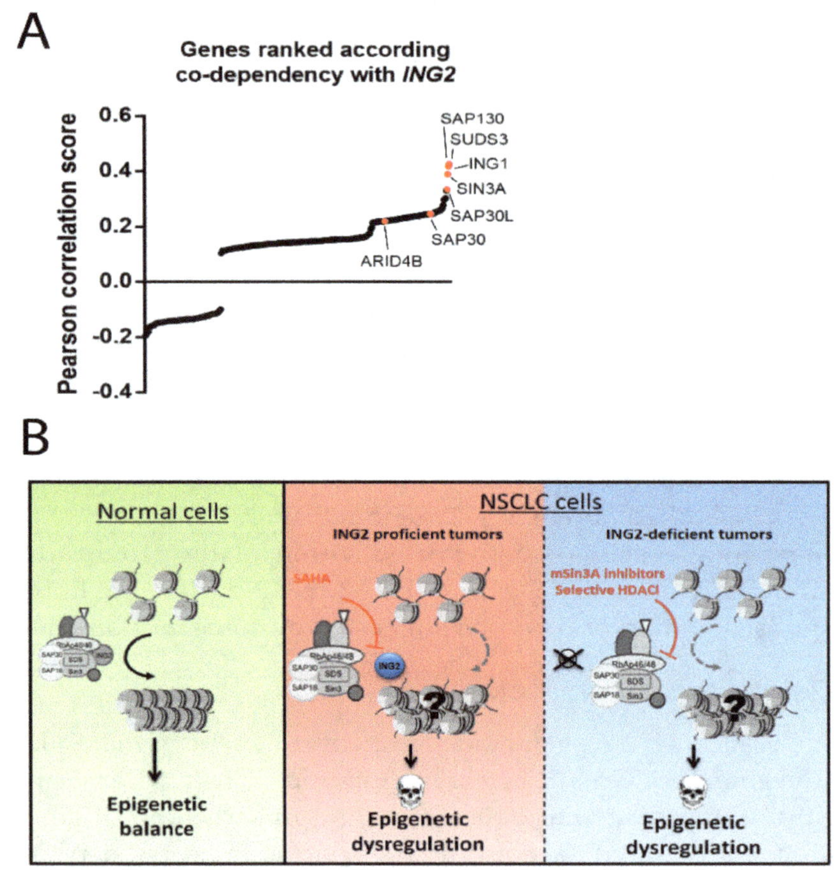

Figure 3. Co-dependency between *ING2* and mSin3A/HDAC complex members in tumor cell lines. (**A**) Graph depicting ranked Pearson correlation score between the CERES dependency score for each tested gene in the Cancer Dependency Map Project and the ING2 CERES dependency score. (**B**) Working model for a ING2 biomarker-based therapeutic strategy in NSCLC. Tumors expressing ING2 are more likely to depend on the oncogenic properties of mSin3A/HDAC for survival and could be targeted by suberoyl anilide hydroxamic acid (SAHA). Tumors that lose ING2 expression cannot be treated by SAHA, but can be treated by mSin3A direct inhibitors (mSin3Ai) or HDAC1/2 inhibitors (s.HDACi).

4.2. Targeting SIN3A-Mediated ING2 Functions in Cancer Cells

Suberoyl anilide hydroxamic acid (SAHA), also called vorinostat, a class I, II, and IV HDAC inhibitor (HDACi), was described as a potent inhibitor of the mSin3A/HDAC complex-mediated functions [37]. More precisely, ING2 protein interaction with the mSin3A-HDAC complex was abrogated in HEK 293T cells treated with SAHA [77]. Interestingly, HDAC inhibitor induced dissociation of ING2 with the mSin3A/HDAC complex was independent from the PHD domain of ING2, suggesting that this drug effect was not dependent on the ING2 chromatin fixation. Similar observations were made with other HDACi molecules (trichostatin A and apicidin). Notably, ING2 and mSin3A/HDAC complex occupancy on the tumor suppressor *p21* promoter was reduced in SAHA treated HEK 293T. Consequently, authors hypothesized that ING2 disruption lead to the induction of *p21* transcription, as it was observed, upon HDACi treatment [78]. Conversely, an independent study showed that *p21* expression was reduced in ING2-downregulated U2OS cells, leading to cell cycle progression, in a p53-independent manner [79]. These contradictory findings might be explained by the broader cellular effects of SAHA, a pan-HDAC inhibitor [80], or by the potential impact of SAHA on ING2 post-translational modification. Notably, as already mentioned above, ING2 sumoylation on Lysine 195 has been described to enhance its interaction with mSin3A [25]. Therefore, whether ING2 disruption induced by SAHA is dependent on its sumoylation status is an interesting question that needs to be explored. Nevertheless, the use of SAHA represents an attractive approach to target ING2-mediated mSin3A/HDAC epigenetic functions.

Interestingly, the Cancer Dependency Map also uncovered a co-dependency between ING1 and ING2 in multiple cancer cell lines (data not shown) suggesting a potential crosstalk between the protein's functions. Coherently, these two members of the ING family share an important structural homology, except for the N-terminal part, and are both stable and exclusive components of the mSin3A/HDAC complex. However, the subscription of ING1 and ING2 to this complex is highly conserved throughout evolution [81], suggesting that some ING1 and ING2 mSin3A/HDAC-mediated functions are biologically important but not redundant. In line with this hypothesis, *ING1* and *ING2* double knock-out mice show embryonic lethality (not published), but not their single knock-out counterparts, which shows distinct phenotypes [9,82]. In terms of therapeutic approach, HDAC inhibitors do not disturb ING1 interaction to mSin3A/HDAC [77], and it is, therefore, unknown if HDAC inhibitors could impact ING1 epigenetic functions. Finally, to our knowledge no study to date has concomitantly explored the status of ING1 and ING2 proteins in human cancers. Altogether, more experimental data are needed to precisely decipher the potential redundant or exclusive mSin3A/HDAC-mediated roles relying on ING1 and ING2.

During the last two decades, many HDAC inhibitors have been developed and were tested in clinical trials due to their pleiotropic antineoplastic properties [83]. Indeed, in various types of cancer, histone deacetylation was found to deeply impact cellular fate [84]. Of note, studies claiming to inactivate mSin3A as a therapeutic target in leukemia are limited to the use of non-selective HDAC inhibitors that do not target mSin3A directly. To date, HDAC inhibitors have only been approved for T cell-lymphoma (vorinostat, romidepsin, and belinostat) and multiple myeloma (panobinostat), but many clinical trials are ongoing in solid tumors [85]. As the specificity of HDAC inhibitors have greatly improved over the last decades, deciphering the biological consequences of these treatments on ING2 epigenetic function is of prime interest in order to explore new therapeutic strategies.

Altogether, these findings lead us to hypothesize a biomarker-based therapeutic strategy, involving ING2 as a tumor predictive factor for SAHA sensitivity in NSCLC (Figure 3, Panel B). In light of the observation of a high frequency of mSin3A/HDAC complex-alteration in cancer, determining if such genomic alteration could make ING2-expressing cells more prone to HDAC inhibitors efficacy is a very interesting hypothesis to elucidate. Conversely, in ING2-non-expressing cells, as this "target" could not be disrupted by SAHA, small molecules that directly inhibit mSin3A or more specific HDAC inhibitors, could represent a more convenient way to circumvent this issue. Experimental studies are actually ongoing to explore this working hypothesis.

5. Conclusions

ING2 protein is a chromatin reader and a stable component of the mSin3A/HDAC complex. Several tumor suppressive functions have been described for ING2 in cancer cell lines, and in accordance with these observations, ING2 expression is lost in many cancer subtypes. Interestingly, genomic alterations of mSin3A/HDAC members occur frequently in NSCLC, mainly through gene amplification. Recent experimental data have revealed that a vast majority of tumor cell lines depend on a functionally active mSin3A/HDAC complex to proliferate. As ING2 can be pharmacologically disrupted from the mSin3A/HDAC complex by SAHA, we built a model based on an ING2 biomarker-guided therapeutic hypothesis. Further research is still warranted to confirm the predictive value of ING2 in clinical practice of NSCLC.

Author Contributions: A.B. (Alice Blondel), A.B. (Amine Benberghout), and C.R. were responsible for literature review and manuscript writing. A.B. (Alice Blondel) and C.R. were responsible for editing the figures. A.B. (Amine Benberghout) was responsible for editing the tables. R.P. was responsible for manuscript design and review. All authors approved the final version of the manuscript.

Acknowledgments: A.B. (Alice Blondel) is a recipient of the doctoral fellowship ARED/INSERM (région Bretagne). C.R. is a recipient of the FHU Camin (CHU Rennes) and Nuovo-Soldati Fundation (CHU Genève) fellowships.

References

1. Molina, J.R.; Yang, P.; Cassivi, S.D.; Schild, S.E.; Adjei, A.A. Non-small cell lung cancer: Epidemiology, risk factors, treatment, and survivorship. *Mayo Clin. Proc.* **2008**, *83*, 584–594. [CrossRef]
2. Shi, X.; Hong, T.; Walter, K.L.; Ewalt, M.; Michishita, E.; Hung, T.; Carney, D.; Peña, P.; Lan, F.; Kaadige, M.R.; et al. ING2 PHD domain links histone H3 lysine 4 methylation to active gene repression. *Nature* **2006**, *442*, 96–99. [CrossRef] [PubMed]
3. Peña, P.V.; Davrazou, F.; Shi, X.; Walter, K.L.; Verkhusha, V.V.; Gozani, O.; Zhao, R.; Kutateladze, T.G. Molecular mechanism of histone H3K4me3 recognition by plant homeodomain of ING2. *Nature* **2006**, *442*, 100–103. [CrossRef] [PubMed]
4. Doyon, Y.; Cayrou, C.; Ullah, M.; Landry, A.-J.; Côté, V.; Selleck, W.; Lane, W.S.; Tan, S.; Yang, X.-J.; Côté, J. ING tumor suppressor proteins are critical regulators of chromatin acetylation required for genome expression and perpetuation. *Mol. Cell* **2006**, *21*, 51–64. [CrossRef] [PubMed]
5. Pile, L.A.; Spellman, P.T.; Katzenberger, R.J.; Wassarman, D.A. The SIN3 deacetylase complex represses genes encoding mitochondrial proteins: Implications for the regulation of energy metabolism. *J. Biol. Chem.* **2003**, *278*, 37840–37848. [CrossRef]
6. Larrieu, D.; Ythier, D.; Binet, R.; Brambilla, C.; Brambilla, E.; Sengupta, S.; Pedeux, R. ING2 controls the progression of DNA replication forks to maintain genome stability. *EMBO Rep.* **2009**, *10*, 1168–1174. [CrossRef]
7. Pedeux, R.; Sengupta, S.; Shen, J.C.; Demidov, O.N.; Saito, S.; Onogi, H.; Kumamoto, K.; Wincovitch, S.; Garfield, S.H.; McMenamin, M.; et al. ING2 regulates the onset of replicative senescence by induction of p300-dependent p53 acetylation. *Mol. Cell. Biol.* **2005**, *25*, 6639–6648. [CrossRef]
8. Wang, J.; Chin, M.Y.; Li, G. The novel tumor suppressor p33ING2 enhances nucleotide excision repair via inducement of histone H4 acetylation and chromatin relaxation. *Cancer Res.* **2006**, *66*, 1906–1911. [CrossRef]
9. Saito, M.; Kumamoto, K.; Robles, A.I.; Horikawa, I.; Furusato, B.; Okamura, S.; Goto, A.; Yamashita, T.; Nagashima, M.; Lee, T.-L.; et al. Targeted disruption of Ing2 results in defective spermatogenesis and development of soft-tissue sarcomas. *PLoS ONE* **2010**, *5*, e15541. [CrossRef]
10. Garkavtsev, I.; Kazarov, A.; Gudkov, A.; Riabowol, K. Suppression of the novel growth inhibitor p33ING1 promotes neoplastic transformation. *Nat. Genet.* **1996**, *14*, 415–420. [CrossRef]
11. Shimada, Y.; Saito, A.; Suzuki, M.; Takahashi, E.; Horie, M. Cloning of a novel gene (ING1L) homologous to ING1, a candidate tumor suppressor. *Cytogenet. Cell Genet.* **1998**, *83*, 232–235. [CrossRef] [PubMed]
12. Nagashima, M.; Shiseki, M.; Miura, K.; Hagiwara, K.; Linke, S.P.; Pedeux, R.; Wang, X.W.; Yokota, J.; Riabowol, K.; Harris, C.C. DNA damage-inducible gene p33ING2 negatively regulates cell proliferation through acetylation of p53. *Proc. Natl. Acad. Sci. USA* **2001**, *98*, 9671–9676. [CrossRef] [PubMed]
13. Nagashima, M.; Shiseki, M.; Pedeux, R.M.; Okamura, S.; Kitahama-Shiseki, M.; Miura, K.; Yokota, J.; Harris, C.C. A novel PHD-finger motif protein, p47ING3, modulates p53-mediated transcription, cell cycle control, and apoptosis. *Oncogene* **2003**, *22*, 343–350. [CrossRef] [PubMed]
14. Shiseki, M.; Nagashima, M.; Pedeux, R.M.; Kitahama-Shiseki, M.; Miura, K.; Okamura, S.; Onogi, H.; Higashimoto, Y.; Appella, E.; Yokota, J.; et al. p29ING4 and p28ING5 bind to p53 and p300, and enhance p53 activity. *Cancer Res.* **2003**, *63*, 2373–2378.
15. Unoki, M.; Kumamoto, K.; Robles, A.I.; Shen, J.C.; Zheng, Z.-M.; Harris, C.C. A novel ING2 isoform, ING2b,

synergizes with ING2a to prevent cell cycle arrest and apoptosis. *FEBS Lett.* **2008**, *582*, 3868–3874. [CrossRef] [PubMed]

16. Luger, K.; Mäder, A.W.; Richmond, R.K.; Sargent, D.F.; Richmond, T.J. Crystal structure of the nucleosome core particle at 2.8 A resolution. *Nature* **1997**, *389*, 251–260. [CrossRef]
17. Murray, K. The occurrence of epsilon-n-methyl lysine in histones. *Biochemistry* **1964**, *3*, 10–15. [CrossRef]
18. Fischle, W.; Franz, H.; Jacobs, S.A.; Allis, C.D.; Khorasanizadeh, S. Specificity of the chromodomain Y chromosome family of chromodomains for lysine-methylated ARK(S/T) motifs. *J. Biol. Chem.* **2008**, *283*, 19626–19635. [CrossRef]
19. Bernstein, B.E.; Kamal, M.; Lindblad-Toh, K.; Bekiranov, S.; Bailey, D.K.; Huebert, D.J.; McMahon, S.; Karlsson, E.K.; Kulbokas, E.J.; Gingeras, T.R.; et al. Genomic maps and comparative analysis of histone modifications in human and mouse. *Cell* **2005**, *120*, 169–181. [CrossRef]
20. Santos-Rosa, H.; Schneider, R.; Bannister, A.J.; Sherriff, J.; Bernstein, B.E.; Emre, N.C.T.; Schreiber, S.L.; Mellor, J.; Kouzarides, T. Active genes are tri-methylated at K4 of histone H3. *Nature* **2002**, *419*, 407–411. [CrossRef]
21. Gozani, O.; Karuman, P.; Jones, D.R.; Ivanov, D.; Cha, J.; Lugovskoy, A.A.; Baird, C.L.; Zhu, H.; Field, S.J.; Lessnick, S.L.; et al. The PHD finger of the chromatin-associated protein ING2 functions as a nuclear phosphoinositide receptor. *Cell* **2003**, *114*, 99–111. [CrossRef]
22. Kaadige, M.R.; Ayer, D.E. The polybasic region that follows the plant homeodomain zinc finger 1 of Pf1 is necessary and sufficient for specific phosphoinositide binding. *J. Biol. Chem.* **2006**, *281*, 28831–28836. [CrossRef] [PubMed]
23. Bua, D.J.; Martin, G.M.; Binda, O.; Gozani, O. Nuclear phosphatidylinositol-5-phosphate regulates ING2 stability at discrete chromatin targets in response to DNA damage. *Sci. Rep.* **2013**, *3*, 2137. [CrossRef] [PubMed]
24. Ohkouchi, C.; Kumamoto, K.; Saito, M.; Ishigame, T.; Suzuki, S.-I.; Takenoshita, S.; Harris, C.C. ING2, a tumor associated gene, enhances PAI-1 and HSPA1A expression with HDAC1 and mSin3A through the PHD domain and C-terminal. *Mol. Med. Rep.* **2017**, *16*, 7367–7374. [CrossRef]
25. Ythier, D.; Larrieu, D.; Binet, R.; Binda, O.; Brambilla, C.; Gazzeri, S.; Pedeux, R. Sumoylation of ING2 regulates the transcription mediated by Sin3A. *Oncogene* **2010**, *29*, 5946–5956. [CrossRef]
26. Zhang, Y.; Iratni, R.; Erdjument-Bromage, H.; Tempst, P.; Reinberg, D. Histone deacetylases and SAP18, a novel polypeptide, are components of a human Sin3 complex. *Cell* **1997**, *89*, 357–364. [CrossRef]
27. Parthun, M.R.; Widom, J.; Gottschling, D.E. The major cytoplasmic histone acetyltransferase in yeast: Links to chromatin replication and histone metabolism. *Cell* **1996**, *87*, 85–94. [CrossRef]
28. Laherty, C.D.; Billin, A.N.; Lavinsky, R.M.; Yochum, G.S.; Bush, A.C.; Sun, J.M.; Mullen, T.M.; Davie, J.R.; Rose, D.W.; Glass, C.K.; et al. SAP30, a component of the mSin3 corepressor complex involved in N-CoR-mediated repression by specific transcription factors. *Mol. Cell* **1998**, *2*, 33–42. [CrossRef]
29. Zhang, Y.; Sun, Z.W.; Iratni, R.; Erdjument-Bromage, H.; Tempst, P.; Hampsey, M.; Reinberg, D. SAP30, a novel protein conserved between human and yeast, is a component of a histone deacetylase complex. *Mol. Cell* **1998**, *1*, 1021–1031. [CrossRef]
30. Alland, L.; David, G.; Shen-Li, H.; Potes, J.; Muhle, R.; Lee, H.-C.; Hou, H.; Chen, K.; DePinho, R.A. Identification of mammalian Sds3 as an integral component of the Sin3/histone deacetylase corepressor complex. *Mol. Cell. Biol.* **2002**, *22*, 2743–2750. [CrossRef]
31. Yang, X.; Zhang, F.; Kudlow, J.E. Recruitment of O-GlcNAc transferase to promoters by corepressor mSin3A: Coupling protein O-GlcNAcylation to transcriptional repression. *Cell* **2002**, *110*, 69–80. [CrossRef]
32. Muñoz, I.M.; MacArtney, T.; Sanchez-Pulido, L.; Ponting, C.P.; Rocha, S.; Rouse, J. Family with sequence similarity 60A (FAM60A) protein is a cell cycle-fluctuating regulator of the SIN3-HDAC1 histone deacetylase complex. *J. Biol. Chem.* **2012**, *287*, 32346–32353. [CrossRef] [PubMed]
33. Fleischer, T.C.; Yun, U.J.; Ayer, D.E. Identification and characterization of three new components of the mSin3A corepressor complex. *Mol. Cell. Biol.* **2003**, *23*, 3456–3467. [CrossRef] [PubMed]
34. Li, J.; Lin, Q.; Wang, W.; Wade, P.; Wong, J. Specific targeting and constitutive association of histone deacetylase complexes during transcriptional repression. *Genes Dev.* **2002**, *16*, 687–692. [CrossRef] [PubMed]
35. Peinado, H.; Ballestar, E.; Esteller, M.; Cano, A. Snail mediates E-cadherin repression by the recruitment of the Sin3A/histone deacetylase 1 (HDAC1)/HDAC2 complex. *Mol. Cell. Biol.* **2004**, *24*, 306–319. [CrossRef]

36. Kumamoto, K.; Fujita, K.; Kurotani, R.; Saito, M.; Unoki, M.; Hagiwara, N.; Shiga, H.; Bowman, E.D.; Yanaihara, N.; Okamura, S.; et al. ING2 is upregulated in colon cancer and increases invasion by enhanced MMP13 expression. *Int. J. Cancer* **2009**, *125*, 1306–1315. [CrossRef]
37. Sardiu, M.E.; Smith, K.T.; Groppe, B.D.; Gilmore, J.M.; Saraf, A.; Egidy, R.; Peak, A.; Seidel, C.W.; Florens, L.; Workman, J.L.; et al. Suberoylanilide hydroxamic acid (SAHA)-induced dynamics of a human histone deacetylase protein interaction network. *Mol. Cell Proteomics* **2014**, *13*, 3114–3125. [CrossRef]
38. Kumamoto, K.; Spillare, E.A.; Fujita, K.; Horikawa, I.; Yamashita, T.; Appella, E.; Nagashima, M.; Takenoshita, S.; Yokota, J.; Harris, C.C. Nutlin-3a activates p53 to both down-regulate inhibitor of growth 2 and up-regulate mir-34a, mir-34b, and mir-34c expression, and induce senescence. *Cancer Res.* **2008**, *68*, 3193–3203. [CrossRef]
39. Serrano, M.; Lin, A.W.; McCurrach, M.E.; Beach, D.; Lowe, S.W. Oncogenic ras provokes premature cell senescence associated with accumulation of p53 and p16INK4a. *Cell* **1997**, *88*, 593–602. [CrossRef]
40. Lotem, J.; Sachs, L. Hematopoietic cells from mice deficient in wild-type p53 are more resistant to induction of apoptosis by some agents. *Blood* **1993**, *82*, 1092–1096. [CrossRef]
41. Yonish-Rouach, E.; Resnitzky, D.; Lotem, J.; Sachs, L.; Kimchi, A.; Oren, M. Wild-type p53 induces apoptosis of myeloid leukaemic cells that is inhibited by interleukin-6. *Nature* **1991**, *352*, 345–347. [CrossRef] [PubMed]
42. Di Leonardo, A.; Linke, S.P.; Clarkin, K.; Wahl, G.M. DNA damage triggers a prolonged p53-dependent G1 arrest and long-term induction of Cip1 in normal human fibroblasts. *Genes Dev.* **1994**, *8*, 2540–2551. [CrossRef] [PubMed]
43. Lu, F.; Dai, D.L.; Martinka, M.; Ho, V.; Li, G. Nuclear ING2 expression is reduced in human cutaneous melanomas. *Br. J. Cancer* **2006**, *95*, 80–86. [CrossRef] [PubMed]
44. Zhang, H.; Pan, K.; Wang, H.; Weng, D.; Song, H.; Zhou, J.; Huang, W.; Li, J.; Chen, M.; Xia, J. Decreased expression of ING2 gene and its clinicopathological significance in hepatocellular carcinoma. *Cancer Lett.* **2008**, *261*, 183–192. [CrossRef] [PubMed]
45. Zhao, S.; Yang, X.-F.; Gou, W.-F.; Lu, H.; Li, H.; Zhu, Z.-T.; Sun, H.-Z.; Zheng, H.-C. Expression profiles of inhibitor of growth protein 2 in normal and cancer tissues: An immunohistochemical screening analysis. *Mol. Med. Rep.* **2016**, *13*, 1881–1887. [CrossRef]
46. Han, X.-R.; Bai, X.-Z.; Sun, Y.; Yang, Y. Nuclear ING2 expression is reduced in osteosarcoma. *Oncol. Rep.* **2014**, *32*, 1967–1972. [CrossRef]
47. Jiang, J.; Liu, Y.; Zhao, Y.; Tian, F.; Wang, G. miR-153-3p Suppresses Inhibitor of Growth Protein 2 Expression to Function as Tumor Suppressor in Acute Lymphoblastic Leukemia. *Technol. Cancer Res. Treat.* **2019**, *18*, 1533033819852990. [CrossRef]
48. Temel, M.; Turkmen, A.; Dokuyucu, R.; Cevik, C.; Oztuzcu, S.; Cengiz, B.; Mutaf, M. A novel tumor suppressor gene in basal cell carcinoma: Inhibition of growth factor-2. *Tumour Biol.* **2015**, *36*, 4611–4616. [CrossRef]
49. Okano, T.; Gemma, A.; Hosoya, Y.; Hosomi, Y.; Nara, M.; Kokubo, Y.; Yoshimura, A.; Shibuya, M.; Nagashima, M.; Harris, C.C.; et al. Alterations in novel candidate tumor suppressor genes, ING1 and ING2 in human lung cancer. *Oncol. Rep.* **2006**, *15*, 545–549. [CrossRef]
50. Walzak, A.A.; Veldhoen, N.; Feng, X.; Riabowol, K.; Helbing, C.C. Expression profiles of mRNA transcript variants encoding the human inhibitor of growth tumor suppressor gene family in normal and neoplastic tissues. *Exp. Cell Res.* **2008**, *314*, 273–285. [CrossRef]
51. Gao, Y.; Ma, H.; Gao, C.; Lv, Y.; Chen, X.; Xu, R.; Sun, M.; Liu, X.; Lu, X.; Pei, X.; et al. Tumor-promoting properties of miR-8084 in breast cancer through enhancing proliferation, suppressing apoptosis and inducing epithelial-mesenchymal transition. *J. Transl. Med.* **2018**, *16*, 38. [CrossRef] [PubMed]
52. Gournay, M.; Paineau, M.; Archambeau, J.; Pedeux, R. Regulat-INGs in tumors and diseases: Focus on ncRNAs. *Cancer Lett.* **2019**, *447*, 66–74. [CrossRef] [PubMed]
53. Sironi, E.; Cerri, A.; Tomasini, D.; Sirchia, S.M.; Porta, G.; Rossella, F.; Grati, F.R.; Simoni, G. Loss of heterozygosity on chromosome 4q32-35 in sporadic basal cell carcinomas: Evidence for the involvement of p33ING2/ING1L and SAP30 genes. *J. Cutan. Pathol.* **2004**, *31*, 318–322. [CrossRef] [PubMed]
54. Borkosky, S.S.; Gunduz, M.; Nagatsuka, H.; Beder, L.B.; Gunduz, E.; Ali, M.A.L.S.; Rodriguez, A.P.; Cilek, M.Z.; Tominaga, S.; Yamanaka, N.; et al. Frequent deletion of ING2 locus at 4q35.1 associates with advanced tumor stage in head and neck squamous cell carcinoma. *J. Cancer Res. Clin. Oncol.* **2009**, *135*, 703–713. [CrossRef]

55. Zhang, H.; Ma, H.; Wang, Q.; Chen, M.; Weng, D.; Wang, H.; Zhou, J.; Li, Y.; Sun, J.; Chen, Y.; et al. Analysis of loss of heterozygosity on chromosome 4q in hepatocellular carcinoma using high-throughput SNP array. *Oncol. Rep.* **2010**, *23*, 445–455. [PubMed]
56. Borkosky, S.S.; Gunduz, M.; Beder, L.; Tsujigiwa, H.; Tamamura, R.; Gunduz, E.; Katase, N.; Rodriguez, A.P.; Sasaki, A.; Nagai, N.; et al. Allelic loss of the ING gene family loci is a frequent event in ameloblastoma. *Oncol. Res.* **2010**, *18*, 509–518. [CrossRef] [PubMed]
57. Cetin, E.; Cengiz, B.; Gunduz, E.; Gunduz, M.; Nagatsuka, H.; Bekir-Beder, L.; Fukushima, K.; Pehlivan, D.; Nishizaki, K.; Shimizu, K.; et al. Deletion mapping of chromosome 4q22-35 and identification of four frequently deleted regions in head and neck cancers. *Neoplasma* **2008**, *55*, 299–304.
58. Mittal, K.R.; Chen, F.; Wei, J.J.; Rijhvani, K.; Kurvathi, R.; Streck, D.; Dermody, J.; Toruner, G.A. Molecular and immunohistochemical evidence for the origin of uterine leiomyosarcomas from associated leiomyoma and symplastic leiomyoma-like areas. *Mod. Pathol.* **2009**, *22*, 1303–1311. [CrossRef]
59. Wang, H.-Q.; Yang, C.-Y.; Wang, S.-Y.; Wang, T.; Han, J.-L.; Wei, K.; Liu, F.-C.; Xu, J.; Peng, X.-Z.; Wang, J.-M. Cell-free plasma hypermethylated CASZ1, CDH13 and ING2 are promising biomarkers of esophageal cancer. *J. Biomed. Res.* **2018**, *32*, 424–433.
60. Cerami, E.; Gao, J.; Dogrusoz, U.; Gross, B.E.; Sumer, S.O.; Aksoy, B.A.; Jacobsen, A.; Byrne, C.J.; Heuer, M.L.; Larsson, E.; et al. The cBio cancer genomics portal: An open platform for exploring multidimensional cancer genomics data. *Cancer Discov.* **2012**, *2*, 401–404. [CrossRef]
61. Gao, J.; Aksoy, B.A.; Dogrusoz, U.; Dresdner, G.; Gross, B.; Sumer, S.O.; Sun, Y.; Jacobsen, A.; Sinha, R.; Larsson, E.; et al. Integrative analysis of complex cancer genomics and clinical profiles using the cBioPortal. *Sci. Signal* **2013**, *6*, pl1. [CrossRef] [PubMed]
62. Ythier, D.; Brambilla, E.; Binet, R.; Nissou, D.; Vesin, A.; de Fraipont, F.; Moro-Sibilot, D.; Lantuejoul, S.; Brambilla, C.; Gazzeri, S.; et al. Expression of candidate tumor suppressor gene ING2 is lost in non-small cell lung carcinoma. *Lung Cancer* **2010**, *69*, 180–186. [CrossRef] [PubMed]
63. Pan, Y.Q.; Zhang, X.; Xu, D.P.; Bao, W.G.; Lin, A.F.; Xu, H.H.; Yan, W.H. Decreased expression of ING2 gene and its clinicopathological significance in Chinese NSCLC patients. *Neoplasma* **2014**, *61*, 468–475. [CrossRef] [PubMed]
64. Al Zeyadi, M.; Dimova, I.; Ranchich, V.; Rukova, B.; Nesheva, D.; Hamude, Z.; Georgiev, S.; Petrov, D.; Toncheva, D. Whole genome microarray analysis in non-small cell lung cancer. *Biotechnol. Biotechnol. Equip.* **2015**, *29*, 111–118. [CrossRef] [PubMed]
65. Nie, J.; Liu, L.; Wu, M.; Xing, G.; He, S.; Yin, Y.; Tian, C.; He, F.; Zhang, L. HECT ubiquitin ligase Smurf1 targets the tumor suppressor ING2 for ubiquitination and degradation. *FEBS Lett.* **2010**, *584*, 3005–3012. [CrossRef]
66. Li, H.; Xiao, N.; Wang, Y.; Wang, R.; Chen, Y.; Pan, W.; Liu, D.; Li, S.; Sun, J.; Zhang, K.; et al. Smurf1 regulates lung cancer cell growth and migration through interaction with and ubiquitination of PIPKIγ. *Oncogene* **2017**, *36*, 5668–5680. [CrossRef]
67. Tan, W.-L.; Jain, A.; Takano, A.; Newell, E.W.; Iyer, N.G.; Lim, W.-T.; Tan, E.-H.; Zhai, W.; Hillmer, A.M.; Tam, W.-L.; et al. Novel therapeutic targets on the horizon for lung cancer. *Lancet Oncol.* **2016**, *17*, e347–e362. [CrossRef]
68. Smolle, E.; Fink-Neuboeck, N.; Lindenmann, J.; Smolle-Juettner, F.; Pichler, M. The Biological and Clinical Relevance of Inhibitor of Growth (ING) Genes in Non-Small Cell Lung Cancer. *Cancers* **2019**, *11*, 1118. [CrossRef]
69. Tsherniak, A.; Vazquez, F.; Montgomery, P.G.; Weir, B.A.; Kryukov, G.; Cowley, G.S.; Gill, S.; Harrington, W.F.; Pantel, S.; Krill-Burger, J.M.; et al. Defining a Cancer Dependency Map. *Cell* **2017**, *170*, 564–576. [CrossRef]
70. Laherty, C.D.; Yang, W.M.; Sun, J.M.; Davie, J.R.; Seto, E.; Eisenman, R.N. Histone deacetylases associated with the mSin3 corepressor mediate mad transcriptional repression. *Cell* **1997**, *89*, 349–356. [CrossRef]
71. Cowley, S.M.; Iritani, B.M.; Mendrysa, S.M.; Xu, T.; Cheng, P.F.; Yada, J.; Liggitt, H.D.; Eisenman, R.N. The mSin3A chromatin-modifying complex is essential for embryogenesis and T-cell development. *Mol. Cell. Biol.* **2005**, *25*, 6990–7004. [CrossRef]
72. Dannenberg, J.-H.; David, G.; Zhong, S.; van der Torre, J.; Wong, W.H.; Depinho, R.A. mSin3A corepressor regulates diverse transcriptional networks governing normal and neoplastic growth and survival. *Genes Dev.* **2005**, *19*, 1581–1595. [CrossRef] [PubMed]
73. Yao, C.; Carraro, G.; Konda, B.; Guan, X.; Mizuno, T.; Chiba, N.; Kostelny, M.; Kurkciyan, A.; David, G.;

McQualter, J.L.; et al. Sin3a regulates epithelial progenitor cell fate during lung development. *Development* **2017**, *144*, 2618–2628. [CrossRef] [PubMed]

74. Bansal, N.; David, G.; Farias, E.; Waxman, S. Emerging Roles of Epigenetic Regulator Sin3 in Cancer. *Adv. Cancer Res.* **2016**, *130*, 113–135. [PubMed]
75. Kwon, Y.-J.; Petrie, K.; Leibovitch, B.A.; Zeng, L.; Mezei, M.; Howell, L.; Gil, V.; Christova, R.; Bansal, N.; Yang, S.; et al. Selective Inhibition of SIN3 Corepressor with Avermectins as a Novel Therapeutic Strategy in Triple-Negative Breast Cancer. *Mol. Cancer Ther.* **2015**, *14*, 1824–1836. [CrossRef] [PubMed]
76. McDonel, P.; Demmers, J.; Tan, D.W.M.; Watt, F.; Hendrich, B.D. Sin3a is essential for the genome integrity and viability of pluripotent cells. *Dev. Biol.* **2012**, *363*, 62–73. [CrossRef]
77. Smith, K.T.; Martin-Brown, S.A.; Florens, L.; Washburn, M.P.; Workman, J.L. Deacetylase inhibitors dissociate the histone-targeting ING2 subunit from the Sin3 complex. *Chem. Biol.* **2010**, *17*, 65–74. [CrossRef]
78. Richon, V.M.; Sandhoff, T.W.; Rifkind, R.A.; Marks, P.A. Histone deacetylase inhibitor selectively induces p21WAF1 expression and gene-associated histone acetylation. *Proc. Natl. Acad. Sci. USA* **2000**, *97*, 10014–10019. [CrossRef]
79. Larrieu, D.; Ythier, D.; Brambilla, C.; Pedeux, R. ING2 controls the G1 to S-phase transition by regulating p21 expression. *Cell Cycle* **2010**, *9*, 3984–3990. [CrossRef]
80. Jones, P.A.; Issa, J.-P.J.; Baylin, S. Targeting the cancer epigenome for therapy. *Nat. Rev. Genet.* **2016**, *17*, 630–641. [CrossRef]
81. Loewith, R.; Meijer, M.; Lees-Miller, S.P.; Riabowol, K.; Young, D. Three yeast proteins related to the human candidate tumor suppressor p33(ING1) are associated with histone acetyltransferase activities. *Mol. Cell. Biol.* **2000**, *20*, 3807–3816. [CrossRef] [PubMed]
82. Kichina, J.V.; Zeremski, M.; Aris, L.; Gurova, K.V.; Walker, E.; Franks, R.; Nikitin, A.Y.; Kiyokawa, H.; Gudkov, A.V. Targeted disruption of the mouse ing1 locus results in reduced body size, hypersensitivity to radiation and elevated incidence of lymphomas. *Oncogene* **2006**, *25*, 857–866. [CrossRef] [PubMed]
83. Roca, M.S.; Di Gennaro, E.; Budillon, A. Implication for Cancer Stem Cells in Solid Cancer Chemo-Resistance: Promising Therapeutic Strategies Based on the Use of HDAC Inhibitors. *J. Clin. Med.* **2019**, *8*, 912. [CrossRef] [PubMed]
84. Patra, S.; Panigrahi, D.P.; Praharaj, P.P.; Bhol, C.S.; Mahapatra, K.K.; Mishra, S.R.; Behera, B.P.; Jena, M.; Bhutia, S.K. Dysregulation of histone deacetylases in carcinogenesis and tumor progression: A possible link to apoptosis and autophagy. *Cell. Mol. Life Sci.* **2019**, *76*, 3263–3282. [CrossRef]
85. Eckschlager, T.; Plch, J.; Stiborova, M.; Hrabeta, J. Histone Deacetylase Inhibitors as Anticancer Drugs. *Int. J. Mol. Sci.* **2017**, *18*, 1414. [CrossRef]

2

Is There an Interplay between Immune Checkpoint Inhibitors, Thromboprophylactic Treatments and Thromboembolic Events? Mechanisms and Impact in Non-Small Cell Lung Cancer Patients

Federico Nichetti [1,*], Francesca Ligorio [1], Emma Zattarin [1], Diego Signorelli [1], Arsela Prelaj [1], Claudia Proto [1], Giulia Galli [1], Antonio Marra [2], Giulia Apollonio [1], Luca Porcu [3], Filippo de Braud [1,4] Giuseppe Lo Russo [1], Roberto Ferrara [1] and Marina Chiara Garassino [1]

1 Department of Medical Oncology, Fondazione IRCCS Istituto Nazionale dei Tumori, 20133 Milan, Italy; francesca.ligorio@istitutotumori.mi.it (F.L.); emma.zattarin@istitutotumori.mi.it (E.Z.); Diego.Signorelli@istitutotumori.mi.it (D.S.); Arsela.Prelaj@istitutotumori.mi.it (A.P.); Claudia.proto@istitutotumori.mi.it (C.P.); giulia.galli@istitutotumori.mi.it (G.G.); Giulia.Apollonio@istitutotumori.mi.it (G.A.); Filippo.DeBraud@istitutotumori.mi.it (F.d.B.); Giuseppe.LoRusso@istitutotumori.mi.it (G.L.R.); Roberto.Ferrara@istitutotumori.mi.it (R.F.); Marina.Garassino@istitutotumori.mi.it (M.C.G.)

2 Department of Medical Oncology, Istituto Europeo di Oncologia, 20141 Milan, Italy; Antonio.marra@ieo.it

3 Department of Oncology, IRCCS Istituto di Ricerche Farmacologiche Mario Negri, 20156 Milan, Italy; luca.porcu@marionegri.it

4 Department of Oncology and Hemato-Oncology, University of Milan, 20122 Milan, Italy

* Correspondence: federico.nichetti@istitutotumori.mi.it

Abstract: PD-1 pathway blockade has been shown to promote proatherogenic T-cell responses and destabilization of atherosclerotic plaques. Moreover, preclinical evidence suggests a potential synergy of antiplatelet drugs with immune checkpoint inhibitors (ICIs). We conducted an analysis within a prospective observational protocol (APOLLO study) to investigate the rates, predictors, and prognostic significance of thromboembolic events (TE) and thromboprophylaxis in patients with advanced NSCLC treated with ICIs. Among 217 patients treated between April 2014 and September 2018, 13.8% developed TE events. Current smoking status (HR 3.61 (95% CI 1.52–8.60), $p = 0.004$) and high (>50%) PD-L1 (HR 2.55 (95% CI 1.05–6.19), $p = 0.038$) resulted in being independent TE predictors. An increased risk of death following a diagnosis of TE (HR 2.93; 95% CI 1.59–5.42; $p = 0.0006$) was observed. Patients receiving antiplatelet treatment experienced longer progression-free survival (PFS) (6.4 vs. 3.4 months, HR 0.67 (95% CI 0.48–0.92), $p = 0.015$) and a trend toward better OS (11.2 vs. 9.6 months, HR 0.78 (95% CI 0.55–1.09), $p = 0.14$), which were not confirmed in a multivariate model. No impact of anticoagulant treatment on patients' outcomes was observed. NSCLC patients treated with ICIs bear a consistent risk for thrombotic complications, with a detrimental effect on survival. The impact of antiplatelet drugs on ICIs efficacy deserves further investigation in prospective trials.

Keywords: immunotherapy; immune checkpoint inhibitors; thromboprophylaxis; aspirin; thromboembolic events; non-small cell lung cancer

1. Introduction

Non-small cell lung cancer (NSCLC) is the leading cause of cancer related death worldwide, with a five year overall survival rate of 10–15% [1]. Thromboembolic (TE) events represent a major complication among NSCLC patients, being reported in up to 14% of cases [2]. Among solid cancers, NSCLC patients are at higher risk of TE events, particularly during anticancer chemotherapy, resulting in worsened quality of life, increased health care costs, and shorter survival [2,3].

In recent years, the advent of immunotherapy has revolutionized the treatment landscape of NSCLC. Several clinical trials demonstrated the superior efficacy of immune checkpoint inhibitors (ICIs) over chemotherapy in the first and more advanced lines of treatment [4–10], with a markedly different toxicity profile. Monoclonal antibodies targeting the programmed cell death 1 (PD-1) and the programmed cell death ligand 1 (PD-L1) axis have been associated with a spectrum of immune related adverse events (irAEs), arising as a results of an aberrant activation of the immune system, thus leaving common chemotherapy associated AEs in the background [11]. Among these, TE events have not been commonly considered as an ICIs drug related toxicity and extremely low rates have been reported in ICI clinical trials, ranging from 0 to less than 5% [4–10]. A recent meta-analysis analyzing single agent PD-1/PD-L1 inhibitors and irAEs across different cancer types did not include thromboembolism as a toxicity outcome, with only single patient cases of TE events reported as treatment related deaths [12]. For these reasons, the incidence of TE events and potential variables able to identify patients at higher risk in this population are currently undefined [13]. Nevertheless, PD-1 pathway blockade has been shown to promote proatherogenic T-cell responses and growth and destabilization of atherosclerotic plaques in mouse models, suggesting that ICIs could potentially foster arterial vascular events [14,15]. Furthermore, despite a partially different pathogenesis, there is an emerging consensus that that venous and arterial TE events are not quite as disparate as previously thought and should be both investigated as a cancer related complication [16].

Given the negative impact of TE events on morbidity and mortality, anticoagulant and antiplatelet agents have been investigated as potential strategies to improve cancer patients' outcome. Experimental evidence suggests that low molecular weight heparin (LMWH) might have antitumor effects via inhibition of angiogenesis and metastatic spread [17]. However, clinical studies evaluating LMWH in lung cancer patients provided modest results [18–20], so that thromboprophylaxis is not routinely recommended in clinical practice. Considering antiplatelet drugs, preclinical data suggest that cyclooxygenase (COX) driven prostaglandin E2 (PGE2) might promote tumor immune escape and regulate PD-L1 expression within the tumor microenvironment [21–24]. Moreover, COX inhibitors (COXi) such as aspirin (ASA) and celecoxib significantly synergized with anti-PD-1 treatment in mouse models of melanoma and colorectal cancer [21,25]. While the addition of COXi to standard chemotherapy failed to improve patient outcomes in NSCLC [26–28], their use was associated with longer time to progression in ICI treated melanoma patients [29], and no data in NSCLC patients are currently available. COX-1/-2 and the microsomal form of human prostaglandin E synthase 1 (mPGES1) are both known to be overexpressed in NSCLC cells, suggesting a potential role for COXi in enhancing ICIs' efficacy also in this scenario [30].

In this study, we aimed at exploring the impact of TE events and anticoagulant and antiplatelet treatments in patients with NSCLC treated with ICIs.

2. Materials and Methods

2.1. Study Population

The present study was an unplanned analysis within a prospective observational protocol approved by the local Institutional Review Board (INT 22_15, APOLLO study) and was conducted in accordance with the Declaration of Helsinki. Medical records of all consecutive patients with locally advanced or metastatic NSCLC who completed at least one treatment cycle with ICIs, at Istituto Nazionale dei Tumori, Milan, Italy, between April 2014 and September 2018 were retrospectively reviewed. All patients signed a written informed consent. ICIs included PD-1 inhibitors (nivolumab and pembrolizumab), PD-L1 inhibitors (atezolizumab, avelumab, and durvalumab), and cytotoxic T-lymphocyte antigen 4 (CTLA-4) inhibitors (ipilimumab and tremelimumab). Treatments were provided until disease progression, unacceptable toxicity, or consent withdrawal. All patients were followed up until death, loss of contact, or time of data lock (31 January 2019). Treatment response was assessed per Response Evaluation Criteria in Solid Tumors (RECIST) v1.1.

2.2. Identification of TE Events and Anticoagulant and Antiplatelet Treatment

Both venous (deep venous thrombosis of the limbs, pulmonary embolism, or venous thrombosis of other districts excluding superficial thrombophlebitis) and arterial (acute coronary syndrome, cerebrovascular accident, or arterial thrombosis of other districts) TE events were identified by retrospective review of medical records including diagnostic imaging results (computerized tomography (CT), CT angiography, doppler ultrasonography), medication history, and review of outside medical records when available. Asymptomatic TE reported as an incidental imaging finding was included as a TE event. TE events were included while on ICI therapy or if they occurred within 90 days after ICI suspension and no other cancer treatment had been initiated by the patient. TE occurring during subsequent treatment lines were not considered as events. Baseline data regarding previous TE events and ongoing prophylactic or therapeutic anticoagulant treatment and antiplatelet treatment were also recorded. For the purpose of the study, patients were defined as receiving thromboprophylaxis if anticoagulant or antiplatelet treatment was ongoing at ICI treatment initiation and was not suspended before the first disease assessment.

2.3. Study Objectives

The main objectives of the study were (1) to evaluate the rates of TE events in NSCLC patients treated with ICIs and (2) to explore the impact of TE events and anticoagulant and antiplatelet treatments on patients' survival. Secondary objectives were to investigate potential risk factors for TE events and to assess the risk assessment capacity of the Khorana score in this population [31].

2.4. Statistical Analysis

Descriptive statistics were used to analyze and report patients' characteristics. Association between categorical or continuous variables and TE events were performed by the Chi-squared or Wilcoxon–Mann–Whitney test, respectively. The thresholds for neutrophil to lymphocyte ratio (NLR) (outside the lung immune prognostic index (LIPI)) and platelet to lymphocyte ratio (PLR) were determined by calculating the area under the curve from the receiver operating characteristic (ROC) curves according to TE event occurrence [32]. Progression-free survival (PFS) was calculated from ICI start to the date of radiological or clinical disease progression, last follow-up, or death for any cause. Overall survival (OS) was calculated from ICI start to the date of death or last follow-up. Survival curves were estimated by the Kaplan–Meier method and compared by log-rank. Duration of follow-up was calculated using the reverse Kaplan–Meier method. To assess the impact of TE events on survival, OS of patients who developed TE events was compared to those who did not. To eliminate the likelihood of immortal time bias (due to the time dependent nature of TE) [33], TE events were tested as a time varying covariate, where patients started in the "no TE event" group and were switched to the "TE event" group at the date of TE diagnosis. To test the biological relationship between TE events and covariates, TE event specific hazards were calculated considering the interval from the date of ICI start to the first date of TE identification, and patients not developing TE before starting any subsequent anticancer treatment were censored at the last date of follow-up or death. Cox's proportional hazards models were used to identify the strongest predictors of TE development and for survival analyses. Hazards ratios (HRs) together with 95% confidence intervals (CI) were provided. Multivariate analysis was calculated for the significant ($p \leq 0.1$) variables by the univariate test or by a priori selection for biological relevance. The statistical significance threshold was set to a two tailed 0.05 value. R software (Version 3.5.3) and RStudio software (Version 1.1.456) were used for statistical analyses.

3. Results

3.1. Patients' Characteristics

A total of 217 patients were included. At the moment of data analysis, 30 patients (13.8%) developed TE events, 181 (83.4%) had progressed, and 166 (76.5%) had died. Median follow up was 37.8 (22.6–43.9) months. Patients' characteristics of the entire study population and according to occurrence of TE events are shown in Table 1. Baseline laboratory values are provided in Table S1. No significant differences in terms of clinical and biological characteristics were observed between patients experiencing TE events or not except for smoking status and PD-L1 expression. Specifically, the percentages of current smokers (42.9% vs. 23.3%, $p = 0.05$) and of patients with tumor PDL-1 expression >50% (43.3 vs. 18.8%, $p = 0.01$) were significantly higher among the TE event group compared to the no TE event group. Regarding blood parameters, TE events occurred more frequently in patients with lower baseline PLR ($p = 0.002$) and lower NLR ($p = 0.053$), with a threshold defined by ROC curves of 181 and 3.2, respectively.

Table 1. Baseline patients' characteristics in the whole case series and according to the presence or absence of TE events.

Characteristic	Overall $n = 217$	Without TE $n = 187$	With TE $n = 30$
Sex, Male	136 (62.7)	115 (61.5)	21 (70.0)
Age, median (range), y	70 (32–90)	70 (32–90)	70 (56–83)
≤65	77 (35.5)	66 (35.3)	11 (36.7)
>65	140 (64.5)	121 (64.7)	19 (63.3)
ECOG PS			
0–1	198 (91.2)	168 (89.8)	30 (100.0)
≥2	19 (8.8)	19 (10.2)	\
Smoking *			
Never or former	154 (71.0)	138 (76.7)	16 (57.1)
Current	54 (24.9)	42 (23.3)	12 (42.9)
Pathologic subtype			
Non-squamous	168 (77.4)	146 (78.1)	22 (73.3)
Squamous	49 (22.6)	41 (21.9)	8 (26.7)
Molecular status [x]			
EGFR mutation	11 (5.1)	10 (6.3)	1 (3.7)
ALK translocation	2 (0.9)	1 (0.7)	1 (3.8)
PD-L1 status #			
≤50%	89 (41.0)	79 (42.2)	10 (33.3)
>50%	48 (22.1)	35 (18.8)	13 (43.3)
Not assessed	80 (36.9)	73 (39.0)	7 (23.4)
Previous Tx with TKI	18 (8.3)	15 (8.0)	3 (10.0)
Disease stage			
Locally advanced	10 (4.6)	8 (4.3)	2 (6.7)
Metastatic	207 (95.4)	179 (95.7)	28 (93.3)
Number of disease sites **			
≤2	98 (45.2)	80 (42.8)	18 (60.0)
>2	109 (50.2)	99 (52.9)	10 (33.3)
Brain metastases	44 (20.3)	39 (20.9)	5 (16.7)
Liver metastases	44 (20.3)	39 (20.9)	5 (16.7)

Table 1. *Cont.*

Characteristic	Overall $n = 217$	Without TE $n = 187$	With TE $n = 30$
Comorbidities			
Arterial hypertension	44 (20.3)	38 (20.3)	6 (20.0)
COPD	25 (11.5)	27 (11.8)	3 (10.0)
Diabetes mellitus	21 (9.7)	18 (9.6)	3 (10.0)
Previous ACS	18 (8.3)	13 (7.0)	5 (16.7)
Previous stroke	9 (4.1)	6 (3.2)	3 (10.0)
Atrial fibrillation	10 (4.6)	10 (5.4)	\
Previous venous TE events	37 (17.1)	31 (16.6)	6 (20.0)
BMI [xx]			
>25	88 (40.6)	71 (47.3)	17 (68.0)
>30	41 (18.9)	34 (18.2)	7 (23.3)
Antiplatelet treatment	69 (31.8)	56 (29.9)	13 (43.3)
ASA based treatment	61 (28.1)	49 (26.2)	12 (40.0)
Anticoagulant treatment	47 (21.7)	42 (22.5)	5 (16.7)
Therapeutic dosage	8 (3.7)	7 (3.7)	1 (3.3)

Data are presented as n (%) except where otherwise noted. * Data were missing for 9 patients. ** Patients with locally advanced disease were excluded from the analysis. [x] No ROS1 rearrangements were detected. EGFR mutations and ALK rearrangements were not assessed in 31 and 39 patients, respectively. [#] Defined positive as a tumor proportion score (TPS) ≥50% using Dako clone 22C3 or Ventana clone SP263 antibodies. [xx] Data were missing for 42 patients. Abbreviations: ACS: acute coronary syndrome; ASA: aspirin; BMI: body mass index; COPD: chronic obstructive pulmonary disease; ECOG PS: Eastern Cooperative Oncology Group Performance Status; LMWH: low molecular weight heparin; TE events: thromboembolic events; TKI: tyrosine kinase inhibitor; Tx: treatment.

Treatment characteristics are reported in Table 2. The majority of patients (151, 69.6%) underwent treatment with anti-PD1 (nivolumab in 117 cases, pembrolizumab in 34 cases), 58 (26.7%) with an anti-PD-L1 (atezolizumab in 16 cases, avelumab in 4 cases, and durvalumab in 38 cases), and 8 (3.7%) patients with combined durvalumab + tremelimumab. The median number of administered treatment cycles and treatment duration were markedly higher in the TE group (20 (9–31) vs. 6 (3–16) cycles ($p < 0.001$) and 9.4 (5.4–21.7) vs. 2.9 (1.4–9.0) months ($p < 0.001$), respectively). ICI treatment was still ongoing at the time of database lock in 31 cases (14.3%). The overall objective response rate was 18.9%, whereas the disease control rate was 54.8% and both were significantly higher in patients experiencing TE events ($p = 0.015$ and 0.001, respectively). No significant differences in terms of irAEs were observed between the two groups.

Table 2. Treatment characteristics in the whole case series and according to the presence or absence of TE events.

Characteristic	Overall $n = 217$	Without TE $n = 187$	With TE $n = 30$
Line of Treatment			
<2	55 (25.4)	51 (27.3)	4 (13.3)
≥2	162 (74.6)	136 (72.7)	26 (86.7)
Drug Class			
Anti-PD-1	151 (69.6)	133 (71.1)	18 (60.0)
Anti-PD-L1	58 (26.7)	46 (24.6)	12 (40.0)
Anti PD-L1 + Anti CTLA-4	8 (3.7)	8 (4.3)	\
No. of administered cycles, median (IQR)	7 (3–19)	6 (3–16)	20 (9–31)
Treatment duration, median (IQR, months)	3.6 (1.5–10.3)	2.9 (1.4–9.0)	9.4 (5.4–21.7)

Table 2. *Cont.*

Characteristic	Overall $n = 217$	Without TE $n = 187$	With TE $n = 30$
Best Response			
Complete Response	5 (2.3)	4 (2.1)	1 (3.3)
Partial Response	36 (16.6)	26 (13.9)	10 (33.3)
Stable Disease	78 (35.9)	64 (34.2)	14 (46.7)
Progressive Disease	98 (45.2)	93 (49.7)	5 (16.7)
Objective Response	41 (18.9)	30 (16.0)	11 (36.7)
Disease Control	119 (54.8)	94 (50.3)	25 (83.3)
Adverse Events ≥2 (other than TE)			
Anemia	6 (2.8)	4 (2.1)	2 (6.7)
Thrombocytopenia	2 (0.9)	2 (1.1)	\
Fatigue	10 (4.6)	9 (4.8)	1 (3.3)
Liver toxicity	10 (4.6)	8 (4.3)	2 (6.7)
Arthralgia	4 (1.8)	4 (2.1)	\
Colitis/diarrhea	7 (3.2)	7 (3.7)	\
Hyper/hypothyroidism	9 (4.1)	7 (3.7)	2 (6.7)
Pneumonitis	9 (4.1)	8 (4.3)	1 (3.3)
Pruritus or skin rash	8 (3.7)	6 (3.2)	2 (6.7)

Data are presented as *n* (%) except where otherwise noted. Abbreviations: CTLA-4: cytotoxic T-lymphocyte antigen 4; IQR: interquartile range; PD-1/PD-L1: programmed death-1/programmed death-ligand 1; TE: thromboembolic events.

3.2. Clinical Characteristics and Risk Factors of TE Events

The detailed description of TE events is provided in Table S2. Thirty (13.8%) patients developed TE events, with 16 venous (5 deep vein thrombosis, 6 pulmonary embolism, 2 portal vein thrombosis, 3 miscellaneous) and 14 arterial (2 acute coronary syndromes, 9 strokes, 3 visceral arterial thromboses) cases. Two venous TE events occurred after definitive ICI suspension for disease progression, but before any other treatment was initiated. Median time to occurrence of TE events was 7.5 months (range 1.2–33.6 months; see Figure 1), with no difference between arterial and venous cases. TE events were never the cause of treatment suspension or death in our population. No patient had more than one TE event during ICIs.

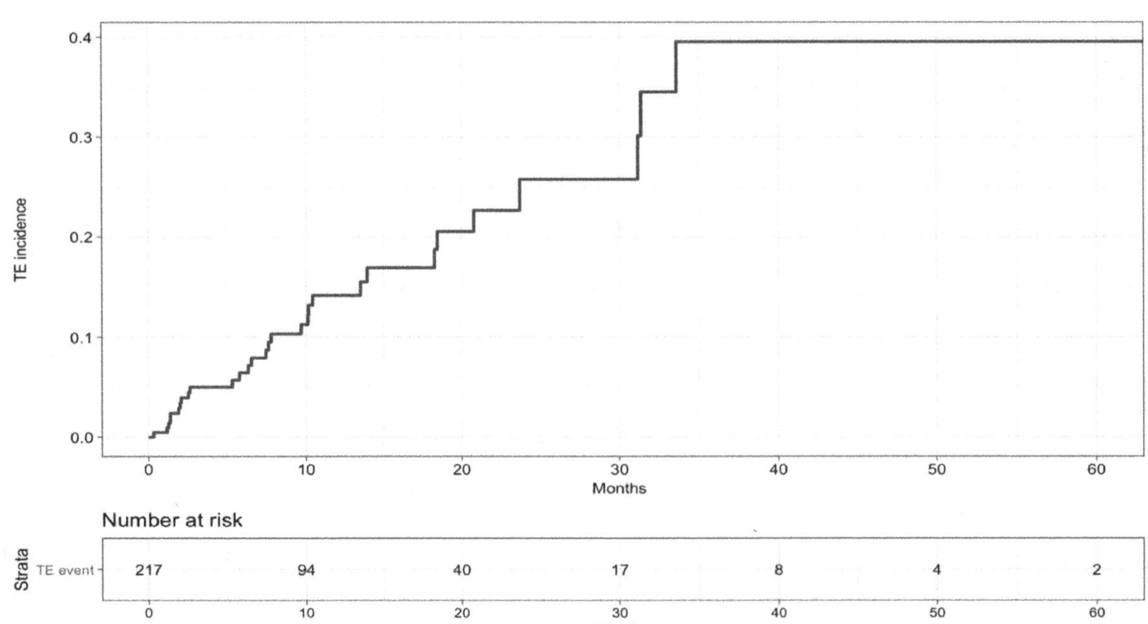

Figure 1. Thromboembolic events' cumulative incidence.

In the whole study population, sixty-nine patients (31.8%) were on antiplatelet treatment, of whom 61 were ASA users, the remaining taking clopidogrel or ticlopidine. Forty-seven (21.7%) patients were under anticoagulant treatment, of whom 44 with LMWH and 8 receiving a therapeutic dosage. No significant difference was observed for anticoagulant or antiplatelet treatment use in TE patients compared to no TE patients.

The Cox regression analysis identified variables affecting the risk of TE events (Table 3): by univariate analysis, the best predictors of TE events were smoking status (HR 2.48; 95% CI 1.17–5.26; $p = 0.02$) and PD-L1 positivity (HR 2.16; 95% CI 0.94–4.95; $p = 0.07$), while high PLR (HR 0.42; 95% CI 0.19–0.92; $p = 0.03$) and presence of >2 metastatic sites (HR 0.52; 95% CI 0.24–1.12; $p = 0.09$) were associated with a reduced TE risk. Kaplan–Meier curves for TE event specific hazards according to these variables are available in Figures S1–S4. Given the number of target events and the biological rationale, only smoking status, PD-L1 status, and PLR were included in the multivariate analysis (Table 4). This model confirmed an independent association between smoking status (HR 3.61; 95% CI 1.52–8.60; $p = 0.004$), PD-L1 positive status (HR 2.55; 95% CI 1.05–6.19; $p = 0.038$), and TE events. Of note, the Khorana score showed only a non-significant trend for TE prediction, and anticoagulant or antiplatelet treatments did not result in a protective effect (Table 3).

Table 3. Univariate analyses of TE event specific hazards according to patients and treatment characteristics.

Variables	Subgroups	HR	95% CI	*p*
Sex	Male vs. female	1.73	0.79–3.79	0.17
Age	>65 vs. ≤65	0.97	0.46–2.03	0.93
Smoking	Current vs. never/former	2.48	1.17–5.26	**0.02**
ECOG PS *	≥1 vs. 0	1.12	0.54–2.35	0.76
PD-L1 status	>50% vs. <50%	2.16	0.94–4.95	**0.07**
Pathologic subtype	Squamous vs. non-squamous	1.52	0.68–3.43	0.31
Number of disease sites	>2 vs. ≤2	0.52	0.24–1.12	**0.09**
Brain metastases	Yes vs. no	0.74	0.28–1.93	0.53
Liver metastases	Yes vs. no	0.74	0.28–1.93	0.53
BMI	>25 vs. ≤25	1.98	0.85–4.59	0.11
	>30 vs. ≤30	1.18	0.49–2.82	0.71
Previous venous TEs	Yes vs. no	1.12	0.46–2.75	0.80
Khorana score	2 vs. 1	1.37	0.58–3.20	0.47
	3 vs. 1	1.75	0.64–4.78	0.28
Antiplatelet treatment	Yes vs. no	1.57	0.76–3.25	0.22
Anticoagulant treatment	Yes vs. no	0.86	0.33–2.25	0.75
Drug class	Anti-PD-1 vs. anti-PD-L1 (+/−anti CTLA4)	1.23	0.59–2.55	0.59
Line of treatment	≥2 vs. <2	2.34	0.81–6.72	0.11
LDH	>480 vs. ≤480 U/L	2.01	0.85–4.73	0.11
NLR	>3.2 vs. ≤3.2	0.80	0.38–1.66	0.54
PLR	>181 vs. ≤181	0.42	0.19–0.92	**0.03**

The *p* value is indicated in bold numbers when statistically significant. * This threshold was set since no patients with baseline ECOG PS ≥ 2 had a TE event. Abbreviations: ASA: aspirin; BMI: body mass index; CI: confidence interval; LDH: lactate dehydrogenase; LMWH: low molecular weight heparin; NLR: neutrophil to lymphocyte ratio; PLR: platelet to lymphocyte ratio; ECOG PS: Eastern Cooperative Oncology Group Performance Status; TE: thromboembolic events.

Table 4. Multivariate analyses of TE event specific hazards according to patients and treatment characteristics.

Variables	Subgroups	HR	95% CI	*p*
Smoking	Current vs. never/former	3.61	1.52–8.60	**0.004**
PD-L1 status	>50% vs. <50%	2.55	1.05–6.19	**0.038**
PLR	> 181 vs. ≤181	0.53	0.21–1.33	0.178

The *p* value is indicated in bold numbers when statistically significant. Abbreviations: CI: confidence interval; PLR: platelet to lymphocyte ratio.

3.3. Impact of TE Events and Anticoagulant and Antiplatelet Treatments on Survival

The impact of TE events and anticoagulant and antiplatelet treatments on patients' OS was first assessed by univariate analysis (Table 5). Given the preliminary associations with a better objective response rate, disease control rate, and treatment duration, the effect of TE diagnosis on OS was first explored as a time independent variable. Patients experiencing TE events showed longer OS compared with those who did not (median, 15.9 vs. 8.8 months, HR 0.59; 95% CI, 0.37–0.93; $p = 0.02$; see Figure S5). However, with TE events defined as a time varying covariate, we observed an increased risk of death following a diagnosis of TE, with an overall univariable HR of 1.70 (95% CI, 1.06–2.72; $p = 0.029$). No significant impact on OS was detected for anticoagulant treatment (median, 7.8 vs. 10.3 months, HR 1.21; 95% CI, 0.84–1.73; $p = 0.31$; Figure 2), considered either prophylactic or therapeutic, nor for antiplatelet therapy, despite an observed favorable trend (median, 11.2 vs. 9.6 months, HR 0.78; 95% CI 0.55–1.09; $p = 0.14$; Figure 3). A multivariate model including other covariates statistically associated with OS (i.e., ECOG PS, PD-L1 status, line of treatment, and LIPI) was performed. Since NLR and PLR positively correlated with each other (Pearson coefficient correlation = 0.68; $p < 0.001$) and NLR was included in the LIPI, PLR was excluded from the multivariate analysis. In this model, TE events kept an independent negative prognostic value in terms of OS (HR 2.93; 95% CI 1.59–5.42; $p = 0.0006$; Table 6).

Table 5. Univariate Cox proportional hazards model for overall survival.

Variables	Subgroups	HR	95% CI	*p*
TE events	Yes vs. no, time independent	0.59	0.37–0.93	**0.023**
	Yes vs. no, time dependent	1.70	1.06–2.72	**0.029**
Anticoagulant treatment	Yes vs. no	1.21	0.84–1.73	0.31
Antiplatelet treatment	Yes vs. no	0.78	0.55–1.09	0.14
Sex	Male vs. female	1.26	0.92–1.73	0.16
Age	>65 vs. ≤65	1.06	0.77–1.45	0.74
Smoking	Current vs. never/former	0.89	0.62–1.28	0.53
ECOG PS	≥2 vs. 0–1	3.71	2.21–6.25	**<0.0001**
PD-L1 status	>50% vs. ≤50%	0.48	0.30–0.76	**0.0016**
Number of disease sites	>2 vs. ≤2	1.05	0.77–1.43	0.74
Brain metastases	Yes vs. no	1.04	0.71–1.51	0.85
Liver metastases	Yes vs. no	1.38	0.95–1.98	0.09
Line of treatment	≥2 vs. <2	1.63	1.09–2.43	**0.018**
BMI	>25 vs. ≤25	0.92	0.65–1.30	0.64
	>30 vs. ≤30	1.20	0.82–1.77	0.35
LIPI	High vs. low	3.44	2.11–5.62	**<0.0001**
	Intermediate vs. low	1.89	1.29–2.75	
PLR	311.18 vs. 145.73	1.17	1.05–1.31	**0.005**

The *p* value is indicated in bold numbers when statistically significant. Abbreviations: ASA: aspirin; BMI: body mass index; CI: confidence interval; LMWH: low molecular weight heparin; PLR: platelet to lymphocyte ratio; ECOG PS: Eastern Cooperative Oncology Group Performance Status; LIPI: lung immune prognostic index, TE events: thromboembolic events.

When looking at PFS (Table 7), antiplatelet drugs users were characterized by a longer PFS compared to nonusers (median, 6.4 vs. 3.4 months, HR 0.67; 95% CI 0.48–0.92; $p = 0.015$; Figure 4). Notably, a comparable difference was observed when restricting the analysis only to patients taking ASA (median, 6.5 vs. 3.4 months, HR 0.67; 95% CI 0.48–0.94; $p = 0.021$; Figure S6). Conversely, baseline anticoagulants use resulted in a trend for worse PFS (median, 2.3 vs. 4.2 months, HR 1.38; 95% CI 0.98–1.96; $p = 0.065$; Figure 5). Patients receiving anticoagulant treatment had significantly worse baseline ECOG PS (see Table S3), which could explain the lower PFS experienced upon ICIs. In the multivariate model including other covariates statistically associated with PFS (i.e., ECOG PS, PD-L1 status, presence of liver metastases, line of treatment, and LIPI), antiplatelet and anticoagulant treatments did not confirm an effect on patients PFS (HR 0.96; 95% CI, 0.59–1.57; $p = 0.88$, and HR 1.38; 95% CI, 0.82–2.32; $p = 0.22$, respectively; Table 8).

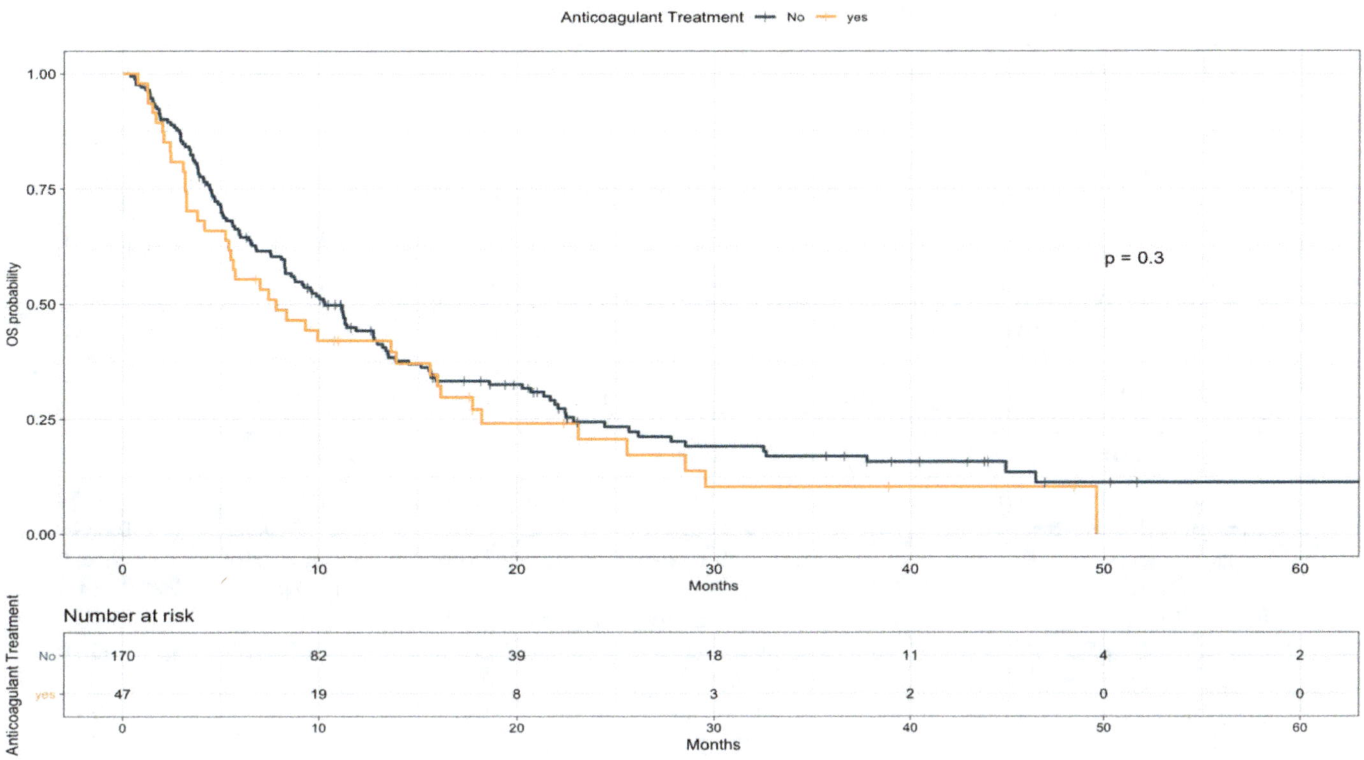

Figure 2. Overall survival according to anticoagulant treatment.

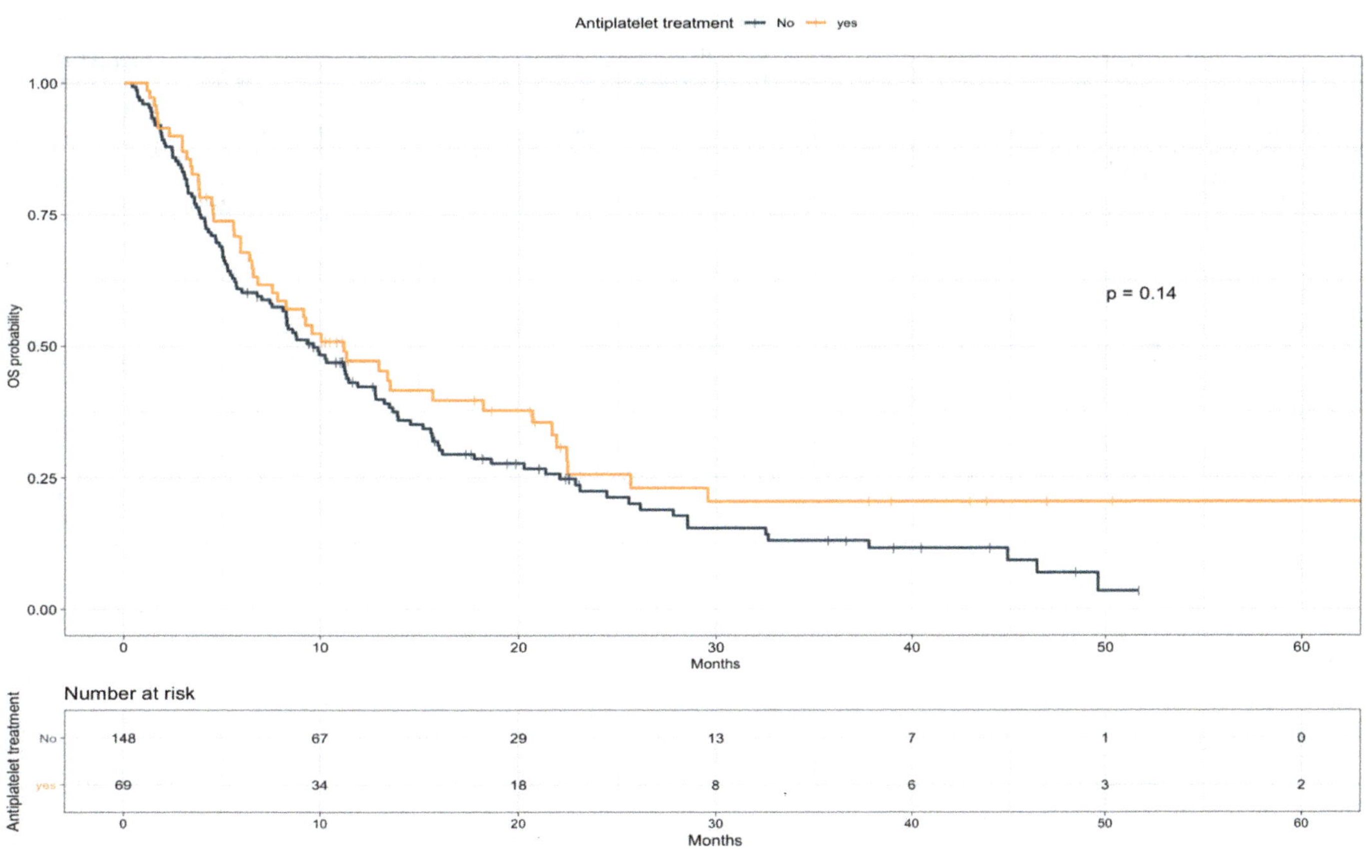

Figure 3. Overall survival according to antiplatelet treatment.

Table 6. Multivariate Cox proportional hazards models for overall survival.

Variables	Subgroups	HR	95% CI	*p*
TE events	Yes vs. no, time dependent	2.93	1.59–5.42	**0.0006**
ECOG PS	≥2 vs. 0–1	3.29	1.50–7.21	**0.0029**
PD-L1 status	>50% vs. ≤50%	0.36	0.21–0.64	**0.0004**
Line of treatment	≥2 vs. <2	1.64	0.93–2.91	0.0889
LIPI	High vs. low	3.14	1.58–6.27	**0.0001**
	Intermediate vs. low	3.14	1.82–5.40	

The *p* value is indicated in bold numbers when statistically significant. Abbreviations: ASA: aspirin; CI: confidence interval; ECOG PS: Eastern Cooperative Oncology Group Performance Status; LIPI: lung immune prognostic index.

Table 7. Univariate Cox proportional hazards model for progression-free survival.

Variables	Subgroups	HR	95% CI	*p*
Anticoagulant treatment	Yes vs. no	1.38	0.98–1.96	**0.065**
Antiplatelet treatment	Yes vs. no	0.67	0.48–0.92	**0.014**
Sex	Male vs. female	1.08	0.80–1.46	0.62
Age	>65 vs. ≤65	0.91	0.67–1.23	0.54
Smoking	Current vs. never/former	0.79	0.56–1.11	0.18
ECOG PS	≥2 vs. 0–1	2.55	1.57–4.13	**0.0001**
PD-L1 status	>50% vs. ≤50%	0.40	0.26–0.61	**<0.0001**
Number of disease sites	>2 vs. ≤2	1.00	0.75–1.35	0.99
Brain metastases	Yes vs. no	1.05	0.73–1.50	0.80
Liver metastases	Yes vs. no	1.44	1.02–2.05	**0.041**
Line of Treatment	≥2 vs. <2	1.78	1.23–2.57	**0.002**
BMI	>25 vs. ≤25	0.78	0.56–1.09	0.15
	>30 vs. ≤30	1.12	0.77–1.63	0.56
LIPI	High vs. low	2.80	1.76–4.47	**0.0001**
	Intermediate vs. low	1.59	1.11–2.26	
PLR	311.18 vs. 145.73	1.35	1.18–1.55	**<0.0001**

The *p* value is indicated in bold numbers when statistically significant. Abbreviations: ASA: aspirin; BMI: body mass index; CI: confidence interval; LMWH: low molecular weight heparin; PLR: platelet to lymphocyte ratio; ECOG PS: Eastern Cooperative Oncology Group Performance Status; LIPI: lung immune prognostic index.

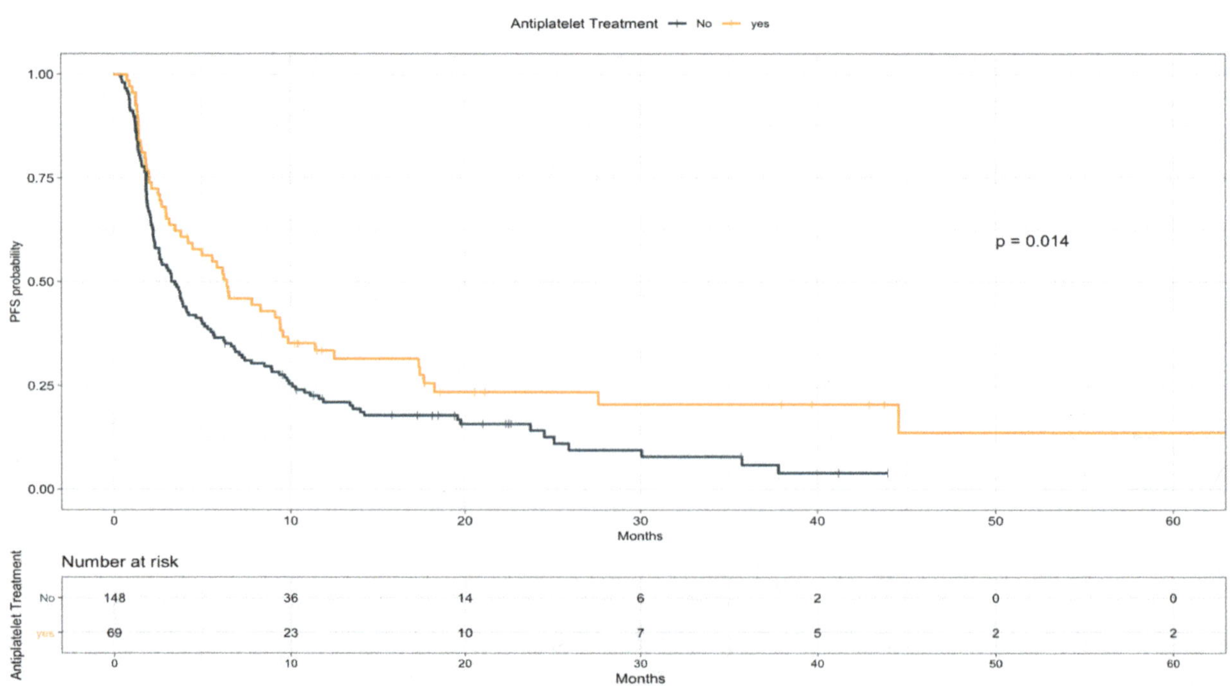

Figure 4. Progression-free survival according to antiplatelet treatment.

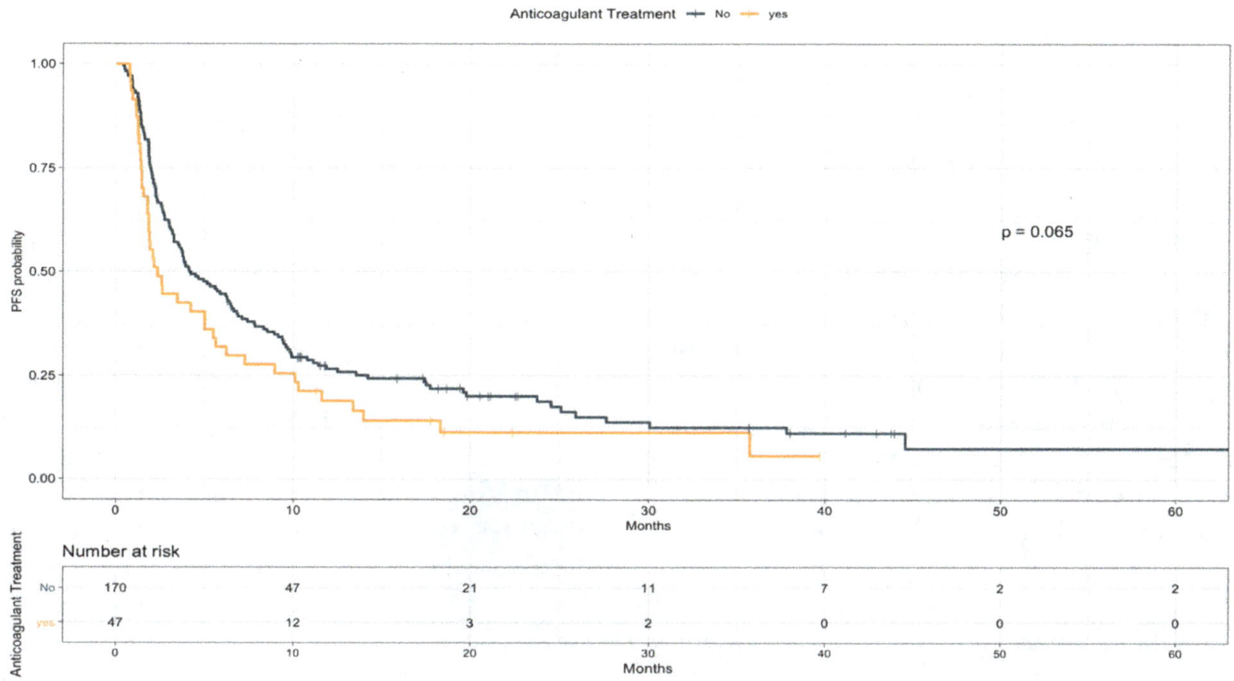

Figure 5. Progression-free survival according to anticoagulant treatment.

Table 8. Multivariate Cox proportional hazards models for progression-free survival.

Variables	Subgroups	HR	95% CI	*p*
Antiplatelet treatment	Yes vs. no	0.96	0.59–1.57	0.88
Anticoagulant treatment	Yes vs. No	1.38	0.82–2.32	0.22
ECOG PS	≥2 vs. 0–1	2.01	0.94–4.32	0.073
Liver metastases	Yes vs. no	1.10	0.64–1.89	0.73
PD-L1 status	>50% vs. ≤50%	0.41	0.25–0.67	**0.0004**
Line of treatment	≥2 vs. <2	1.79	1.07–2.98	**0.025**
LIPI	High vs. low	2.74	1.41–5.31	**0.0039**
	Intermediate vs. low	2.04	1.25–3.32	

The *p* value is indicated in bold numbers when statistically significant. Abbreviations: ASA: aspirin; BMI: body mass index; CI: confidence interval; PLR: derived platelet to lymphocyte ratio; ECOG PS: Eastern Cooperative Oncology Group Performance Status; LIPI: lung immune prognostic index.

4. Discussion

Thromboembolic events are a common complication in patients with lung cancer, contributing to increased morbidity and mortality [34,35]. To date, the incidence of TE events in cancer patients receiving immunotherapy is unknown. Preclinical data showed that the PD-1/PD-L1 pathway plays an important role in downregulating proatherogenic T-cell responses, so that its blockade may lead to increased levels of pro-inflammatory cytokines and T-cell driven progression and destabilization of atherosclerotic plaques [14,15]. In the clinical setting, only a few isolated reports described thrombotic events as possible irAEs, mostly as arterial cases [36–38]. Tomita et al. presented a first report of acute coronary syndrome in a PD-L1 high, NSCLC patient who achieved complete response with nivolumab, suggesting it as a possible immune related adverse event [37]. Boutros and colleagues described four TE cases during ICI treatment, highlighting the presence of large amounts of entrapped leucocytes in a patient's thrombus after embolectomy [38]. Finally, in a large series including patients with different cancer subtypes receiving ICIs, an unexpected high rate of TE events (30.3%) was reported, with a potential association with worsened survival [39].

In the present study, we described for the first time the rates and characteristics of TE events in NSCLC patients receiving ICIs. We showed that the risk is not negligible, as the percentage of patients developing thrombosis was in line with previous literature data in the overall NSCLC patients' population [2]. Moreover, while TE risk is particularly high in the first few months following the start of chemotherapy [40], here we showed that TE events occurred throughout the course of ICI treatment, with two thirds of cases reported after the first six months. Of note, about half of the cases were represented by arterial events. In our opinion, these data raise two hypotheses: ICIs may directly increase the risk of arterial events (as suggested by mouse models) or these events may be linked to risk factors independent of patients' cancer treatment. In this latter scenario, ICI long responders develop TE events as a result of longer survival, longer exposure to "other-than-cancer" risk factors (e.g., lifestyle, comorbidities), and thus longer time at risk for incident TE. In our series, the increased TE risk associated with smoking status and high PD-L1 expression agreed with both of these hypotheses, as these factors may promote atherogenesis, but also contribute to better patient outcome during ICI treatment. In particular, PGE2 concentration in lung cancer tissue significantly correlates with PD-1 expression on $CD8^+$ tumor infiltrating lymphocytes, suggesting PGE2 related inflammation as a possible link between TE events and T-cells' exhaustion [41]. Furthermore, we observed that the development of TE events during ICIs is an independent prognostic factor associated with worse survival when considered as a time dependent variable [39].

Overall, these observations raise the problem of how to predict and prevent TE events effectively in this population. Most risk assessment models for cancer associated thrombosis were developed on patients treated with chemotherapy and only for venous events [31,42], justifying why we did not observe a good prediction power for the Khorana score in our series.

Regarding thromboprophylaxis, randomized trials have shown that LMWH and direct oral anticoagulants approximately halve the risk of venous TE events in cancer patients [43–45]. However, most studies did not consider arterial events and did not include a relevant number of patients treated with ICIs. In our study, we did not observe a significant difference in TE rates according to anticoagulant or antiplatelet treatment. Moreover, LMWH users experienced worse PFS and a trend toward worse OS. Due to the lack of rationale for a detrimental effect of LMWH on ICIs' efficacy, we hypothesize that thromboprophylaxis was prescribed in patients in worse clinical conditions, with higher disease burden and reduced mobility.

Intriguingly, patients receiving antiplatelet treatment, and in particular ASA users, experienced longer PFS and a non-significant trend toward better OS. This benefit might also be underestimated in our series, since patients might have been receiving antiplatelet drugs for multiple comorbidities (e.g., hypertension, diabetes, previous cardiovascular accidents; see Table S4) that represent negative prognostic indicators themselves. Preclinical studies showed that the COX-2/mPGES1 pathway is able to promote tumor immune escape mechanisms by increasing the number of T regulatory cells [46] and myeloid derived suppressor cells [47], as well as by driving increased expression of indoleamine 2,3-dioxygenase 1 [48] and PD-L1 [24,49,50] by cancer cells. Moreover, a potential synergic effect between COX inhibition and anti-PD/PD-L1 immunotherapy has been demonstrated in mouse tumor models [21,22]. Our findings support these hypotheses, showing for the first time in a clinical scenario that COX inhibition with ASA is associated with better outcome in NSCLC patients treated with ICIs. Of note, prospective, randomized trials testing COX inhibitors (NCT03638297, NCT03245489) and PGE2 receptor 4 antagonists (NCT03696212, NCT03658772) in combination with ICIs are ongoing [23]. However, the effect of COX-2/mPGES1 pathway inhibition on PD-L1 expression and the impact of this modulation on ICIs efficacy are still controversial. While some in vitro studies reported that COX-2 inhibition reduced the expression of PD-L1 [24,49,51] and may potentially reduce exhaustion of T-cells in the tumor microenvironment [41], others highlighted that treatment with celecoxib did not affect PD-L1 levels in melanoma and NSCLC cells [22,52], and PD-L1 staining was also shown to be dramatically greater in mPGES1 knock out derived tumor tissues compared to controls [22]. Furthermore, the effect of other COXi (e.g., nonsteroidal anti-inflammatory drugs and paracetamol) on

ICI treatment outcome might differ from that of low dose ASA due to the different COX selectivity and reversibility of the binding. Finally, an alternative way to reduce PGE2 through reprogramming the fatty acid metabolism of tumor infiltrating myeloid derived suppressor cells has been shown to synergize with PD-1 blockade in murine models [53].

Our study had clearly some limitations. In particular, the retrospective, monocentric nature of the investigation, the lack of a statistical power calculation, the limited number of events, the heterogeneity of treatment lines and ICIs administered (e.g., anti-PD-1 and anti-PD-L1), and the missing data like PD-L1 status for several cases might have affected our results. Likewise, we included patients receiving variable anticoagulant and antiplatelet compounds, with different treatment schedules (e.g., prophylactic or therapeutic dosages) and affecting different biological pathways (e.g., aspirin as a COX inhibitor vs. clopidogrel targeting $P2Y_{12}$ on platelets). Future investigations should include prospective homogenous cohorts to prevent any bias on this issue. Despite a strong preclinical rationale, the initial association between antiplatelet agents' use and ICIs' efficacy was not confirmed when other factors were considered. A control arm (e.g., NSCLC patients treated with chemotherapy) with a propensity matching to compare the outcomes of patients with comparable baseline characteristics will be necessary to elucidate a potential synergy in future studies. Similarly, in order to demonstrate a direct correlation between ICIs and TE events, a control arm of patients with similar characteristics not receiving immunotherapy would have been optimal. However, this comparison is hard to perform, since NSCLC patients treated with chemotherapy are at even higher risk of TE events, as are patients with driver mutations receiving targeted therapies [54–56]. Moreover, if tested, lower rates of PD-L1 positivity would be found in these populations, as this might represent the reason to omit ICIs. Finally, given the partially different pathogenesis of arterial and venous TE events, future studies conducted on larger series analyzing these events separately could be useful.

5. Conclusions

In conclusion, we aimed at evaluating the clinical relevance of TE events and antithrombotic treatments in NSCLC patients treated with immunotherapy. To our knowledge, this is the first study to show to that these patients bear a consistent risk for thrombotic complications.

Our study was exploratory in its nature and clearly prevented definitive conclusions. Nevertheless, our data serve as a first report on this topic and deserve further investigation in prospective studies to better define patients at high risk for TE events as candidates for thromboprophylaxis. Our aim was to raise awareness on this issue, which might become even more significant as immunotherapy-chemotherapy combinations enter clinical practice in the near future [57,58].

Lastly, we investigated a potential association between the use of antiplatelet agents and ICI treatment outcomes. Together with previous preclinical evidence, our data provide an additional rationale to implement novel clinical trials testing COX-2 inhibitors' potential to prevent NSCLC immune evasion, as well as to enhance the anti-tumor activity of PD-1/PD-L1 based immunotherapy. If these findings are confirmed, these compounds may represent a valid, low cost option to increase ICIs' efficacy and patients' outcomes.

Supplementary Materials:
Table S1: Baseline laboratory values in the whole case series and according to the presence or absence of TE events, Table S2: Characteristics of Thromboembolic Events occurred during treatment with Immune-Checkpoint Inhibitors, Table S3. Use of anticoagulant treatment according to patients' baseline ECOG PS, Table S4: Baseline patients' characteristics in the whole case series and according to antiplatelet use, Figure S1: TE-specific hazard according to smoking status, Figure S2: TE-specific hazard according to PD-L1 status, Figure S3: TE-specific hazard according to Platelet to Lymphocyte Ratio (PLR), Figure S4: TE-specific hazard according to number of disease sites, Figure S5: Overall Survival Among Patients with or without TE Events considered as a time-independent variable, Figure S6: Progression Free Survival according to Aspirin (ASA) treatment.

Author Contributions: Conceptualization, F.N. and M.C.G.; methodology, F.N., A.M., C.P., G.L.R. and G.G.; recruiting NSCLC cases, R.F., D.S., C.P., G.L.R., A.P. and G.G.; collection and assembly of data F.N., E.Z., F.L., G.A. and D.S., data analysis and interpretation L.P., F.N., E.Z. and F.L., writing, original draft preparation, F.N.; writing, review and editing, A.M., F.L., E.Z., R.F. and G.L.R.; supervision, R.F., D.S., C.P., G.L.R., A.P., M.C.G. and F.d.B. All authors have read and agreed to the published version of the manuscript.

Abbreviations and Acronyms

ASA	Aspirin
BMI	Body mass index
CI	Confidence interval
COX	Cyclooxygenase
COXi	COX Inhibitors
CT	Computerized tomography
CTLA-4	Cytotoxic T-lymphocyte antigen 4
ECOG PS	Eastern Cooperative Oncology Group Performance Status
HR	Hazards ratio
ICIs	Immune checkpoint inhibitors
irAEs	Immune-related adverse events
LDH	Lactate dehydrogenase
LIPI	Lung immune prognostic index
LMWH	Low molecular weight heparin
mPGES1	Human prostaglandin E synthase 1
NLR	Neutrophil to lymphocyte ratio
NSCLC	Non-small cell lung cancer
OS	Overall Survival
PD-1/PD-L1	Programmed death-1/programmed death-ligand 1
PFS	Progression-free survival
PGE2	Prostaglandin E2
PLR	Platelet to lymphocyte ratio
ROC	Receiver operating characteristic
TE	Thromboembolic

References

1. Siegel, R.L.; Miller, K.D.; Jemal, A. Cancer statistics. *CA Cancer J. Clin.* **2018**, *68*, 7–30. [CrossRef]
2. Connolly, G.C.; Dalal, M.; Lin, J.; Khorana, A.A. Incidence and predictors of venous thromboembolism (VTE) among ambulatory patients with lung cancer. *Lung Cancer* **2012**, *78*, 253–258. [CrossRef]
3. Lyman, G.H.; Eckert, L.; Wang, Y.; Wang, H.; Cohen, A. Venous thromboembolism risk in patients with cancer receiving chemotherapy: A real-world analysis. *Oncologist* **2013**, *18*, 1321–1329. [CrossRef]
4. Antonia, S.J.; Villegas, A.; Daniel, D.; Vicente, D.; Murakami, S.; Hui, R.; Yokoi, T.; Chiappori, A.; Lee, K.H.; de Wit, M.; et al. Durvalumab after Chemoradiotherapy in Stage III Non-Small-Cell Lung Cancer. *N. Engl. J. Med.* **2017**, *377*, 1919–1929. [CrossRef]
5. Rittmeyer, A.; Barlesi, F.; Waterkamp, D.; Park, K.; Ciardiello, F.; von Pawel, J.; Gadgeel, S.M.; Hida, T.; Kowalski, D.M.; Dols, M.C.; et al. Atezolizumab versus docetaxel in patients with previously treated non-small-cell lung cancer (OAK): A phase 3, open-label, multicentre randomised controlled trial. *Lancet* **2017**, *389*, 255–265. [CrossRef]
6. Garassino, M.C.; Cho, B.C.; Kim, J.H.; Mazieres, J.; Vansteenkiste, J.; Lena, H.; Corral Jaime, J.; Gray, J.E.; Powderly, J.; Chouaid, C.; et al. Durvalumab as third-line or later treatment for advanced non-small-cell lung cancer (ATLANTIC): An open-label, single-arm, phase 2 study. *Lancet Oncol.* **2018**, *19*, 521–536. [CrossRef]

7. Borghaei, H.; Paz-Ares, L.; Horn, L.; Spigel, D.R.; Steins, M.; Ready, N.E.; Chow, L.Q.; Vokes, E.E.; Felip, E.; Holgado, E.; et al. Nivolumab versus Docetaxel in Advanced Nonsquamous Non-Small-Cell Lung Cancer. *N. Engl. J. Med.* **2015**, *373*, 1627–1639. [CrossRef]
8. Brahmer, J.; Reckamp, K.L.; Baas, P.; Crino, L.; Eberhardt, W.E.; Poddubskaya, E.; Antonia, S.; Pluzanski, A.; Vokes, E.E.; Holgado, E.; et al. Nivolumab versus Docetaxel in Advanced Squamous-Cell Non-Small-Cell Lung Cancer. *N. Engl. J. Med.* **2015**, *373*, 123–135. [CrossRef]
9. Herbst, R.S.; Baas, P.; Kim, D.W.; Felip, E.; Perez-Gracia, J.L.; Han, J.Y.; Molina, J.; Kim, J.H.; Arvis, C.D.; Ahn, M.J.; et al. Pembrolizumab versus docetaxel for previously treated, PD-L1-positive, advanced non-small-cell lung cancer (KEYNOTE-010): A randomised controlled trial. *Lancet* **2016**, *387*, 1540–1550. [CrossRef]
10. Reck, M.; Rodriguez-Abreu, D.; Robinson, A.G.; Hui, R.; Csoszi, T.; Fulop, A.; Gottfried, M.; Peled, N.; Tafreshi, A.; Cuffe, S.; et al. Pembrolizumab versus Chemotherapy for PD-L1-Positive Non-Small-Cell Lung Cancer. *N. Engl. J. Med.* **2016**, *375*, 1823–1833. [CrossRef]
11. Martins, F.; Sofiya, L.; Sykiotis, G.P.; Lamine, F.; Maillard, M.; Fraga, M.; Shabafrouz, K.; Ribi, C.; Cairoli, A.; Guex-Crosier, Y.; et al. Adverse effects of immune-checkpoint inhibitors: Epidemiology, management and surveillance. *Nat. Rev. Clin. Oncol.* **2019**. [CrossRef]
12. Wang, Y.; Zhou, S.; Yang, F.; Qi, X.; Wang, X.; Guan, X.; Shen, C.; Duma, N.; Vera Aguilera, J.; Chintakuntlawar, A.; et al. Treatment-Related Adverse Events of PD-1 and PD-L1 Inhibitors in Clinical Trials: A Systematic Review and Meta-analysis. *JAMA Oncol.* **2019**. [CrossRef]
13. Lyon, A.R.; Yousaf, N.; Battisti, N.M.L.; Moslehi, J.; Larkin, J. Immune checkpoint inhibitors and cardiovascular toxicity. *Lancet Oncol.* **2018**, *19*, e447–e458. [CrossRef]
14. Bu, D.X.; Tarrio, M.; Maganto-Garcia, E.; Stavrakis, G.; Tajima, G.; Lederer, J.; Jarolim, P.; Freeman, G.J.; Sharpe, A.H.; Lichtman, A.H. Impairment of the programmed cell death-1 pathway increases atherosclerotic lesion development and inflammation. *Arterioscler. Thromb. Vasc. Biol.* **2011**, *31*, 1100–1107. [CrossRef]
15. Cochain, C.; Chaudhari, S.M.; Koch, M.; Wiendl, H.; Eckstein, H.H.; Zernecke, A. Programmed cell death-1 deficiency exacerbates T cell activation and atherogenesis despite expansion of regulatory T cells in atherosclerosis-prone mice. *PLoS ONE* **2014**, *9*, e93280. [CrossRef]
16. Navi, B.B.; Reiner, A.S.; Kamel, H.; Iadecola, C.; Okin, P.M.; Tagawa, S.T.; Panageas, K.S.; DeAngelis, L.M. Arterial thromboembolic events preceding the diagnosis of cancer in older persons. *Blood* **2019**, *133*, 781–789. [CrossRef]
17. Niers, T.M.; Klerk, C.P.; DiNisio, M.; Van Noorden, C.J.; Buller, H.R.; Reitsma, P.H.; Richel, D.J. Mechanisms of heparin induced anti-cancer activity in experimental cancer models. *Crit. Rev. Oncol. Hematol.* **2007**, *61*, 195–207. [CrossRef]
18. Zhang, J.; Zhang, Y.L.; Ma, K.X.; Qu, J.M. Efficacy and safety of adjunctive anticoagulation in patients with lung cancer without indication for anticoagulants: A systematic review and meta-analysis. *Thorax* **2013**, *68*, 442–450. [CrossRef]
19. Macbeth, F.; Noble, S.; Evans, J.; Ahmed, S.; Cohen, D.; Hood, K.; Knoyle, D.; Linnane, S.; Longo, M.; Moore, B.; et al. Randomized Phase III Trial of Standard Therapy Plus Low Molecular Weight Heparin in Patients With Lung Cancer: FRAGMATIC Trial. *J. Clin. Oncol.* **2016**, *34*, 488–494. [CrossRef]
20. Ek, L.; Gezelius, E.; Bergman, B.; Bendahl, P.O.; Anderson, H.; Sundberg, J.; Wallberg, M.; Falkmer, U.; Verma, S.; Belting, M.; et al. Randomized phase III trial of low-molecular-weight heparin enoxaparin in addition to standard treatment in small-cell lung cancer: The RASTEN trial. *Ann. Oncol.* **2018**, *29*, 398–404. [CrossRef]
21. Zelenay, S.; van der Veen, A.G.; Bottcher, J.P.; Snelgrove, K.J.; Rogers, N.; Acton, S.E.; Chakravarty, P.; Girotti, M.R.; Marais, R.; Quezada, S.A.; et al. Cyclooxygenase-Dependent Tumor Growth through Evasion of Immunity. *Cell* **2015**, *162*, 1257–1270. [CrossRef]
22. Kim, S.H.; Roszik, J.; Cho, S.N.; Ogata, D.; Milton, D.R.; Peng, W.; Menter, D.G.; Ekmekcioglu, S.; Grimm, E.A. The COX2 Effector Microsomal PGE2 Synthase 1 is a Regulator of Immunosuppression in Cutaneous Melanoma. *Clin. Cancer Res.* **2019**, *25*, 1650–1663. [CrossRef]
23. Li, X.; Wenes, M.; Romero, P.; Huang, S.C.; Fendt, S.M.; Ho, P.C. Navigating metabolic pathways to enhance antitumour immunity and immunotherapy. *Nat. Rev. Clin. Oncol.* **2019**. [CrossRef]
24. Botti, G.; Fratangelo, F.; Cerrone, M.; Liguori, G.; Cantile, M.; Anniciello, A.M.; Scala, S.; D'Alterio, C.;

Trimarco, C.; Ianaro, A.; et al. COX-2 expression positively correlates with PD-L1 expression in human melanoma cells. *J. Transl. Med.* **2017**, *15*, 46. [CrossRef]

25. Hamada, T.; Cao, Y.; Qian, Z.R.; Masugi, Y.; Nowak, J.A.; Yang, J.; Song, M.; Mima, K.; Kosumi, K.; Liu, L.; et al. Aspirin Use and Colorectal Cancer Survival According to Tumor CD274 (Programmed Cell Death 1 Ligand 1) Expression Status. *J. Clin. Oncol.* **2017**, *35*, 1836–1844. [CrossRef]
26. Edelman, M.J.; Wang, X.; Hodgson, L.; Cheney, R.T.; Baggstrom, M.Q.; Thomas, S.P.; Gajra, A.; Bertino, E.; Reckamp, K.L.; Molina, J.; et al. Phase III Randomized, Placebo-Controlled, Double-Blind Trial of Celecoxib in Addition to Standard Chemotherapy for Advanced Non-Small-Cell Lung Cancer With Cyclooxygenase-2 Overexpression: CALGB 30801 (Alliance). *J. Clin. Oncol.* **2017**, *35*, 2184–2192. [CrossRef]
27. Groen, H.J.; Sietsma, H.; Vincent, A.; Hochstenbag, M.M.; van Putten, J.W.; van den Berg, A.; Dalesio, O.; Biesma, B.; Smit, H.J.; Termeer, A.; et al. Randomized, placebo-controlled phase III study of docetaxel plus carboplatin with celecoxib and cyclooxygenase-2 expression as a biomarker for patients with advanced non-small-cell lung cancer: The NVALT-4 study. *J. Clin. Oncol.* **2011**, *29*, 4320–4326. [CrossRef]
28. Edelman, M.J.; Tan, M.T.; Fidler, M.J.; Sanborn, R.E.; Otterson, G.; Sequist, L.V.; Evans, T.L.; Schneider, B.J.; Keresztes, R.; Rogers, J.S.; et al. Randomized, double-blind, placebo-controlled, multicenter phase II study of the efficacy and safety of apricoxib in combination with either docetaxel or pemetrexed in patients with biomarker-selected non-small-cell lung cancer. *J. Clin. Oncol.* **2015**, *33*, 189–194. [CrossRef]
29. Wang, S.-J.; Khullar, K.; Yegya-Raman, N.; Kim, S.; Silk, A.W.; Malhotra, J.; Gentile, M.A.; Mehnert, J.M.; Jabbour, S.K. Cyclooxygenase inhibitor use during checkpoint blockade immunotherapy and effect on time to progression for metastatic melanoma patients. *J. Clin. Oncol.* **2019**, *37*. [CrossRef]
30. Yoshimatsu, K.; Altorki, N.K.; Golijanin, D.; Zhang, F.; Jakobsson, P.J.; Dannenberg, A.J.; Subbaramaiah, K. Inducible prostaglandin E synthase is overexpressed in non-small cell lung cancer. *Clin. Cancer Res.* **2001**, *7*, 2669–2674.
31. Khorana, A.A.; Kuderer, N.M.; Culakova, E.; Lyman, G.H.; Francis, C.W. Development and validation of a predictive model for chemotherapy-associated thrombosis. *Blood* **2008**, *111*, 4902–4907. [CrossRef]
32. Grilz, E.; Posch, F.; Konigsbrugge, O.; Schwarzinger, I.; Lang, I.M.; Marosi, C.; Pabinger, I.; Ay, C. Association of Platelet-to-Lymphocyte Ratio and Neutrophil-to-Lymphocyte Ratio with the Risk of Thromboembolism and Mortality in Patients with Cancer. *Thromb. Haemost.* **2018**, *118*, 1875–1884. [CrossRef]
33. Conner, S.C.; Trinquart, L. Survivorship Bias in Analyses of Immune Checkpoint Inhibitor Trials. *JAMA Oncol.* **2019**. [CrossRef]
34. Blom, J.W.; Osanto, S.; Rosendaal, F.R. The risk of a venous thrombotic event in lung cancer patients: Higher risk for adenocarcinoma than squamous cell carcinoma. *J. Thromb. Haemost.* **2004**, *2*, 1760–1765. [CrossRef]
35. Walker, A.J.; Baldwin, D.R.; Card, T.R.; Powell, H.A.; Hubbard, R.B.; Grainge, M.J. Risk of venous thromboembolism in people with lung cancer: A cohort study using linked UK healthcare data. *Br. J. Cancer* **2017**, *116*, e1. [CrossRef]
36. Ferreira, M.; Pichon, E.; Carmier, D.; Bouquet, E.; Pageot, C.; Bejan-Angoulvant, T.; Campana, M.; Vermes, E.; Marchand-Adam, S. Coronary Toxicities of Anti-PD-1 and Anti-PD-L1 Immunotherapies: A Case Report and Review of the Literature and International Registries. *Target. Oncol.* **2018**, *13*, 509–515. [CrossRef]
37. Tomita, Y.; Sueta, D.; Kakiuchi, Y.; Saeki, S.; Saruwatari, K.; Sakata, S.; Jodai, T.; Migiyama, Y.; Akaike, K.; Hirosako, S.; et al. Acute coronary syndrome as a possible immune-related adverse event in a lung cancer patient achieving a complete response to anti-PD-1 immune checkpoint antibody. *Ann. Oncol.* **2017**, *28*, 2893–2895. [CrossRef]
38. Boutros, C.; Scoazec, J.Y.; Mateus, C.; Routier, E.; Roy, S.; Robert, C. Arterial thrombosis and anti-PD-1 blockade. *Eur. J. Cancer* **2018**, *91*, 164–166. [CrossRef]
39. Roopkumar, J.; Kim, A.S.; Bicky, T.; Hobbs, B.P.; Khorana, A.A. Venous Thromboembolism in Cancer Patients Receiving Immunotherapy. *Blood* **2018**, *132*, 2510. [CrossRef]
40. Chew, H.K.; Wun, T.; Harvey, D.; Zhou, H.; White, R.H. Incidence of venous thromboembolism and its effect on survival among patients with common cancers. *Arch. Int. Med.* **2006**, *166*, 458–464. [CrossRef]
41. Wang, J.; Zhang, L.; Kang, D.; Yang, D.; Tang, Y. Activation of PGE2/EP2 and PGE2/EP4 signaling pathways positively regulate the level of PD-1 in infiltrating CD8+ T cells in patients with lung cancer. *Oncol. Lett.* **2018**, *15*, 552–558. [CrossRef] [PubMed]
42. Verso, M.; Agnelli, G.; Barni, S.; Gasparini, G.; LaBianca, R. A modified Khorana risk assessment score for

venous thromboembolism in cancer patients receiving chemotherapy: The Protecht score. *Int. Emerg. Med.* **2012**, *7*, 291–292. [CrossRef] [PubMed]

43. Agnelli, G.; Gussoni, G.; Bianchini, C.; Verso, M.; Mandala, M.; Cavanna, L.; Barni, S.; Labianca, R.; Buzzi, F.; Scambia, G.; et al. Nadroparin for the prevention of thromboembolic events in ambulatory patients with metastatic or locally advanced solid cancer receiving chemotherapy: A randomised, placebo-controlled, double-blind study. *Lancet Oncol.* **2009**, *10*, 943–949. [CrossRef]
44. Carrier, M.; Abou-Nassar, K.; Mallick, R.; Tagalakis, V.; Shivakumar, S.; Schattner, A.; Kuruvilla, P.; Hill, D.; Spadafora, S.; Marquis, K.; et al. Apixaban to Prevent Venous Thromboembolism in Patients with Cancer. *N. Engl. J. Med.* **2019**, *380*, 711–719. [CrossRef]
45. Khorana, A.A.; Soff, G.A.; Kakkar, A.K.; Vadhan-Raj, S.; Riess, H.; Wun, T.; Streiff, M.B.; Garcia, D.A.; Liebman, H.A.; Belani, C.P.; et al. Rivaroxaban for Thromboprophylaxis in High-Risk Ambulatory Patients with Cancer. *N. Engl. J. Med.* **2019**, *380*, 720–728. [CrossRef]
46. Sharma, S.; Yang, S.C.; Zhu, L.; Reckamp, K.; Gardner, B.; Baratelli, F.; Huang, M.; Batra, R.K.; Dubinett, S.M. Tumor cyclooxygenase-2/prostaglandin E2-dependent promotion of FOXP3 expression and CD4+ CD25+ T regulatory cell activities in lung cancer. *Cancer Res.* **2005**, *65*, 5211–5220. [CrossRef]
47. Veltman, J.D.; Lambers, M.E.; van Nimwegen, M.; Hendriks, R.W.; Hoogsteden, H.C.; Aerts, J.G.; Hegmans, J.P. COX-2 inhibition improves immunotherapy and is associated with decreased numbers of myeloid-derived suppressor cells in mesothelioma. Celecoxib influences MDSC function. *BMC Cancer* **2010**, *10*, 464. [CrossRef]
48. Hennequart, M.; Pilotte, L.; Cane, S.; Hoffmann, D.; Stroobant, V.; Plaen, E.; Van den Eynde, B.J. Constitutive IDO1 Expression in Human Tumors Is Driven by Cyclooxygenase-2 and Mediates Intrinsic Immune Resistance. *Cancer Immunol. Res.* **2017**, *5*, 695–709. [CrossRef]
49. Prima, V.; Kaliberova, L.N.; Kaliberov, S.; Curiel, D.T.; Kusmartsev, S. COX2/mPGES1/PGE2 pathway regulates PD-L1 expression in tumor-associated macrophages and myeloid-derived suppressor cells. *Proc. Natl. Acad. Sci. USA* **2017**, *114*, 1117–1122. [CrossRef]
50. Shimizu, K.; Okita, R.; Saisho, S.; Maeda, A.; Nojima, Y.; Nakata, M. Prognostic value of Cox-2 and PD-L1 expression and its relationship with tumor-infiltrating lymphocytes in resected lung adenocarcinoma. *Cancer Manag. Res.* **2017**, *9*, 741–750. [CrossRef]
51. Tang, H.; Liu, Y.; Wang, C.; Zheng, H.; Chen, Y.; Liu, W.; Chen, X.; Zhang, J.; Chen, H.; Yang, Y.; et al. Inhibition of COX-2 and EGFR by Melafolone Improves Anti-PD-1 Therapy through Vascular Normalization and PD-L1 Downregulation in Lung Cancer. *J. Pharmacol. Exp. Ther.* **2019**, *368*, 401–413. [CrossRef] [PubMed]
52. Shimizu, K.; Okita, R.; Saisho, S.; Maeda, A.I.; Nojima, Y.; Nakata, M. Impact of COX2 Inhibitor for Regulation of PD-L1 Expression in Non-small Cell Lung Cancer. *Anticancer Res.* **2018**, *38*, 4637–4644. [CrossRef] [PubMed]
53. Veglia, F.; Tyurin, V.A.; Blasi, M.; De Leo, A.; Kossenkov, A.V.; Donthireddy, L.; To, T.K.J.; Schug, Z.; Basu, S.; Wang, F.; et al. Fatty acid transport protein 2 reprograms neutrophils in cancer. *Nature* **2019**, *569*, 73–78. [CrossRef]
54. Ng, T.L.; Smith, D.E.; Mushtaq, R.; Patil, T.; Dimou, A.; Yang, S.; Liu, Q.; Li, X.; Zhou, C.; Jones, R.T.; et al. ROS1 Gene Rearrangements Are Associated With an Elevated Risk of Peridiagnosis Thromboembolic Events. *J. Thorac. Oncol.* **2019**, *14*, 596–605. [CrossRef]
55. Dou, F.; Li, H.; Zhu, M.; Liang, L.; Zhang, Y.; Yi, J.; Zhang, Y. Association between oncogenic status and risk of venous thromboembolism in patients with non-small cell lung cancer. *Respir. Res.* **2018**, *19*, 88. [CrossRef]
56. Zugazagoitia, J.; Biosca, M.; Oliveira, J.; Olmedo, M.E.; Domine, M.; Nadal, E.; Ruffinelli, J.C.; Munoz, N.; Luna, A.M.; Hernandez, B.; et al. Incidence, predictors and prognostic significance of thromboembolic disease in patients with advanced ALK-rearranged non-small cell lung cancer. *Eur. Respir. J.* **2018**, *51*. [CrossRef]
57. Gandhi, L.; Rodriguez-Abreu, D.; Gadgeel, S.; Esteban, E.; Felip, E.; De Angelis, F.; Domine, M.; Clingan, P.; Hochmair, M.J.; Powell, S.F.; et al. Pembrolizumab plus Chemotherapy in Metastatic Non-Small-Cell Lung Cancer. *N. Engl. J. Med.* **2018**, *378*, 2078–2092. [CrossRef]
58. Paz-Ares, L.; Luft, A.; Vicente, D.; Tafreshi, A.; Gumus, M.; Mazieres, J.; Hermes, B.; Cay Senler, F.; Csoszi, T.; Fulop, A.; et al. Pembrolizumab plus Chemotherapy for Squamous Non-Small-Cell Lung Cancer. *N. Engl. J. Med.* **2018**, *379*, 2040–2051. [CrossRef]

3

A Small Compound KJ-28d Enhances the Sensitivity of Non-Small Cell Lung Cancer to Radio- and Chemotherapy

Hwani Ryu [1,2], Hyo Jeong Kim [1], Jie-Young Song [1], Sang-Gu Hwang [1], Jae-Sung Kim [1], Joon Kim [2], Thi Hong Nhung Bui [3], Hyun-Kyung Choi [3,*] and Jiyeon Ahn [1,*]

1 Division of Radiation Biomedical Research, Korea Institute of Radiological & Medical Sciences (KIRAMS), Seoul 01812, Korea; hwanya85@kirams.re.kr (H.R.); hjkim@kirams.re.kr (H.J.K.); immu@kirams.re.kr (J.-Y.S.); sgh63@kirams.re.kr (S.-G.H.); jaesung@kirams.re.kr (J.-S.K.)

2 Department of Biology, Korea University, Seoul 02841, Korea; joonkim@korea.ac.kr

3 Department of Medicinal Chemistry, Jungwon University, Goesan 28024, Korea; buihongnhung103@gmail.com

* Correspondence: hkchoi45@jwu.ac.kr (H.-K.C.); ahnjy@kirams.re.kr (J.A.)

Abstract: We previously reported on a poly (ADP-ribose) polymerase (PARP) 1/2 inhibitor *N*-(3-(hydroxycarbamoyl)phenyl)carboxamide (designated KJ-28d), which increased the death of human ovarian cancer *BRCA1*-deficient SNU-251 cells. In the present study, we further investigated the antitumor activities of KJ-28d in *BRCA*-proficient non-small cell lung cancer (NSCLC) cells to expand the use of PARP inhibitors. KJ-28d significantly inhibited the growth of NSCLC cells in vitro and in vivo, and induced DNA damage and reactive oxygen species in A549 and H1299 cells. Combined treatment with KJ-28d and ionizing radiation led to increased DNA damage responses in A549 and H1299 cells compared to KJ-28d or ionizing radiation alone, resulting in apoptotic cell death. Moreover, the combination of KJ-28d plus a DNA-damaging therapeutic agent (carboplatin, cisplatin, paclitaxel, or doxorubicin) synergistically inhibited cell proliferation, compared to either drug alone. Taken together, the findings demonstrate the potential of KJ-28d as an effective anti-cancer therapeutic agent for *BRCA*-deficient and -proficient cancer cells. KJ-28d might have potential as an adjuvant when used in combination with radiotherapy or DNA-damaging agents, pending further investigations.

Keywords: poly (ADP-ribose) polymerase inhibitor; non-small cell lung cancer; DNA damage; radiotherapy; chemotherapy; combination therapy

---

1. Introduction

Lung cancer is one of the most commonly occurring cancers worldwide. Non-small cell lung cancer (NSCLC) accounts for more than 84% of all lung cancers [1]. Despite recent advances in our understanding of the molecular and genetic basis of lung cancer and improvements in therapy, the 5-year survival rate of patients with NSCLC in both Korea (23.7%) and the United States (23%) is lower than that for many other leading cancers [1,2]. The standard chemotherapy treatment used for NSCLC is either the platinum-based (cisplatin, carboplatin, etc.) or taxane-based (paclitaxel, docetaxel, etc.) regimens, or epidermal growth factor receptor (EGFR) inhibitors. However, because of the lack of response or resistance to those therapies, many patients with NSCLC consider new alternative therapies or receive combination therapies [3]. Therefore, the development of novel drugs or strategies of combination therapy with existing drugs is urgently required.

Ionizing radiation (IR) is directly cytotoxic through the induction of DNA single- or double-strand breaks (DSB) and indirectly cytotoxic through the generation of reactive oxygen species (ROS), leading to tumor cell death and thus cancer treatment. Similarly, platinum- or taxane-based chemotherapeutic agents inhibit cell mitosis through the induction of DNA damage. DNA lesions induced by IR or cytotoxic agents can be repaired by six major DNA repair pathways: base excision repair, nucleotide excision repair, direct repair (i.e., O^6-alkylguanine DNA alkyltransferase directly repairs DNA damaged lesions by removing O^6-methylguanine), mismatch repair, homologous recombination (HR), and non-homologous end-joining pathways. NSCLC is characterized by genomic instability with mutations and translocations in oncogenes, such as the *Ki-ras2 Kirsten rat sarcoma viral oncogene homolog proto-oncogene* (*KRAS*), *EGFR*, *ALK receptor tyrosine kinase* (*ALK*), *ataxia-telangiectasia mutated* (*ATM*) or *phosphatidylinositol-4,5-bisphosphate 3-kinase catalytic subunit alpha* (*PIK3CA*), and tumor suppressor genes, such as the *tumor protein p53* (*TP53*), *liver kinase B1* (*LKB1*), or *Kelch-like ECH-associated protein 1* (*KEAP1*) [4–11].

Poly (ADP-ribose) polymerases (PARPs) are a family of 18 protein members that function as catalytic enzymes by adding ADP-ribose polymers to lysine residues of themselves and target proteins, a process termed poly (ADP-ribosyl)ation (PARylation). Among the proteins of the PARP family, PARP-1 and -2 are abundant nuclear enzymes involved in DNA damage repair, which involves binding to DNA breaks and facilitating the localization of repair enzymes, such as breast cancer 1/2 (BRCA1/2), to the sites of DNA damage [12,13]. Olaparib, rucaparib, niraparib, and talazoparib targeting PARP1/2 have been approved by the United States Food and Drug Administration (FDA) for the treatment of breast or ovarian cancer in patients harboring HR mutations that induce synthetic lethality in the *BRCA1* or *BRCA2* gene.

Evidence is accumulating that PARP inhibitors (PARPi) have therapeutic efficacy in cancer cells with high genomic instability by inducing synthetic lethality of cells with deficient or insufficient DNA repair [14–16]. Briefly, in this scenario, IR, or radiotherapy or cytotoxic chemotherapeutic agents that induce severe DNA damage could lead to insufficient DNA repair in targeted tumor cells. Consecutively, cells that adopt the "BRCAness" state could be treated with PARP inhibitor (PARPi) [17–20].

We have previously identified a potential novel PARPi, termed *N*-(3-(hydroxycarbamoyl)phenyl) carboxamide (designated KJ-28d). KJ-28d inhibited PARP-1/2 activities and displayed significant antitumor activity in human ovarian cancer *BRCA1*-deficient (*BRCA1* mutation at 5564G>A) SNU-251 cells [21]. In this study, we further investigated the antitumor activity of KJ-28d in *BRCA*-proficient cell lines, as well as the combination of KJ-28d and DNA damage-inducing radiotherapy or cytotoxic chemotherapeutics in human NSCLC cells.

2. Results

2.1. *KJ-28d Inhibits Growth of Human NSCLC Cells In Vitro and In Vivo*

Among the reported novel PARP-1 inhibitors, we examined KJ-28d, as shown in Figure 1A, based on the prior demonstrations of its significant inhibitory activity against PARP-1, as well as antitumor activity in *BRCA*-deficient ovarian cancer cells [21]. Specifically, we assessed whether KJ-28d can inhibit the growth of *BRCA*-proficient cancer cells. Human NSCLC cells were treated with KJ-28d and growth inhibition was determined using the 3-(4,5-dimethylthiazol-2-yl)-2,5- diphenyltetrazolium bromide (MTT) assay. KJ-28d significantly inhibited the growth of A549, H1299, H460, and H1650 human NSCLC cells with a determined IC_{50} value, as shown in Figure 1B, and induced the sub-G1 phase (apoptotic cell) in A549 and H1299 cells, as shown in Supplementary Figure S1.

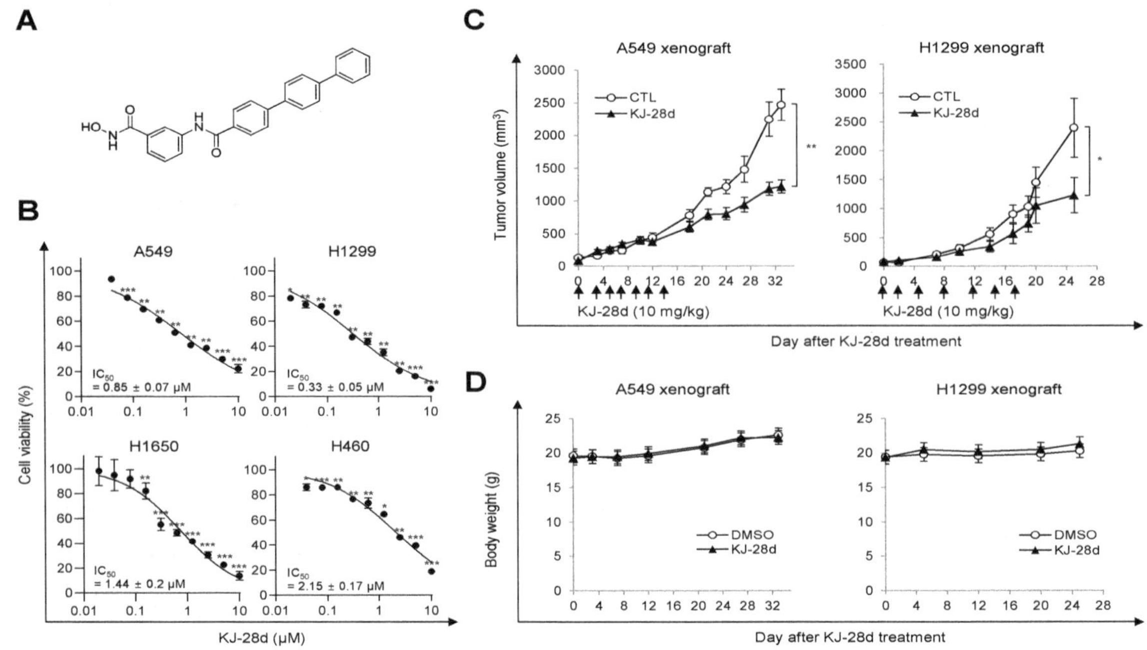

Figure 1. KJ-28d inhibits tumor growth of A549 and H1299 xenografts in nude mice. (**A**) The chemical structure of the KJ-28d compound. (**B**) A549, H1299, H1650, and H460 human non-small cell lung cancer (NSCLC) cells were treated with KJ-28d at the indicated concentrations for 5 days, and cell viabilities were determined by the MTT assay. Data are presented as means ± standard deviation (SD) from at least three independent experiments. * $p < 0.05$, ** $p < 0.01$, *** $p < 0.001$ versus DMSO-treated control. (**C,D**) A549 cells and H1299 cells were subcutaneously injected into the thigh of the right hind leg of BALB/c nu/nu mice ($n = 3$ per group, A549; $n = 4$ per group, H1299). Two weeks after tumor cell injection, KJ-28d (10 mg/kg) or DMSO (control) was intraperitoneally administered once every 2 or 3 days for seven times in total. (**C**) Longest (L) and shortest (W) tumor axes were measured, and tumor volume (mm^3) was calculated as $L \times W^2/2$. Data shown represent average tumor volume (* $p < 0.05$, ** $p < 0.01$). Results are shown as means ± SD. (**D**) The body weights of A549 and H1299 xenograft mice were determined once a week during the experiments. Data are shown as means ± SD.

We next determined whether the antitumor effect associated with the in vitro KJ-28d treatment could be translated into a similar effect in an in vivo xenograft mouse model. BALB/c-nu/nu mice were subcutaneously (*s.c.*) implanted with A549 or H1299 cells in the right hind leg, and when tumors were palpable (average diameter approximately 150 mm^3; 10 days post-implantation), mice were intraperitoneally (*i.p.*) administered a dose of 10 mg/kg KJ-28d or DMSO (control vehicle) once every 2 or 3 days for a total of seven times. KJ-28d treatment inhibited A549 or H1299 cell-derived tumor growth by 51% and 49%, respectively, as compared with the respective vehicle, as shown in Figure 1C. Additionally, to determine the toxicity of KJ-28d, we measured the body weight of mice. Mice treated with KJ-28d did not show any difference in body weight as compared with control mice, as shown in Figure 1D. The results suggested that KJ-28d has antitumor activity for NSCLC cells in vitro and in vivo.

2.2. *KJ-28d Induces DNA Damage and Generation of ROS in NSCLC Cells*

Since PARPi induce accumulation of DNA damage [22,23], we sought to determine whether KJ-28d could induce DNA damage in NSCLC cells. The DNA damage was measured in A549 and H1299 cells at different time points after KJ-28d treatment by detecting the phosphorylation on Ser139 of the H2AX (γ-H2AX) histone protein, which is an indicator of the presence of DNA double-strand damage. KJ-28d induced γ-H2AX in both cell types at the latest time point (24 h), as shown in Figure 2A. As treatment with KJ-28d resulted in inducing a DNA damage response, we also investigated whether KJ-28d could augment ROS generation in NSCLC cells. Flow cytometry analysis showed that treatment of A549 and H1299 cells with 5 μM KJ-28d led to distinctly increased ROS levels, which were then reduced following treatment with *N*-acetyl-L-cysteine (NAC), a general free radical scavenger, as shown in Figure 2B,C. These results suggested that KJ-28d is able to exhibit antitumor activities in NSCLC cells through the accumulation of DNA damage and the generation of ROS.

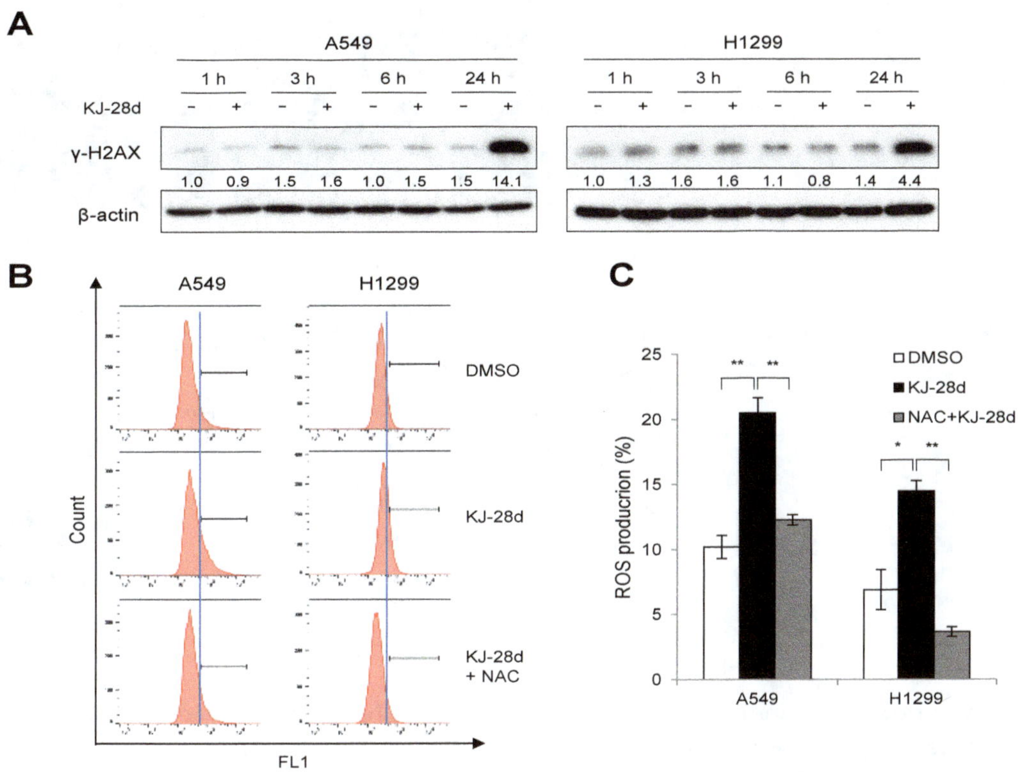

Figure 2. KJ-28d induces DNA damage and generation of reactive oxygen species (ROS). (**A**) A549 and H1299 cells were treated with 5 μM KJ-28d at indicated time points and immunoblotted for the detection of expression of γ-H2AX. (**B**,**C**) A549 and H1299 cells were treated with 5 mM NAC for 1 h, followed by KJ-28d for 24 h after incubation with 2′,7′-dichlorodihydrofluorescein diacetate (CM-H_2DCFHDA) for 30 min. Total cellular ROS production was measured using flow cytometry. Data are representative of three independent experiments (**B**). The bar graph shows the quantitative analysis of flow cytometer data (**C**). Data are presented as the mean ± SD of three independent experiments. * $p < 0.05$, ** $p < 0.01$ versus corresponding values.

2.3. *KJ-28d Potentiated Ionizing Radiation-Induced DNA Damage and Radiosensitized NSCLC Cells*

As IR induces severe DNA damage, which can lead to overloading DNA repair capacity, it has been reported that PARP inhibitors enhance IR-induced DNA damage [14,17,20,22]. To examine whether KJ-28d could induce increased DNA damage in combination with IR, DNA damage was measured in A549 and H1299 cells treated with KJ-28d and IR by detecting the presence of γ-H2AX. Immunoblot analysis revealed a significant increase in the phosphorylation levels of H2AX protein as compared with KJ-28d or IR alone. Similarly, we observed high levels of staining of γ-H2AX foci in A549 and H1299 cells treated with both KJ-28d and IR, as shown in Figure 3A–C. PARylation by PARP-1 catalytic activity is a post-translational modification involved in DNA damage repair. To determine whether KJ-28d suppresses cellular PARylation, H1299 cells were treated with the indicated concentrations of either KJ-28d or olaparib, and A549 cells were treated with 5 μM KJ-28d with or without IR. We observed that 10 μM KJ-28d and 5 and 10 μM olaparib inhibited protein PARylation in H1299, as shown in Figure 3D, and 5 μM of KJ-28d inhibited IR-induced PARylation in A549 cells, as shown in Figure 3E.

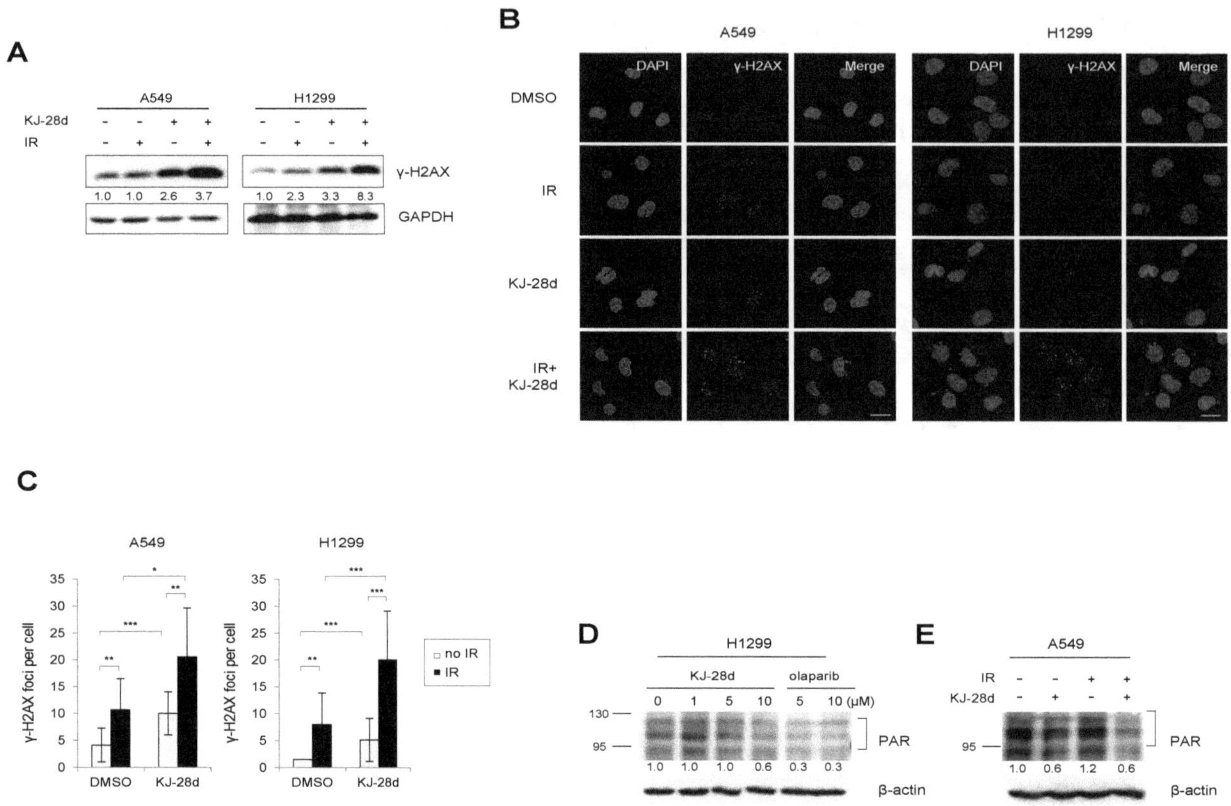

Figure 3. KJ-28d potentiates ionizing radiation (IR)-induced DNA damage responses. A549 and H1299 cells were treated with 5 μM KJ-28d 2 h before IR (4 Gy) and incubated for 24 h. The cell lysates were subjected to immunoblotting for detection of γ-H2AX (**A**), whereas cells were immunostained for γ-H2AX foci (red) and nuclei (DAPI: blue). Images were captured at 400× magnification. Scale bar: 20 μm (**B**). Quantification of the number of γ-H2AX foci per cell (**C**). Data represent the mean ± SD of three independent experiments. * $p < 0.05$, ** $p < 0.01$, *** $p < 0.001$ versus corresponding cells. (**D**) H1299 cells were treated with KJ-28d at indicated concentrations for 1 h. (**E**) A549 cells were treated with 5 μM KJ-28d and IR (4 Gy) and incubated for 1 h. The cell lysates were immunoblotted for the detection of expression of PAR. β-actin was used as a loading control.

Since KJ-28d potentiated IR-induced DNA damage in NSCLC cells, we further examined whether KJ-28d inhibited IR-induced cell growth. A549 and H1299 cells were treated with KJ-28d 2 h before IR. The clonogenic survival assay revealed that KJ-28d radiosensitized both cell lines, as shown in Figure 4A. Dose enhancement ratios (DER) of 0.75 μM KJ-28d-treated (at a surviving fraction of 0.37) to DMSO-treated cells were 1.5 and 1.23 in A549 and H1299 cells, respectively. We next determined whether treatment with KJ-28d could induce apoptotic cell death in A549 and H1299 cells. Apoptotic cell populations of these cell lines were detected using flow cytometer analysis with annexin /propidium iodide (PI) staining. Following treatment with 5 μM of KJ-28d and IR, the number of A549 and H1299 cells undergoing both early-stage (annexin V-positive/PI-negative) and late-stage (annexin V-positive/PI-positive) apoptosis increased significantly by 1.5-fold compared to KJ-28d alone, respectively, as shown in Figure 4B. In addition, KJ-28d plus IR treatment increased the cleavage of caspase-3 in both cell lines, as shown in Figure 4C. Taken together, these results indicated that KJ-28d enhanced both IR-induced DNA damage and apoptotic cell death in A549 and H1299 human NSCLC cells.

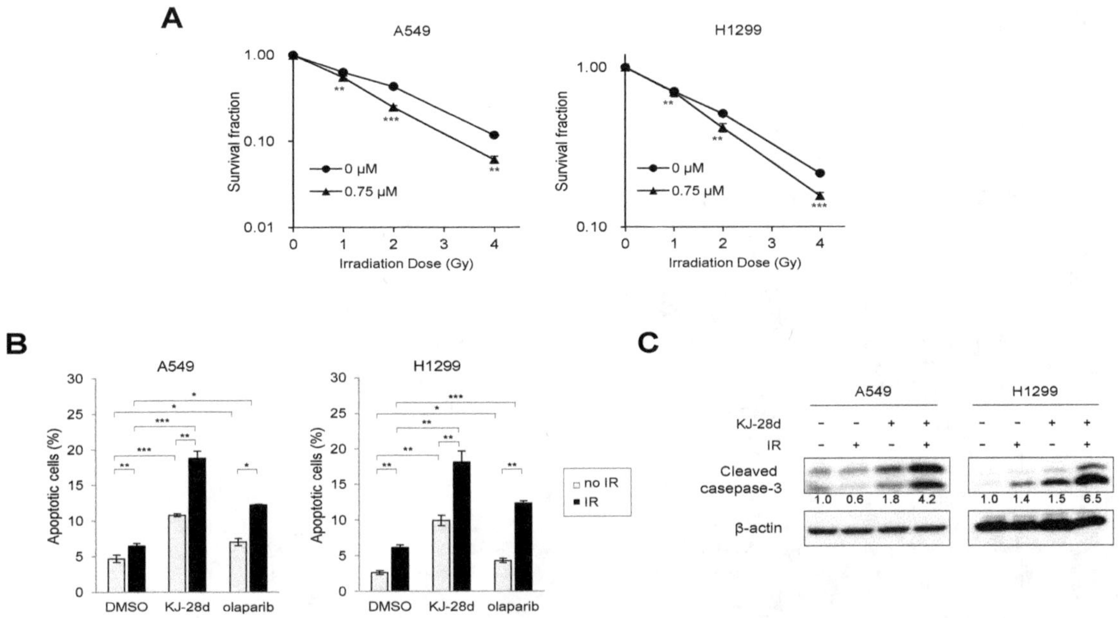

Figure 4. KJ-28d enhances the radiosensitivity of A549 and H1299 cells. (**A**) A549 and H1299 cells were treated with 0.75 μM KJ-28d for 2 h before IR (0, 1, 2, and 4 Gy). Clonogenic survival was measured 10 days after IR. Data are expressed as mean ± SD ($n = 3$) of the surviving fraction compared to non-irradiated cells. Colonies consisting of more than 50 cells were scored as survival colonies. (**B**) A549 and H1299 cells were treated with either 5 μM KJ-28d or 5 μM olaparib plus IR (4 Gy) for 48 h. Apoptotic cells were determined using the APC-conjugated annexin V/PI staining. Cell populations were gated into four groups, as described in Section 4. Bar graphs represent the mean percentage of early (annexin V-positive/PI-negative) and late apoptotic cells (annexin V-positive/PI-positive). Data represent the mean ± SD of three independent experiments. * $p < 0.05$, ** $p < 0.01$, *** $p < 0.001$ versus corresponding cells. (**C**) A549 and H1299 cells were treated with 5 μM KJ-28d plus IR (4 Gy), and the cell lysates were subjected to immunoblotting for detection of cleaved caspase-3. β-actin was used as a loading control.

2.4. The Combination of KJ-28d and DNA Damage-Inducing Chemotherapeutic Agents Synergistically Inhibits NSCLC Cell Growth

In preclinical and clinical studies of advanced NSCLC treatment, administration of PARPi in combination with DNA-damaging therapeutic agents, such as platinum-based compounds, taxane-based compounds, and topoisomerase inhibitors, has demonstrated enhanced cytotoxicity [24–26]. As KJ-28d enhanced radiosensitivity of A549 and H1299 cells, we expected that KJ-28d could increase cytotoxicity when combined with treatment with DNA DSB-inducing agents. A549 and H1299 cells were treated with KJ-28d and carboplatin, cisplatin, paclitaxel, or doxorubicin and evaluation of the synergistic effect of each pair-compound on cell viability was assessed using the MTT assay. Compared to treatment with KJ-28d or each compound alone, combination treatments showed a strong synergistic effect in both A549 and H1299 cells, decreasing cell viability in a dose-dependent manner, as shown in Figure 5A,C. To interpret the effects of all drug combinations, cell viability observed with each concentration of a KJ-28d-compound pair was converted to a combination index (CI) score using the CompuSyn software by Chou–Talalay [27]. CI scores were categorized as synergistic (CI < 0.9, green), additive (1.1 > CI ≥ 0.9, blue), or antagonistic (CI > 1.1, gray). We observed synergistic growth inhibition with a wide range of concentrations of KJ-28d and DSB-inducing agents in both cell lines, as shown in Figure 5B,D. Taken together, these results supported the conclusion that KJ-28d enhances the sensitivity of NSCLC cells to IR or chemotherapeutic agents of DNA-induced damage.

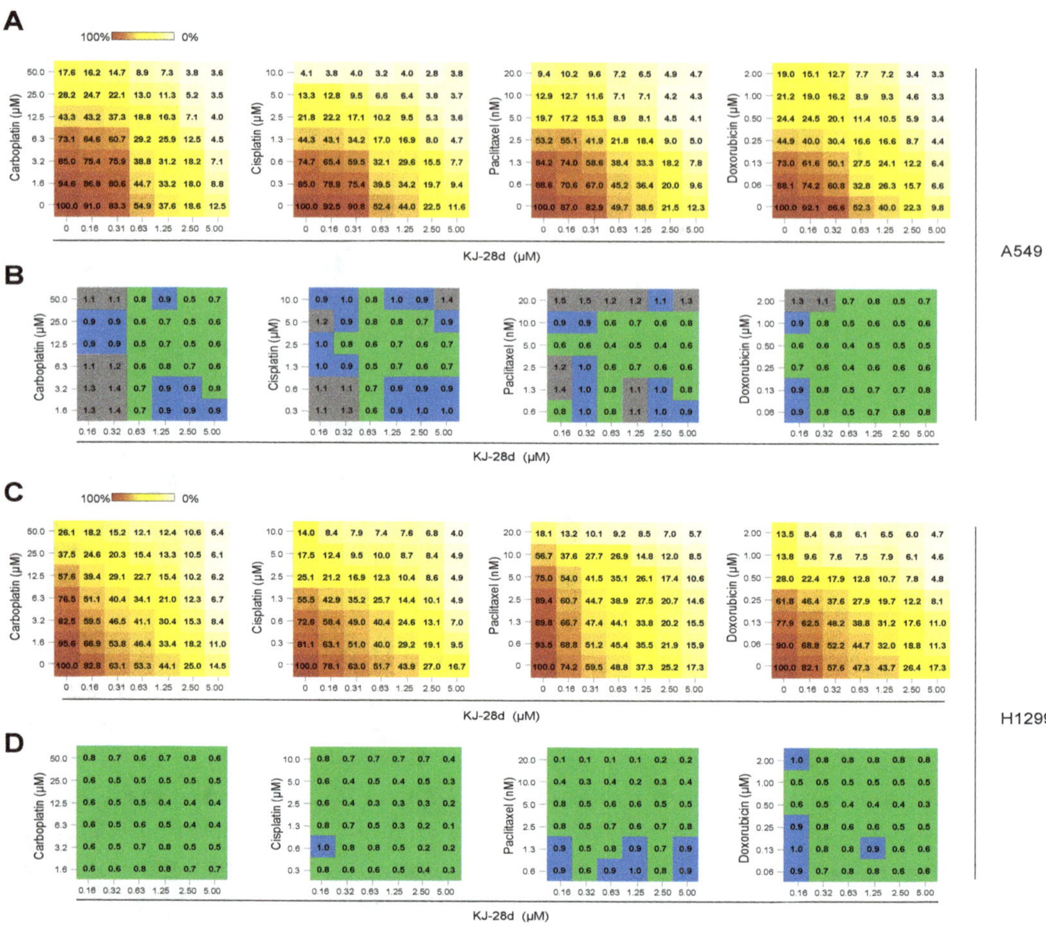

Figure 5. The combination of KJ-28d and DNA damage-inducing chemotherapeutic agents synergistically inhibits growth of A549 and H1299 cells. A549 (**A**) and H1299 (**C**) cells were treated with the single or combined administration of KJ-28d and carboplatin, cisplatin, paclitaxel, or doxorubicin at indicated concentrations. Cell viability was determined 5 days after the treatment by MTT assay. Relative viability (normalized to DMSO-treated cells) is shown for each combination at indicated concentrations. Data are from one representative experiment of three independently repeated experiments. (**B**,**D**) Summary of tables showing combination index (CI) scores of KJ-28d and each chemotherapeutic drug combined at indicated concentrations in A549 (**B**) and H1299 cells (**D**). CI scores were calculated using the CompuSyn software and categorized as synergistic (CI < 0.9, green), additive (1.1 > CI ≥ 0.9, blue), or antagonistic (CI ≥ 1.1, gray). Each CI score was one representative datum from treatment with the indicated concentrations of single- and paired compounds from more than three independent experiments.

3. Discussion

We previously identified KJ-28d as a novel PARP inhibitor that leads to increased cytotoxicity in human ovarian cancer *BRCA-1*-deficient SNU-251 (*BRCA1* mutation at 5564G>A) cells, as well as in triple-negative human ovarian cancer *BRCA1* heterozygous (*BRCA1*+/−) MDA-MB-231 cells [21]. In this study, we further investigated the antitumor activity of KJ-28d on *BRCA*-proficient NSCLC cancer cells, as well as a combination approach with DNA damage-inducing agents to evaluate the synergistic therapeutic efficacy in human NSCLC cells.

NSCLC is a type of cancer with a high mortality rate. Most patients with NSCLC receive treatment with platinum-based drugs, such as cisplatin or carboplatin, as first-line standard therapy. However, many patients who initially benefit from such chemotherapies gradually acquire chemoresistance. Thus, the development of novel therapies and strategies, including combination therapies, is needed. KJ-28d can inhibit the growth of various cancer cells, including NSCLC, breast, and colorectal cancer cells, as shown in Supplementary Figure S2. We specifically focused on NSCLC and revealed its antitumor effects on A549 and H1299 cells both in vitro and in vivo. A549 cells have a *KRAS* oncogenic mutation with c-Myc amplification, while H1299 cells are *TP53* mutant cells, as shown in Supplementary Table S1. Many studies have shown that KRAS-driven c-Myc amplification and TP53 correlate with genomic instability, thereby compromising DNA damage repair (DDR), causing the cells to be vulnerable to DDR inhibiting agents [28]. We observed that KJ-28d induced DNA damage and ROS generation in A549 and H1299 cells, which may facilitate cell death of NSCLC cells. The suppressed cellular PARylation might contribute to inducing DNA damage responses. Recent studies have suggested that PARPi can induce ROS generation due to DNA double stranded breaks. This is considered a characteristic of PARP inhibitors in DNA repair-deficient cells, as well as tumor suppressors or oncogene-mutated cells. Thus, PARPi may crosstalk with other signals [20,29]. In that regard, FDA-approved PARPi compounds have been studied to expand clinical use of PARPi in NSCLC [26,30,31].

Although the rationale for the use of PARPi was based on the reported induced synthetic lethality shown in *BRCA*-deficient cancer cells, preclinical and clinical studies suggested that PARPi could potentially be used as a combination partner with DNA-damaging agents in *BRCA*-proficient cancer cells [26,32,33]. Approximately 50% of patients with NSCLC receive radiotherapy during their treatment course [34]. Radiotherapy is an effective treatment modality, causing severe DNA damage. However, it can only treat tumors at defined doses because of the side effects to surrounding normal tissues. Although PARPi is not yet considered as a radiosensitizer in patients with ovarian cancer harboring *BRCA1/2* mutations in the clinic, the combination of radiotherapy with PARPi could provide promising synergistic therapeutic effects. For that reason, it has been studied in human NSCLC xenografts [35–37]. Olaparib is the first PARPi approved for the treatment of refractory ovarian cancer harboring *BRCA1* or *BRCA2* mutations. We have previously shown that treatment with KJ-28d induced more frequent apoptotic cell death in *BRCA* mutated ovarian cancer cells than olaparib did. It was noteworthy in this study that the combination of KJ-28d and IR also induced significantly more apoptotic cell deaths in NSCLC cells compared to combination treatment with olaparib and IR. Since we initially identified KJ-28d as a PARPi, further studies need to be conducted to elucidate other modes of action, as they may be cytotoxic. Platinum-based agents are widely used for a broad range of solid tumors, including NSCLC, and are the most commonly studied combination partners of PARPi [26,31,38]. Likewise, our results demonstrated that KJ-28d significantly enhanced the sensitivity of A549 and H1299 cells to carboplatin or cisplatin. In addition, we observed synergistic cell growth inhibitions of both cell populations when treated with a combination of KJ-28d with either paclitaxel or doxorubicin that constitute strong DNA-damaging therapeutic agents.

Besides the demonstrated inhibitory PARP activity of KJ-28d, the mechanisms responsible for KJ-28d-induced cytotoxicity in wild-type *BRCA* cancer cells have not been fully uncovered in this study. We suggest that KJ-28d might be involved in the antitumor activity exhibited in NSCLC cells with wild-type *BRCA* based on the experimentally exhibited markedly induced DNA DSBs and ROS generation at the latest examined time point (24 h). Structurally, KJ-28d contains the hydroxamic acid moiety found in histone deacetylase inhibitors (HDACi), including suberoylanilide hydroxamic acid. The hydroxamic acid moiety of HDACi acts as a chelator for zinc ions in the active site of histone deacetylases. To elucidate the possibility of HDAC inhibition, we examined the inhibitory activities of 1–11 HDAC isoforms using in vitro enzyme assays but observed little inhibitory activities of HDACs at KJ-28d concentrations under 5 μM, as shown in Supplementary Table S2. Further structure–activity relationship studies are required to understand the inhibitory activities of PARP-1/2 as a PARPi and to investigate the mechanisms associated with KJ-28d-induced growth inhibition and apoptotic cell death in NSCLC cells.

In summary, KJ-28d was cytotoxic to *BRCA*-proficient cancer cells, including NSCLC cells. Treatment with KJ-28d before IR led to increased DNA damage responses compared to treatment with KJ-28d or IR alone, resulting in the induction of apoptotic cell death. The combination of KJ-28d with carboplatin, cisplatin, paclitaxel, or doxorubicin considerably inhibited cell proliferation. In this context, KJ-28d might act as an effective anti-cancer therapeutic agent against both *BRCA*-deficient and -proficient cancer cells and might have further potential as an adjuvant when used in combination with radiotherapy or DNA-damaging agents. However, further investigations into the mechanisms of action of KJ-28d in cancer cells are warranted.

4. Materials and Methods

4.1. Cell Culture

Human lung cancer cells (A549, H1299, H460, and H1650) were obtained from American Type Culture Collection (ATCC, Manassas, VA, USA). Cells were maintained in Roswell Park Memorial Institute (RPMI) 1640 medium (Welgene, Gyeongsangbuk-do, Korea) supplemented with 10% fetal bovine serum (Welgene) and 100 units/mL penicillin–streptomycin solution (Gibco, Grand Island, NY, USA) at 37 °C in a humidified 5% CO_2 atmosphere.

4.2. Reagents

The PARPi olaparib (AZD2281) was purchased from Selleckchem (Houston, TX, USA). Doxorubicin was purchased from Sigma-Aldrich (St. Louis, MO, USA). All reagents, including carboplatin (Dong-A ST, Seoul, Korea), cisplatin (JW Pharmaceutical, Seoul, Korea), and paclitaxel (Samyang Biopharm, Gyeonggi-do, Korea) were dissolved in dimethyl sulfoxide (DMSO; Sigma-Aldrich). MTT was purchased from Amresco (Solon, OH, USA). Primary antibodies used in this study included the following; anti-cleaved caspase 3 (D175, #9661; Cell Signaling Technology; Danvers, MA, USA), phospho-histone H2AX (Ser 139, sc-517348), and glyceraldehyde 3-phosphate dehydrogenase (GAPDH, sc-47724; Santa Cruz Biotechnology; Dallas, TX, USA), and anti-β-actin (A5441; Sigma-Aldrich) antibodies.

4.3. Cell Viability Assay

Cell viability was assessed using the MTT colorimetric assay. Cells ($6 \sim 8 \times 10^2$ cells/well) were seeded into 96-well plates and treated with various concentrations of KJ-28d or a combination of anti-cancer drugs or IR. After 5 days of treatment, 10 μL MTT (0.5 mg/mL) was added, and cells were further incubated for 3 h. After removal of the supernatant, the resultant pellet was dissolved in DMSO. The absorbance of the resultant formazan was measured at 540 nm using a Multiskan EX plate reader (Thermo LabSystems, Waltham, MA, USA).

4.4. Tumor Xenograft Mouse Models

A549 and H1299 human lung cancer cell xenografts were established by *s.c.* implantation of 2×10^6 cultured cells into the thigh of the right hind leg of six-week-old mice. When tumor volumes had reached approximately 100 mm^3, KJ-28d (10 mg/kg) was administered *i.p.* once per 2 or 3 days for seven times in total. All animal experiments were reviewed and approved by the Institutional Animal Care and Use Committee of Korea Institute of Radiological and Medical Sciences (kirams2018-0063, 2018).

4.5. Detection of Intracellular ROS

Either DMSO- or KJ-28d-treated cells (5×10^5) were further treated with 10 μM CM-H_2DCFH-DA (Thermo Fisher Scientific, Rockford, IL, USA) for 30 min and then washed with phosphate-buffered saline (PBS). After trypsinization, cells were collected, washed, and resuspended in PBS. Inhibition of ROS was evaluated by treating cells with 5 mM NAC 2 h prior to KJ-28d treatment. Intracellular ROS levels were detected using a CyFlow cube 6 flow cytometer (Sysmex Partec, Gorlitz, Germany) at excitation/emission wavelengths of 488/525 nm.

4.6. Immunoblot Analysis

A549 and H1299 cells (1×10^6) were seeded onto a 60 mm dish. Cell lysates were prepared by extracting proteins with radioimmunoprecipitation assay (RIPA) lysis buffer (Millipore, Billerica, MA, USA) supplemented with a protease inhibitor cocktail (Thermo Fisher Scientific). Equal amounts of proteins were separated using SDS-PAGE on 8%–13% gels and transferred to nitrocellulose membranes (Bio-Rad, Hercules, CA, USA). Membranes were blocked with 5% skim milk in Tris-buffered saline-Tween 20 (TBST; 150 mM NaCl, 10 mM Tris, 0.2% Tween 20; Sigma-Aldrich), followed by overnight incubation with primary antibodies at 4 °C. Blots were developed using peroxidase-conjugated secondary antibody, and immunoreactive proteins were visualized using enhanced chemiluminescence reagents, according to the manufacturer's recommendations (Amersham, GE Healthcare, Buckinghamshire, UK). Protein bands were visualized using an ImageQuant LAS 4000 mini digital imaging system (GE Healthcare). Protein levels were analyzed using Image J software (National Institutes of Health, Bethesda, MD, USA). Experiments were repeated at least three times.

4.7. Clonogenic Assay

Cells were seeded on 60 mm culture dishes at various densities and then treated with DMSO or KJ-28d (0.75 μM). After 2 h, cells were treated with the indicated doses of 137Cs γ-radiation. After 10 d, colonies were fixed and stained with 1.5% methylene blue (Sigma-Aldrich) in methanol solution. Colonies containing >50 cells were counted. DER was calculated as the dose (Gy) of radiation that yielded a surviving fraction of 0.1 for DMSO-treated cells divided by that dose for KJ-28d-treated cells. The experiment was performed in triplicate.

4.8. Annexin V/PI-Based Flow Cytometric Analysis

Annexin V assays were performed according to the manufacturer's protocol (BD Pharmingen, San Diego, CA, USA). Briefly, 10,000 cells were plated into 60 mm plates and treated with KJ-28d (10 μM) for 48 h. Cells were harvested and incubated with 4 μL allophycocyanin (APC)-conjugated annexin V (20 μg/mL) and 4 μL PI (50 μg/mL) for 15 min. Fluorescence analyses were performed using flow cytometry (CyFlow cube 6). Cells were classified as early apoptotic (annexin V-positive/PI-negative), late apoptotic/necrotic (annexin V-positive/PI-positive), necrotic/dead (annexin V-negative/PI-positive), and live (annexin V-negative/PI-negative). Flow cytometry data were analyzed using FlowJo software (TreeStar Inc., Ashland, OR, USA).

4.9. Combination Index

CI scores were calculated using the CompuSyn software by Chou (CompuSyn Inc., Paramus, NJ, USA) [27] based on cell viability after treatment with single and paired drug concentrations. The CI equation for two drugs used is given below:

$$\mathrm{CI} = \frac{(\mathrm{D})\mathrm{A}}{(\mathrm{Dx})\mathrm{A}} + \frac{(\mathrm{D})\mathrm{B}}{(\mathrm{Dx})\mathrm{B}}$$

where (Dx)A is the concentration of drug A alone that inhibits x%, (Dx)B is the concentration of drug B alone that inhibits x%, (D)A or (D)B is the portion of drug A or drug B in the combination (D)A + (D)B that inhibits x%. Thus, (D)A + (D)B also inhibits x%.

4.10. Statistical Analyses

Results are shown as means ± SD. Data were analyzed using the two-tailed Student's t-test. Analysis of variance (ANOVA) and Tukey's post hoc test were used for 2 or 3 group comparisons. Differences between groups with p values < 0.05 were considered statistically significant.

Author Contributions: Conceptualization: J.A., H.-K.C., and J.-S.K.; funding acquisition: J.A.; investigation: H.R., H.J.K., and T.H.N.B.; resources: S.-G.H. and J.K.; writing—original draft: J.A. and H.R.; writing—review and editing: J.-Y.S. and H.-K.C.

Abbreviations

PARP-1	Poly (ADP-ribose) polymerase-1
PARPi	PARP inhibitor(s)
PARylation	Poly ADP-ribosylation
NSCLC	non-small cell lung cancer
DSB	double-strand breaks
IR	ionizing radiation
ROS	reactive oxygen species
CI	combination index

References

1. American-Cancer-Society. *Cancer Facts & Figures 2019*; American Cancer Society: Atlanta, GA, USA, 2019.
2. Korea, N.C.C. *Annual Report of Cancer Statistics in Korea in 2016*; Ntational Cancer Center Korea: Gyeonggi-do, Korea, 2016. Available online: https://www.cancer.go.kr/lay1/bbs/S1T674C680/B/26/list.do (accessed on 29 November 2019).
3. Liu, C.Y.; Wang, C.L.; Li, S.H.; Hsu, P.C.; Chen, C.H.; Lin, T.Y.; Kuo, C.H.; Fang, Y.F.; Ko, H.W.; Yu, C.T.; et al. The efficacy of 40 mg versus dose de-escalation to less than 40 mg of afatinib (Giotrif) as the first-line therapy for patients with primary lung adenocarcinoma harboring favorable epidermal growth factor mutations. *Oncotarget* **2017**, *8*, 97602–97612. [CrossRef]
4. Jinesh, G.G.; Sambandam, V.; Vijayaraghavan, S.; Balaji, K.; Mukherjee, S. Molecular genetics and cellular events of K-Ras-driven tumorigenesis. *Oncogene* **2018**, *37*, 839–846. [CrossRef]
5. Chen, Y.; Chen, G.; Li, J.; Huang, Y.Y.; Li, Y.; Lin, J.; Chen, L.Z.; Lu, J.P.; Wang, Y.Q.; Wang, C.X.; et al. Association of Tumor Protein p53 and Ataxia-Telangiectasia Mutated Comutation With Response to Immune Checkpoint Inhibitors and Mortality in Patients With Non-Small Cell Lung Cancer. *JAMA Netw. Open* **2019**, *2*, e1911895. [CrossRef] [PubMed]
6. Fan, Y.; Zhu, X.; Xu, Y.; Lu, X.; Xu, Y.; Wang, M.; Xu, H.; Ding, J.; Ye, X.; Fang, L.; et al. Cell-Cycle and DNA-Damage Response Pathway Is Involved in Leptomeningeal Metastasis of Non-Small Cell Lung Cancer. *Clin. Cancer Res.* **2018**, *24*, 209–216. [CrossRef] [PubMed]
7. Alidousty, C.; Baar, T.; Martelotto, L.G.; Heydt, C.; Wagener, S.; Fassunke, J.; Duerbaum, N.; Scheel, A.H.; Frank, S.; Holz, B.; et al. Genetic instability and recurrent MYC amplification in ALK-translocated NSCLC: A central role of TP53 mutations. *J. Pathol.* **2018**, *246*, 67–76. [CrossRef] [PubMed]
8. Postel-Vinay, S.; Vanhecke, E.; Olaussen, K.A.; Lord, C.J.; Ashworth, A.; Soria, J.C. The potential of exploiting DNA-repair defects for optimizing lung cancer treatment. *Nat. Rev. Clin. Oncol.* **2012**, *9*, 144–155. [CrossRef] [PubMed]
9. Wang, Y.S.; Chen, J.; Cui, F.; Wang, H.; Wang, S.; Hang, W.; Zeng, Q.; Quan, C.S.; Zhai, Y.X.; Wang, J.W.; et al. LKB1 is a DNA damage response protein that regulates cellular sensitivity to PARP inhibitors. *Oncotarget* **2016**, *7*, 73389–73401. [CrossRef] [PubMed]
10. Singh, A.; Misra, V.; Thimmulappa, R.K.; Lee, H.; Ames, S.; Hoque, M.O.; Herman, J.G.; Baylin, S.B.; Sidransky, D.; Gabrielson, E.; et al. Dysfunctional KEAP1-NRF2 interaction in non-small-cell lung cancer. *PLoS Med.* **2006**, *3*, e420. [CrossRef] [PubMed]
11. Rojo de la Vega, M.; Chapman, E.; Zhang, D.D. NRF2 and the Hallmarks of Cancer. *Cancer Cell* **2018**, *34*, 21–43. [CrossRef]
12. Virag, L.; Szabo, C. The therapeutic potential of poly(ADP-ribose) polymerase inhibitors. *Pharmacol. Rev.* **2002**, *54*, 375–429. [CrossRef]
13. Dantzer, F.; Ame, J.C.; Schreiber, V.; Nakamura, J.; Menissier-de Murcia, J.; de Murcia, G. Poly(ADP-ribose) polymerase-1 activation during DNA damage and repair. *Methods Enzymol.* **2006**, *409*, 493–510. [PubMed]

14. Kalimutho, M.; Bain, A.L.; Mukherjee, B.; Nag, P.; Nanayakkara, D.M.; Harten, S.K.; Harris, J.L.; Subramanian, G.N.; Sinha, D.; Shirasawa, S.; et al. Enhanced dependency of KRAS-mutant colorectal cancer cells on RAD51-dependent homologous recombination repair identified from genetic interactions in Saccharomyces cerevisiae. *Mol. Oncol.* **2017**, *11*, 470–490. [CrossRef] [PubMed]
15. Kawahara, N.; Ogawa, K.; Nagayasu, M.; Kimura, M.; Sasaki, Y.; Kobayashi, H. Candidate synthetic lethality partners to PARP inhibitors in the treatment of ovarian clear cell cancer. *Biomed. Rep.* **2017**, *7*, 391–399. [CrossRef] [PubMed]
16. Sizemore, S.T.; Mohammad, R.; Sizemore, G.M.; Nowsheen, S.; Yu, H.; Ostrowski, M.C.; Chakravarti, A.; Xia, F. Synthetic Lethality of PARP Inhibition and Ionizing Radiation is p53-dependent. *Biomed. Rep.* **2017**, *7*, 391–399. [CrossRef] [PubMed]
17. Alli, E.; Sharma, V.B.; Sunderesakumar, P.; Ford, J.M. Defective repair of oxidative dna damage in triple-negative breast cancer confers sensitivity to inhibition of poly(ADP-ribose) polymerase. *Cancer Res.* **2009**, *69*, 3589–3596. [CrossRef] [PubMed]
18. Hastak, K.; Alli, E.; Ford, J.M. Synergistic chemosensitivity of triple-negative breast cancer cell lines to poly(ADP-Ribose) polymerase inhibition, gemcitabine, and cisplatin. *Cancer Res.* **2010**, *70*, 7970–7980. [CrossRef] [PubMed]
19. Turner, N.; Tutt, A.; Ashworth, A. Hallmarks of 'BRCAness' in sporadic cancers. *Nat. Rev. Cancer* **2004**, *4*, 814–819. [CrossRef]
20. Liu, Q.; Gheorghiu, L.; Drumm, M.; Clayman, R.; Eidelman, A.; Wszolek, M.F.; Olumi, A.; Feldman, A.; Wang, M.; Marcar, L.; et al. PARP-1 inhibition with or without ionizing radiation confers reactive oxygen species-mediated cytotoxicity preferentially to cancer cells with mutant TP53. *Oncogene* **2018**, *37*, 2793–2805. [CrossRef]
21. Ryu, H.; Ahn, J.; Choi, H.K. Novel Benzamide Derivatives: Synthesis and Bioactivity as Potent PARP-1 Inhibitors. *Bull. Korean Chem. Soc.* **2017**, *38*, 935–943. [CrossRef]
22. Nile, D.L.; Rae, C.; Hyndman, I.J.; Gaze, M.N.; Mairs, R.J. An evaluation in vitro of PARP-1 inhibitors, rucaparib and olaparib, as radiosensitisers for the treatment of neuroblastoma. *BMC Cancer* **2016**, *16*, 621. [CrossRef]
23. Gill, S.J.; Travers, J.; Pshenichnaya, I.; Kogera, F.A.; Barthorpe, S.; Mironenko, T.; Richardson, L.; Benes, C.H.; Stratton, M.R.; McDermott, U.; et al. Combinations of PARP Inhibitors with Temozolomide Drive PARP1 Trapping and Apoptosis in Ewing's Sarcoma. *PLoS ONE* **2015**, *10*, e0140988. [CrossRef] [PubMed]
24. Donawho, C.K.; Luo, Y.; Luo, Y.; Penning, T.D.; Bauch, J.L.; Bouska, J.J.; Bontcheva-Diaz, V.D.; Cox, B.F.; DeWeese, T.L.; Dillehay, L.E.; et al. ABT-888, an orally active poly(ADP-ribose) polymerase inhibitor that potentiates DNA-damaging agents in preclinical tumor models. *Clin. Cancer Res.* **2007**, *13*, 2728–2737. [CrossRef]
25. Palma, J.P.; Wang, Y.C.; Rodriguez, L.E.; Montgomery, D.; Ellis, P.A.; Bukofzer, G.; Niquette, A.; Liu, X.; Shi, Y.; Lasko, L.; et al. ABT-888 confers broad in vivo activity in combination with temozolomide in diverse tumors. *Clin. Cancer Res.* **2009**, *15*, 7277–7290. [CrossRef] [PubMed]
26. Ramalingam, S.S.; Blais, N.; Mazieres, J.; Reck, M.; Jones, C.M.; Juhasz, E.; Urban, L.; Orlov, S.; Barlesi, F.; Kio, E.; et al. Randomized, Placebo-Controlled, Phase II Study of Veliparib in Combination with Carboplatin and Paclitaxel for Advanced/Metastatic Non-Small Cell Lung Cancer. *Clin. Cancer Res.* **2017**, *23*, 1937–1944. [CrossRef] [PubMed]
27. Chou, T.C. Drug combination studies and their synergy quantification using the Chou-Talalay method. *Cancer Res.* **2010**, *70*, 440–446. [CrossRef] [PubMed]
28. Kastenhuber, E.R.; Lowe, S.W. Putting p53 in Context. *Cell* **2017**, *170*, 1062–1078. [CrossRef] [PubMed]
29. Yin, Z.X.; Hang, W.; Liu, G.; Wang, Y.S.; Shen, X.F.; Sun, Q.H.; Li, D.D.; Jian, Y.P.; Zhang, Y.H.; Quan, C.S.; et al. PARP-1 inhibitors sensitize HNSCC cells to APR-246 by inactivation of thioredoxin reductase 1 (TrxR1) and promotion of ROS accumulation. *Oncotarget* **2018**, *9*, 1885–1897. [CrossRef] [PubMed]
30. Reck, M.; Blais, N.; Juhasz, E.; Gorbunova, V.; Jones, C.M.; Urban, L.; Orlov, S.; Barlesi, F.; Kio, E.; Keilholz, U.; et al. Smoking History Predicts Sensitivity to PARP Inhibitor Veliparib in Patients with Advanced Non-Small Cell Lung Cancer. *J. Thorac. Oncol.* **2017**, *12*, 1098–1108. [CrossRef] [PubMed]
31. Mizugaki, H.; Yamamoto, N.; Nokihara, H.; Fujiwara, Y.; Horinouchi, H.; Kanda, S.; Kitazono, S.; Yagishita, S.; Xiong, H.; Qian, J.; et al. A phase 1 study evaluating the pharmacokinetics and preliminary efficacy of

veliparib (ABT-888) in combination with carboplatin/paclitaxel in Japanese subjects with non-small cell lung cancer (NSCLC). *Cancer Chemother. Pharmacol.* **2015**, *76*, 1063–1072. [CrossRef] [PubMed]

32. Tuli, R.; Surmak, A.J.; Reyes, J.; Armour, M.; Hacker-Prietz, A.; Wong, J.; DeWeese, T.L.; Herman, J.M. Radiosensitization of Pancreatic Cancer Cells In Vitro and In Vivo through Poly (ADP-ribose) Polymerase Inhibition with ABT-888. *Transl. Oncol.* **2014**, *7*, 439–445. [CrossRef]
33. Tuli, R.; Shiao, S.L.; Nissen, N.; Tighiouart, M.; Kim, S.; Osipov, A.; Bryant, M.; Ristow, L.; Placencio-Hickok, V.; Hoffman, D.; et al. A phase 1 study of veliparib, a PARP-1/2 inhibitor, with gemcitabine and radiotherapy in locally advanced pancreatic cancer. *EBioMedicine* **2019**, *40*, 375–381. [CrossRef]
34. Tyldesley, S.; Boyd, C.; Schulze, K.; Walker, H.; Mackillop, W.J. Estimating the need for radiotherapy for lung cancer: An evidence-based, epidemiologic approach. *Int. J. Radiat. Oncol. Biol. Phys.* **2001**, *49*, 973–985. [CrossRef]
35. Wang, L.; Mason, K.A.; Ang, K.K.; Buchholz, T.; Valdecanas, D.; Mathur, A.; Buser-Doepner, C.; Toniatti, C.; Milas, L. MK-4827, a PARP-1/-2 inhibitor, strongly enhances response of human lung and breast cancer xenografts to radiation. *Invest. New Drugs* **2012**, *30*, 2113–2120. [CrossRef]
36. Senra, J.M.; Telfer, B.A.; Cherry, K.E.; McCrudden, C.M.; Hirst, D.G.; O'Connor, M.J.; Wedge, S.R.; Stratford, I.J. Inhibition of PARP-1 by olaparib (AZD2281) increases the radiosensitivity of a lung tumor xenograft. *Mol. Cancer Ther.* **2011**, *10*, 1949–1958. [CrossRef]
37. Albert, J.M.; Cao, C.; Kim, K.W.; Willey, C.D.; Geng, L.; Xiao, D.; Wang, H.; Sandler, A.; Johnson, D.H.; Colevas, A.D.; et al. Inhibition of poly(ADP-ribose) polymerase enhances cell death and improves tumor growth delay in irradiated lung cancer models. *Clin. Cancer Res.* **2007**, *13*, 3033–3042. [CrossRef]
38. Hu, X.L.; Feng, J.H.; Pham, T.A.; Ma, H.Y.; Ma, M.X.; Song, R.; Shen, W.; Xiong, F.; Zhang, X.Q.; Ye, W.C.; et al. Identification of amentoflavone as a potent highly selective PARP-1 inhibitor and its potentiation on carboplatin in human non-small cell lung cancer. *Phytomedicine* **2018**, *50*, 88–98. [CrossRef]

4

Prediction of Anti-Cancer Drug-Induced Pneumonia in Lung Cancer Patients: Novel High-Resolution Computed Tomography Fibrosis Scoring

Hiroshi Gyotoku [1], Hiroyuki Yamaguchi [1,*], Hiroshi Ishimoto [1], Shuntaro Sato [2], Hirokazu Taniguchi [1], Hiroaki Senju [1], Tomoyuki Kakugawa [1,3], Katsumi Nakatomi [1], Noriho Sakamoto [1], Minoru Fukuda [1,4], Yasushi Obase [1], Hiroshi Soda [5], Kazuto Ashizawa [4] and Hiroshi Mukae [1]

1 Department of Respiratory Medicine, Nagasaki University Graduate School of Biomedical Sciences, Nagasaki University, Nagasaki 852-8523, Japan; hirokazu_pc@hotmail.co.jp
2 Clinical Research Center, Nagasaki University Hospital, Nagasaki 852-8501, Japan
3 Department of Pulmonology and Gerontology, Yamaguchi University Graduate School of Medicine, Ube 755-0046, Japan
4 Clinical Oncology Center, Nagasaki University Hospital, Nagasaki 852-8501, Japan
5 Department of Respiratory Medicine, Sasebo City General Hospital, Nagasaki 857-8511, Japan
* Correspondence: yamaguchi-hiroyuki@umin.ac.jp

Abstract: Background and objective: Pre-existing interstitial lung disease (ILD) in lung cancer patients is considered a risk factor for anti-cancer drug-induced pneumonia; however, a method for evaluating ILD, including mild cases, has not yet been established. We aimed to elucidate whether the quantitative high-resolution computed tomography fibrosis score (HFS) is correlated with the risk of anti-cancer drug-induced pneumonia in lung cancer patients, even in those with mild pre-existing ILD. Methods: The retrospective single-institute study cohort comprised 214 lung cancer patients who underwent chemotherapy between April 2013 and March 2016. The HFS quantitatively evaluated the grade of pre-existing ILD. We extracted data regarding age, sex, smoking history, and coexisting factors that could affect the incidence of anti-cancer drug-induced pneumonia. Cox proportional hazard models were used to analyze the effects of the HFS and other factors on the risk of anti-cancer drug-induced pneumonia. Results: Pre-existing ILD was detected in 61 (29%) of 214 patients, while honeycombing and traction bronchiectasis were observed in only 15 (7.0%) and 10 (4.7%) patients, respectively. Anti-cancer drug-induced pneumonia developed in 19 (8.9%) patients. The risk of anti-cancer drug-induced pneumonia increased in proportion to the HFS (hazard ratio, 1.16 per point; 95% confidence interval, 1.09–1.22; $p < 0.0001$). Conclusions: The quantitative HFS was correlated with the risk of developing anti-cancer drug-induced pneumonia in lung cancer patients, even in the absence of honeycombing or traction bronchiectasis. The quantitative HFS may lead to better management of lung cancer patients with pre-existing ILD.

Keywords: lung cancer; interstitial lung disease; pulmonary fibrosis; radiology and other imaging

1. Introduction

Anti-cancer drug-induced pneumonia is a potentially fatal disease in lung cancer patients. Pre-existing chronic interstitial lung disease (ILD) is considered a risk factor for anti-cancer drug-induced pneumonia, as is being male, being elderly, having a poor Eastern Cooperative Oncology Group performance status (ECOG-PS), a history of smoking, and low forced vital capacity [1–4]. The American Thoracic Society/European Respiratory Society/Japanese Respiratory Society/Latin American Thoracic

Association guidelines for the classification of idiopathic interstitial pneumonia (IIP) are often employed for evaluating ILD [5–7]. Several clinical trials of anti-cancer drugs have included lung cancer patients with ILD, which was evaluated according to the IIP guidelines [8–12].

However, the IIP guidelines do not include and evaluate mild pre-existing ILD without honeycombing or traction bronchiectasis. The 2018 idiopathic pulmonary fibrosis (IPF) guidelines define mild ILD as "indeterminate for usual interstitial pneumonia (UIP) HRCT pattern" [13]. Nevertheless, few studies regarding anti-cancer drug-induced pneumonia have referred to mild pre-existing ILD [1,2]. Thus, a quantitative method for evaluating pre-existing ILD, including mild ILD, has not yet been established.

The quantitative high-resolution computed tomography (HRCT) scores of acute interstitial pneumonia and acute respiratory distress syndrome (ARDS) have been reported to correlate with pathology and prognosis [14–17]. The HRCT fibrosis score (HFS) was modified from this score in order to evaluate lung fibrosis easily, with an increased HFS over the course of 6 months indicating poor prognosis [18]. We hypothesized that the HFS could reflect the degree of the lung fibrosing process, resulting in the exact evaluation of the risk of anti-cancer drug-induced pneumonia in lung cancer patients with pre-existing ILD. This retrospective cohort study was designed to determine whether the quantitative HFS correlates with the risk of anti-cancer drug-induced pneumonia in lung cancer patients, including those with mild pre-existing ILD.

2. Methods

2.1. Study Design

This retrospective, single-institute, cohort study was performed at the Department of Respiratory Medicine, Nagasaki University Hospital. Patients were enrolled based on the following three inclusion criteria: admitted to our department between April 2013 and March 2016; pathologically diagnosed with lung cancer; and receiving anti-cancer drugs, including cytotoxic drugs and molecular-target agents. Patients were excluded from the analysis if they irregularly received adjuvant chemotherapy with oral tegafur–uracil alone or if >50% of the lung fields could not be evaluated primarily due to the extensive cancer lesions or postoperative status.

Eligible patients were extracted from lung cancer patients using the hospital's electronic medical record system. Anti-cancer drugs were administered in various clinical conditions, including conventional or adjuvant chemotherapy, and concurrent or sequential radiotherapy. All patients were followed up with until December 2017. A systemic follow-up survey of the lesions was performed by physical examination, chest radiography, and blood tests at least once a month. Chest HRCT was routinely conducted as scheduled for outpatient follow-up. The censored cases were defined as death, transferring hospital, lost to follow-up, or the initiation of immune checkpoint inhibitors.

2.2. Chest HRCT Scoring System

HRCT (Aquilion ONE^{TM}, Canon Medical Systems, Ohtawara, Japan) scans were obtained with 0.5 mm collimation and a 1 mm slice thickness at 1 mm intervals from the lung apices to the bases in the supine position at full inspiration. Two experienced pulmonologists (H.G. and H.I. with 11 and 19 years of experience, respectively), who were blinded to the clinical data, individually assessed the degree of pre-existing ILD using the HFS.

In detail, the HFS was calculated in three areas of each lung before the first administration of anti-cancer drugs: the level of the carina, the level of the right inferior pulmonary vein, and the middle of the two levels. First, the HRCT findings were scored as follows: normal attenuation (score 1), reticular abnormality (score 2), both reticular abnormality and traction bronchiectasis (score 3), and honeycombing (score 4). We did not evaluate extensive pure ground glass opacity, and we organized the lesions after pneumonia, operation, and radiotherapy. Second, the extent of the interstitial abnormalities was estimated as the percentage of the 5% intervals. We multiplied the score and the extent percentage and summed the points for each of the six areas. Finally, we averaged the summed points of the six areas. ILD was categorized as no ILD (HFS = 100), mild ILD (HFS = 101–200), moderate ILD (HFS = 201–300), and severe ILD (HFS = 301–400).

Furthermore, the two independent pulmonologists also evaluated the degree of emphysema using the Goddard score (GS) for the six areas analyzed above [19]. The extent of LAA (low-attenuation areas) was scored as follows: < 5% LAA (score of 0), 6%–25% LAA (score of 1), 26%–50% LAA (score of 2), 51%–75% (score of 3), and > 75% LAA (score of 4). The six scores were summed, and emphysema was graded as no emphysema (GS = 0), mild emphysema (GS = 1–7), moderate emphysema (GS = 8–15), and severe emphysema (GS = 16–24).

2.3. Examples of HFS and GS in Lung Cancer Patients with Pre-Existing ILD

Two representative patients were evaluated using the HFS (Figure 1). Regarding the HFS, Patient A scored 104 points, and patient B scored 122.5 points. The details are provided in Figure 1. Regarding the GS, patient A scored 0 points according to the two pulmonologists. Patient B was awarded 18 points by Dr. H.G. Each of six lung fields was evaluated as score 3; 3 × 6 = 18. In contrast, Patient B was awarded 15 points by Dr. H.I. Overall, patient B received an average GS of 16.5, indicating severe emphysema.

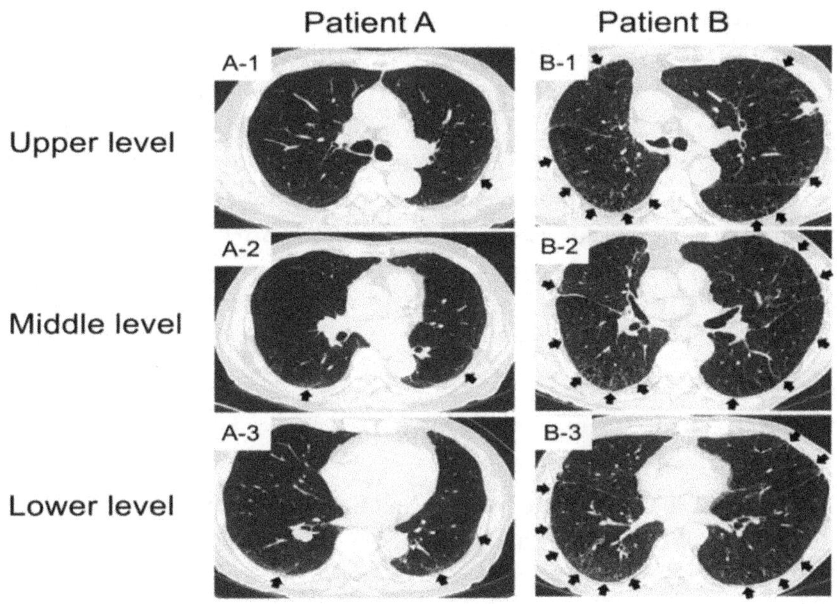

Figure 1. Imaging findings in two representative patients evaluated using the high-resolution computed tomography fibrosis score. The black arrows indicate reticular abnormality (score 2). Patient A scored 104 points, and patient B scored 122.5 points. The scoring of each patient was as follows: Patient A scored 105 points, as evaluated by Dr. H.G. In detail, the (**A-1**) right field was evaluated as 100% of score 1; 100 × 1 = 100. The A-1 left, (**A-2**) right, (**A-2**) left, and (**A-3**) right fields were evaluated as 95% of score 1 and 5% of score 2; (95 × 1) + (5 × 2) = 105. The (**A-3**) left field was evaluated as 90% of score 1 and 10% of score 2; (90 × 1) + (10 × 2) = 110. Thus, the HFS was (100 × 1 + 105 × 4 + 110 × 1)/6 = 105. In contrast, patient A scored 103 points, as evaluated by Dr. H.I. Overall, patient A received an average high-resolution computed tomography fibrosis score (HFS) of 104. Patient B scored 125 points, as evaluated by Dr. H.G. In detail, the (**B-1**) left were evaluated as 80% of score 1 and 20% of score 2; (80 × 1) + (20 × 2) = 120. The (**B-1**) right, (**B-2**) right and left, and (**B-3**) left were evaluated as 75% of score 1 and 25% of score 2; (75 × 1) + (25 × 2) = 125. The (**B-3**) right was evaluated as 70% of score 1 and 30% of score 2; (70 × 1) + (30 × 2) = 130. Thus, the HFS was (120 × 1 + 125 × 4 + 130 × 1)/6 = 125. In contrast, patient B scored 120 points, as evaluated by Dr. H.I. Overall, patient A received an average HFS of 122.5.

2.4. *Anti-Cancer Drug-Induced Pneumonia*

The definition of anti-cancer drug-induced pneumonia was interstitial lung disease developed from anti-cancer drug exposure to 60 days after the final anti-cancer treatment. We determined the diagnosis based on clinical and radiological findings and excluded apparent pulmonary infection, radiation-induced lung injury, and heart failure. The evaluation of anti-cancer drug-induced pneumonia was defined according to the Common Terminology Criteria for Adverse Events (CTCAE) version 4.0 from the National Cancer Institute (Bethesda, MD) [20]. The time to onset of anti-cancer drug-induced pneumonia was defined as the interval between the first administration of anti-cancer drugs and the diagnosis of anti-cancer drug-induced pneumonia.

2.5. *Clinical Data Collection*

We collected other clinical data, including age; sex; ECOG-PS; smoking history; tumor histology; clinical stage; epidermal growth factor receptor mutations; anaplastic lymphoma kinase rearrangements; and previous chemotherapy, thoracic surgery, and thoracic radiation.

2.6. *Statistical Analysis*

The inter-observer variations in the HFS and GS were assessed using intra-class correlation coefficients (ICC). The prevalence of pre-existing ILD and anti-cancer drug-induced pneumonia was accompanied by 95% confidence intervals (CIs), and the difference was evaluated by chi-square test. The cumulative incidence of anti-cancer drug-induced pneumonia, which was stratified by HFS of >110, $110 \geq \text{HFS} > 100$, and $\text{HFS} = 100$, was assessed via the Kaplan–Meier method and the trend log-rank test. We evaluated the hazard ratio (HR) and 95% CI of each potential risk factor for anti-cancer drug-induced pneumonia by simple Cox proportional hazard analysis. We selected variables according to a literature review and clinical expertise. We confirmed whether HFS (per point) may be affected by another potential risk factor using replaced multiple Cox proportional hazards analyses.

The plotting of Kaplan–Meier curves and the trend log-rank test were conducted using GraphPad Prism version 7 (GraphPad Software Inc., La Jolla, CA, USA). The other statistical analyses were performed using JMP pro version 14 (SAS Institute, Cary, NC, USA). A two-tailed p value of < 0.05 was considered statistically significant.

2.7. *Ethical Considerations*

This study was performed in accordance with the Declaration of Helsinki. The institutional review board of Nagasaki University Hospital approved this study protocol (approval number 17032713-3). Informed consent was obtained from the patients by an opt-out system on the hospital website, in accordance with the ethical guideline presented by the Ministry of Health, Labor, and Welfare in Japan. This trial was registered with the University Hospital Medical Information Network in Japan (UMIN), registry number UMIN000026964.

3. Results

3.1. *Patient Characteristics and HFS*

A total of 214 lung cancer patients were extracted and analyzed from 1280 patients with respiratory diseases (Figure 2). The study population was composed of approximately 70% males and ever smokers (Table 1). The inter-observer agreement on the HRCT findings was high for the HFS (ICC = 0.96) and GS (ICC = 0.97) between the two pulmonologists. The prevalence of pre-existing ILD was 28.5% (61/214 cases; 95% CI, 22.5–34.5) in lung cancer patients undergoing anti-cancer drug therapy. Incidentally, all pre-existing ILDs scored by the HFS were mild grade. Honeycombing and traction bronchiectasis were observed in only 15 (7.0%) and 10 (4.7%) of 214 cases, respectively.

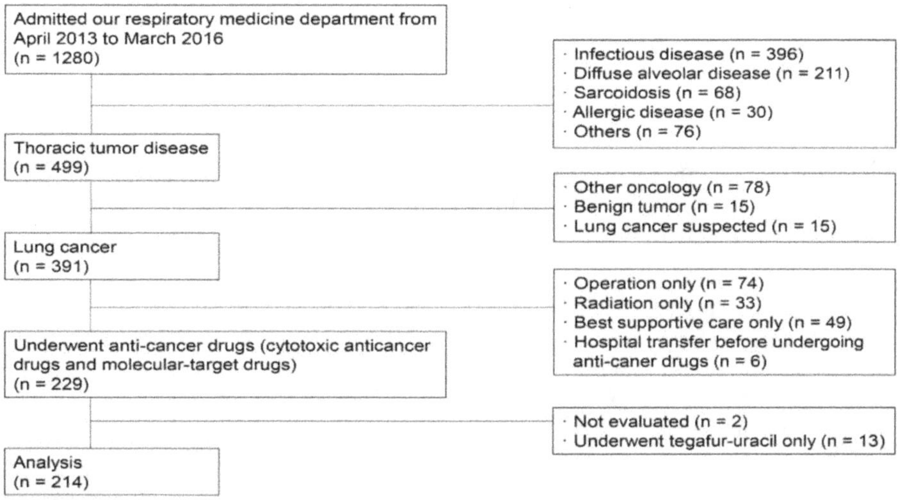

Figure 2. Study flow diagram.

Table 1. Characteristics of lung cancer patients who underwent anti-cancer drugs.

	Total (*n* = 214)
Age, range	67 (25–85)
Gender	
Male	144 (67%)
Female	70 (33%)
Smoking history	
Ever-smoker	148 (69%)
Never-smoker	66 (31%)
ECOG-PS	
0–1	209 (98%)
2–4	5 (2%)
Histology	
Adenocarcinoma	136 (64%)
Squamous cell carcinoma	35 (16%)
Small-cell lung cancer	31 (14%)
Others	12 (6%)
Clinical stage	
I	4 (2%)
II	14 (7%)
III	53 (25%)
IV, Recurrence	143 (67%)
Genetic abnormalities	
Wild type	151 (71%)
EGFR mutations	56 (26%)
ALK rearrangements	7 (3%)
GS	
Normal	93 (43%)
Mild	77 (36%)
Moderate	36 (17%)
Severe	8 (4%)

ECOG-PS, Eastern Cooperative Oncology Group performance status; EGFR, epidermal growth factor receptor; ALK, anaplastic lymphoma kinase; GS, Goddard score.

The prevalence of anti-cancer drug-induced pneumonia was 8.9% (19/214 cases; 95% CI: 5.0–12.8). Anti-cancer drug-induced pneumonia was likely to develop in patients with pre-existing ILD (Figure 3). Although anti-cancer drug-induced pneumonia occurred twice in two patients with mild ILD, we analyzed the first event only. The prevalence of anti-cancer drug-induced pneumonia was 24.6% (15/61 cases; 95% CI, 13.9–35.3) in patients with pre-existing ILD, and 2.6% (4/153 cases; 95% CI, −0.4–5.6) in those without ILD. The development of anti-cancer drug-induced pneumonia was more frequent in patients with pre-existing ILD than in those without ILD ($p < 0.0001$).

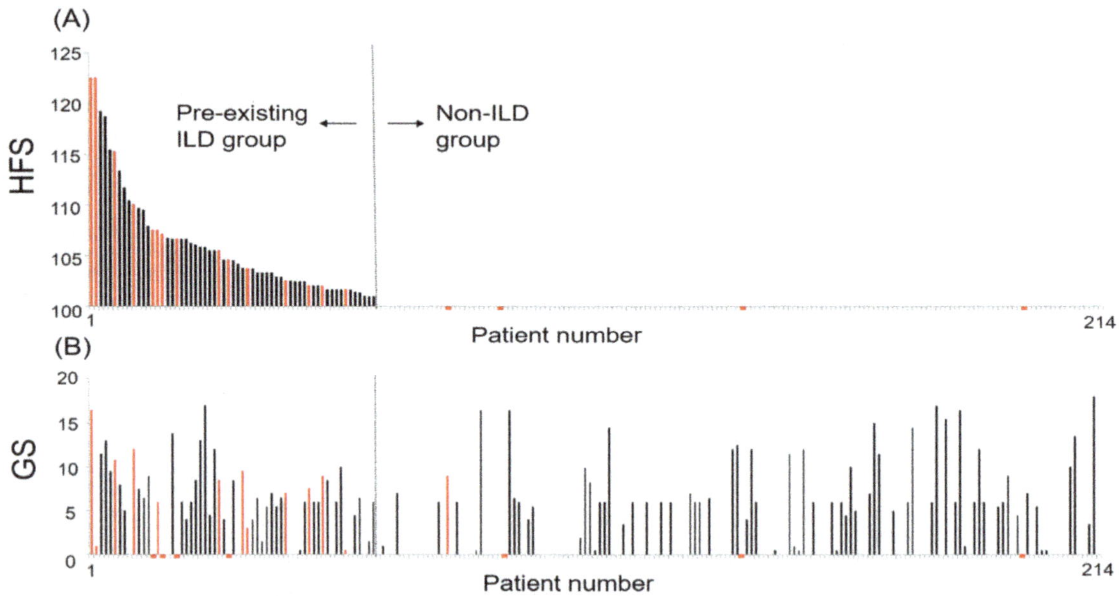

Figure 3. Bar graph of the incidence of anti-cancer drug induced pneumonia according to the high-resolution computed tomography fibrosis score and Goddard score. (**A**) Relationship between the high-resolution computed tomography fibrosis score (HFS) and the development of anti-cancer drug-induced pneumonia in 214 patients with lung cancer. The red bars represent the patients with anti-cancer drug-induced pneumonia, and the black bars represent those without. An HFS of >100 indicates the presence of pre-existing interstitial lung disease (ILD). (**B**) Relationship between the Goddard score (GS) and the development of anti-cancer drug-induced pneumonia in lung cancer patients. The red and black bars are defined as described above. Each pair of upper and lower panels represents the same patient.

3.2. Potential Risk Factors of Anti-Cancer Drug-Induced Pneumonia

The cumulative risk of anti-cancer drug-induced pneumonia was significantly increased in patients with a higher HFS ($p < 0.0001$, Figure 4). The simple Cox proportional hazard analysis showed a risk factor for anti-cancer drug-induced pneumonia (Table 2A); a high HFS and being male were significant risk factors for anti-cancer drug-induced pneumonia. The HFS in particular was a prominent risk factor; an increase of one HFS point was associated with a 16% increased risk of developing anti-cancer drug-induced pneumonia (HR, 1.16; 95% CI, 1.09–1.22; $p < 0.001$). Smoking history and high GS (indicating severe emphysema) were not associated with a risk of anti-cancer drug-induced pneumonia. The robustness of the HFS as a risk factor remained constant in the replaced multiple Cox proportional hazard analyses of other potential risk factors (Table 2B). A multivariate Cox proportional hazard analysis was not performed, because the simple and replaced multiple Cox proportional hazards analyses revealed that the HFS was a prominent risk factor of anti-cancer drug-induced pneumonia.

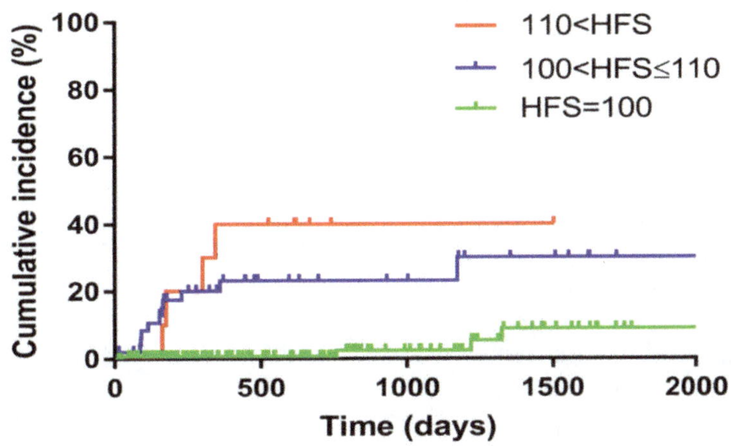

No. at Risk	0	500	1000	1500	2000
110<HFS	10	7	2	2	1
100<HFS≤110	51	18	14	8	3
HFS=100	153	85	45	21	11

Figure 4. Kaplan–Meier estimated curves of the incidence of anti-cancer drug-induced pneumonia stratified by the high-resolution computed tomography fibrosis score. The Kaplan–Meier estimated curves indicated that the incidence of anti-cancer drug-induced pneumonia is increased in patients with higher high-resolution computed tomography fibrosis scores (HFSs) ($p < 0.0001$ according to the log-rank test).

Table 2. (**A**) Potential risk factors for anti-cancer drug induced pneumonia ($n = 214$) by the simple Cox proportional hazards analysis. (**B**) Influence of other clinical factors to the hazard ratio of HFS by the simple and replaced multiple Cox proportional hazards analyses.

	HR	95% CI	*p*-value
Age			
< 70	1.00		
≥ 70	1.37	0.51–3.42	0.51
Gender			
Female	1.00		
Male	3.29	1.09-14.18	0.034
ECOG-PS			
0–1	1.00		
2–4	3.61	0.20–17.67	0.30
Histology			
Adenocarcinoma	1.00		
Squamous-cell carcinoma	0.70	0.11–2.53	0.62
Small-cell carcinoma	0.72	0.11–2.62	0.65
Others	1.03	0.06–5.22	0.97
Clinical Stage			
I–II	n/c		
III	1.00		
IV, Recurrence	0.91	0.36–2.60	0.86

Table 2. *Cont.*

	HR	95% CI	*p*-value
Smoking history			
No	1		
Yes	2.97	0.99-12.80	0.053
Genetic abnormalities †			
No	1		
Yes	0.65	0.21–1.73	0.40
GS (per point)	1.06	0.97–1.15	0.20
HFS (per point)	1.16	1.09–1.22	< 0.0001
Operation			
No	1		
Yes	0.49	0.16–1.30	0.16
Radiation			
No	1		
Yes	1.66	0.66–4.14	0.28

(A) † Gene abnormalities includes anaplastic lymphoma kinase (ALK) and epidermal growth factor receptor (EGFR). HR, hazard ratio; CI, confidence interval; ECOG-PS, Eastern Cooperative Oncology Group performance status; n/c, not calculated; GS, Goddard score; HFS, HRCT fibrosis score.

	HFS		
Variables	**HR**	**95% CI**	***p***
Simple			
HFS	1.16	1.09–1.22	< 0.0001
Replaced multiple			
Variable to adjust the effect of HFS			
Age	1.15	1.08–1.22	<0.0001
Gender	1.14	1.07–1.21	0.0002
ECOG-PS	1.16	1.09–1.22	<0.0001
Histology	1.16	1.09–1.23	<0.0001
Clinical stage	1.15	1.08–1.22	<0.0001
Smoking history	1.15	1.08–1.22	0.0001
Gene abnormalities	1.16	1.08–1.23	<0.0001
GS	1.16	1.08–1.23	<0.0001
Operation	1.16	1.09–1.22	<0.0001
Radiation	1.16	1.09–1.23	<0.0001

(B) HFS, HRCT fibrosis score; HR, hazard ratio; CI, confidence interval; ECOG-PS, Eastern Cooperative Oncology Group performance status; GS, Goddard score.

3.3. *Characteristics of Patients with Anti-Cancer Drug-Induced Pneumonia*

The characteristics of the 19 patients with anti-cancer drug-induced pneumonia are listed in Table S1. Although previous radiotherapy did not confer a risk for anti-cancer drug-induced pneumonia (Table 2A), 10 of 19 these patients had received radiotherapy. The development of radiological interstitial abnormalities in the ten patients did not correspond to the exposure to radiation. The HFS did not correlate with the grade of anti-cancer drug-induced pneumonia. Specific regimens were not associated with the risk of anti-cancer drug-induced pneumonia.

4. Discussion

To the best of our knowledge, the present study is the first to provide the following important findings. The quantitative HFS is positively correlated with the risk of anti-cancer drug-induced pneumonia in lung cancer patients. In particular, the HFS was associated with a risk of anti-cancer drug-induced pneumonia in patients with mild pre-existing ILD, even in the absence of honeycombing or traction bronchiectasis.

The current IIP guidelines do not assess the severity of pre-existing ILD, particularly mild ILD. IPF diagnosed using the IIP guidelines was observed in 2%–8% of lung cancer patients [21–23]. In contrast, 28.5% of lung cancer patients that were administered anti-cancer drugs had mild pre-existing ILD confirmed by the HFS in the present study. In two computed tomography lung cancer screening trials that defined the patterns of mild interstitial lung abnormalities, ILD was detected in 15.7%–21.2% of patients with a history of smoking [24,25]. Since the IIP guidelines do not necessarily consider the radiological process of pulmonary fibrosis, mild ILD may have been overlooked. Precise evaluation of the risk of anti-cancer drug-induced pneumonia requires a quantitative method capable of detecting all levels of ILD, including mild ILD.

In the present study, the quantitative HFS was significantly correlated with the risk of anti-cancer drug-induced pneumonia. Little is known of the relationship between anti-cancer drugs and mild pre-existing ILD [1,2]. A nested case-control study investigated the risk factors for pre-existing ILD associated with chemotherapy and gefitinib [1]. Although this study referred to the severity of ILD, including mild grade, the severity was not clearly defined. The adjusted odds ratios indicated that patients with mild and moderate–severe ILD had an approximately five-fold increased risk of developing acute ILD compared to patients without ILD, suggesting no difference between mild and moderate–severe ILD. Another prospective cohort study identified the risk factors for pre-existing ILD associated with erlotinib [2]. This study evaluated only the extent of interstitial abnormalities, but not the fibrous pattern on HRCT. The study population of patients with pre-existing ILD predominantly comprised patients with mild ILD, in which abnormalities involved <5% of the bilateral lower lobes. The multivariate logistic regression analysis yielded an odds ratio of 4.0 (95% CI, 1.3–12.1) between the presence and absence of ILD. Thus, the present study first revealed that an increase of HFS point was associated with a 16% increased risk of anti-cancer drug-induced pneumonia, even in mild ILD without honeycombing and traction bronchiectasis.

Pre-existing mild ILD might induce drug-induced pneumonia because a histological UIP pattern may be involved. The 2018 IPF guidelines categorize mild ILD as an indeterminate for the UIP HRCT pattern (early UIP pattern) [13]. This category includes the subset of patients with reticular patterns in the absence of honeycombing and traction bronchiectasis, predominantly in the subpleural and basal fields. Lung cancer patients with UIP HRCT patterns exhibited exacerbation of ILD more frequently than did those with non-UIP HRCT patterns [3]. In precision medicine, many novel anti-cancer drugs have been developed, some of which are likely to cause drug-induced pneumonia. The early recognition of the subtle fibrosing findings on HRCT may enable physicians to provide better management of lung cancer patients receiving anti-cancer drugs.

The present study had several limitations. First, all cases of pre-existing ILD incidentally included mild cases. Thus, we did not necessarily verify the utility of the HFS for moderate and severe ILD. However, a previous case-control study revealed that the odds ratio of the development of anti-cancer drug-induced pneumonia was high in patients with moderate/severe pre-existing ILD as well as those with mild ILD [1]. Second, the pulmonary function test results could not be evaluated, due to missing values in clinical practice. Another quantitative HRCT scoring system has been replaced by the diffusion capacity of carbon monoxide test for the prognosis with IPF patients [26]. Third, this was a single institutional analysis, and the number of anti-cancer drug-induced pneumonia cases was small. The present findings are therefore potentially subject to selection bias. Further prospective investigations involving large cohorts are required to confirm our findings.

In conclusion, HFS may correlate with the risk of anti-cancer drug-induced pneumonia in lung cancer patients, even in the absence of honeycombing or traction bronchiectasis. This quantitative HFS could be a predictor of anti-cancer drug-induced pneumonia, which could improve the management of lung cancer patients with ILD.

Author Contributions: Conceptualization, H.G., H.Y. and H.M.; Data curation, S.S. and K.A.; Formal analysis, H.G., H.I. and K.A.; Investigation, H.G., H.S. and M.F.; Methodology, H.Y., H.T., T.K., K.N., N.S. and H.S.; Supervision, H.Y., K.N., Y.O., H.S. and H.M.; Writing —original draft, H.G.; Writing—review & editing, H.Y., N.S., Y.O. and H.S. All authors have read and agreed to the published version of the manuscript.

Acknowledgments: We would like to thank Editage (www.editage.jp) for English language editing.

References

1. Kudoh, S.; Kato, H.; Nishiwaki, Y.; Fukuoka, M.; Nakata, K.; Ichinose, Y.; Tsuboi, M.; Yokota, S.; Nakagawa, K.; Suga, M.; et al. Interstitial Lung Disease in Japanese Patients with Lung Cancer. *Am. J. Respir. Crit. Care Med.* **2008**, *177*, 1348–1357. [CrossRef] [PubMed]
2. Johkoh, T.; Sakai, F.; Kusumoto, M.; Arakawa, H.; Harada, R.; Ueda, M.; Kudoh, S.; Fukuoka, M. Association Between Baseline Pulmonary Status and Interstitial Lung Disease in Patients With Non–Small-Cell Lung Cancer Treated With Erlotinib—A Cohort Study. *Clin. Lung Cancer* **2014**, *15*, 448–454. [CrossRef] [PubMed]
3. Kenmotsu, H.; Naito, T.; Kimura, M.; Ono, A.; Shukuya, T.; Nakamura, Y.; Tsuya, A.; Kaira, K.; Murakami, H.; Takahashi, T.; et al. The Risk of Cytotoxic Chemotherapy-Related Exacerbation of Interstitial Lung Disease with Lung Cancer. *J. Thorac. Oncol.* **2011**, *6*, 1242–1246. [CrossRef] [PubMed]
4. Kobayashi, H.; Naito, T.; Omae, K.; Omori, S.; Nakashima, K.; Wakuda, K.; Ono, A.; Kenmotsu, H.; Murakami, H.; Endo, M.; et al. ILD-NSCLC-GAP index scoring and staging system for patients with non-small cell lung cancer and interstitial lung disease. *Lung Cancer* **2018**, *121*, 48–53. [CrossRef] [PubMed]
5. American Thoracic, S.; European Respiratory, S. American Thoracic Society/European Respiratory Society International Multidisciplinary Consensus Classification of the Idiopathic Interstitial Pneumonias. This joint statement of the American Thoracic Society (ATS), and the European Respiratory Society (ERS) was adopted by the ATS board of directors, June 2001 and by the ERS Executive Committee, June 2001. *Am. J. Respir. Crit. Care Med.* **2002**, *165*, 277–304.
6. Raghu, G.; Collard, H.R.; Egan, J.J.; Martinez, F.J.; Behr, J.; Brown, K.K.; Colby, T.V.; Cordier, J.F.; Flaherty, K.R.; Lasky, J.A.; et al. An official ATS/ERS/Japanese Respiratory Society (JRS)/ Latin American Thoracic Association (ALAT) statement: Idiopathic pulmonary fibrosis: Evidence-based guidelines for diagnosis and management. *Am. J. Respir. Crit. Care Med.* **2011**, *183*, 788–824. [CrossRef]
7. Travis, W.D.; Costabel, U.; Hansell, D.M.; King, T.E.; Jr Lynch, D.A.; Nicholson, A.G.; Ryerson, C.J.; Ryu, J.H.; Selman, M.; Wells, A.U.; et al. An official ATS/ERS statement: Update of the international multidisciplinary classification of the idiopathic interstitial pneumonias. *Am. J. Respir. Crit. Care Med.* **2013**, *188*, 733–748. [CrossRef]
8. Minegishi, Y.; Sudoh, J.; Kuribayasi, H.; Mizutani, H.; Seike, M.; Azuma, A.; Yoshimura, A.; Kudoh, S.; Gemma, A. The safety and efficacy of weekly paclitaxel in combination with carboplatin for advanced non-small cell lung cancer with idiopathic interstitial pneumonias. *Lung Cancer* **2011**, *71*, 70–74. [CrossRef]
9. Minegishi, Y.; Kuribayashi, H.; Kitamura, K.; Mizutani, H.; Kosaihira, S.; Okano, T.; Seike, M.; Azuma, A.; Yoshimura, A.; Kudoh, S.; et al. The Feasibility Study of Carboplatin Plus Etoposide for Advanced Small Cell Lung Cancer with Idiopathic Interstitial Pneumonias. *J. Thorac. Oncol.* **2011**, *6*, 801–807. [CrossRef]
10. Sekine, A.; Satoh, H.; Baba, T.; Ikeda, S.; Okuda, R.; Shinohara, T.; Komatsu, S.; Hagiwara, E.; Iwasawa, T.; Ogura, T.; et al. Safety and efficacy of S-1 in combination with carboplatin in non-small cell lung cancer patients with interstitial lung disease: A pilot study. *Cancer Chemother. Pharmacol.* **2016**, *77*, 1245–1252. [CrossRef]
11. Yasuda, Y.; Hattori, Y.; Tohnai, R.; Ito, S.; Kawa, Y.; Kono, Y.; Urata, Y.; Nogami, M.; Takenaka, D.; Negoro, S.; et al. The safety and efficacy of carboplatin plus nanoparticle albumin-bound paclitaxel in the treatment of non-small cell lung cancer patients with interstitial lung disease. *Jpn. J. Clin. Oncol.* **2017**, *48*, 89–93. [CrossRef] [PubMed]
12. Shimizu, R.; Fujimoto, D.; Kato, R.; Otoshi, T.; Kawamura, T.; Tamai, K.; Matsumoto, T.; Nagata, K.; Otsuka, K.; Nakagawa, A.; et al. The safety and efficacy of paclitaxel and carboplatin with or without bevacizumab for treating patients with advanced nonsquamous non-small cell lung cancer with interstitial lung disease. *Cancer Chemother. Pharmacol.* **2014**, *74*, 1159–1166. [CrossRef] [PubMed]
13. Raghu, G.; Remy-Jardin, M.; Myers, J.L.; Richeldi, L.; Ryerson, C.J.; Lederer, D.; Behr, J.; Cottin, V.; Danoff, S.K.; Morell, F.; et al. Diagnosis of Idiopathic Pulmonary Fibrosis. An Official ATS/ERS/JRS/ALAT Clinical Practice Guideline. *Am. J. Respir. Crit. Care Med.* **2018**, *198*, e44–e68. [CrossRef] [PubMed]

14. Ichikado, K.; Johkoh, T.; Ikezoe, J.; Takeuchi, N.; Kohno, N.; Arisawa, J.; Nakamura, H.; Nagareda, T.; Itoh, H.; Ando, M. Acute interstitial pneumonia: High-resolution CT findings correlated with pathology. *Am. J. Roentgenol.* **1997**, *168*, 333–338. [CrossRef]
15. Ichikado, K.; Suga, M.; Gushima, Y.; Johkoh, T.; Iyonaga, K.; Yokoyama, T.; Honda, O.; Shigeto, Y.; Tomiguchi, S.; Takahashi, M.; et al. Hyperoxia-induced Diffuse Alveolar Damage in Pigs: Correlation between Thin-Section CT and Histopathologic Findings. *Radiology* **2000**, *216*, 531–538. [CrossRef]
16. Ichikado, K.; Suga, M.; Müller, N.L.; Taniguchi, H.; Kondoh, Y.; Akira, M.; Johkoh, T.; Mihara, N.; Nakamura, H.; Takahashi, M.; et al. Acute Interstitial Pneumonia. *Am. J. Respir. Crit. Care Med.* **2002**, *165*, 1551–1556. [CrossRef]
17. Ichikado, K.; Suga, M.; Muranaka, H.; Gushima, Y.; Miyakawa, H.; Tsubamoto, M.; Johkoh, T.; Hirata, N.; Yoshinaga, T.; Kinoshita, Y.; et al. Prediction of Prognosis for Acute Respiratory Distress Syndrome with Thin-Section CT: Validation in 44 Cases. *Radiol.* **2006**, *238*, 321–329. [CrossRef]
18. Oda, K.; Ishimoto, H.; Yatera, K.; Naito, K.; Ogoshi, T.; Yamasaki, K.; Imanaga, T.; Tsuda, T.; Nakao, H.; Kawanami, T.; et al. High-resolution CT scoring system-based grading scale predicts the clinical outcomes in patients with idiopathic pulmonary fibrosis. *Respir. Res.* **2014**, *15*, 10. [CrossRef]
19. Goddard, P.R.; Nicholson, E.; Laszlo, G.; Watt, I. Computed tomography in pulmonary emphysema. *Clin. Radiol.* **1982**, *33*, 379–387. [CrossRef]
20. US Department of Health and Human Services. Common terminology criteria for adverse events (CTCAE). In *NIH publication. no. 10-5410*; US Department of Health and Human Services, National Institutes of Health, National Cancer Institute: Bethesda, MD, USA, 2010.
21. Isobe, K.; Hata, Y.; Sakamoto, S.; Takai, Y.; Shibuya, K.; Homma, S. Clinical characteristics of acute respiratory deterioration in pulmonary fibrosis associated with lung cancer following anti-cancer therapy. *Respirol.* **2010**, *15*, 88–92. [CrossRef]
22. Hironaka, M.; Fukayama, M. Pulmonary fibrosis and lung carcinoma: A comparative study of metaplastic epithelia in honeycombed areas of usual interstitial pneumonia with or without lung carcinoma. *Pathol. Int.* **1999**, *49*, 1060–1066. [CrossRef] [PubMed]
23. Kawasaki, H.; Nagai, K.; Yoshida, J.; Nishimura, M.; Nishiwaki, Y. Postoperative morbidity, mortality, and survival in lung cancer associated with idiopathic pulmonary fibrosis. *J. Surg. Oncol.* **2002**, *81*, 33–37. [CrossRef] [PubMed]
24. Jin, G.Y.; Lynch, D.; Chawla, A.; Garg, K.; Tammemagi, M.; Sahin, H.; Misumi, S.; Kwon, K.S. Interstitial lung abnormalities in a CT lung cancer screening population: Prevalence and progression rate. *Radiol.* **2013**, *268*, 563–571. [CrossRef] [PubMed]
25. Sverzellati, N.; Guerci, L.; Randi, G.; Calabrò, E.; La Vecchia, C.; Marchianò, A.; Pesci, A.; Zompatori, M.; Pastorino, U. Interstitial lung diseases in a lung cancer screening trial. *Eur. Respir. J.* **2011**, *38*, 392–400. [CrossRef] [PubMed]
26. Ley, B.; Elicker, B.M.; Hartman, T.E.; Ryerson, C.J.; Vittinghoff, E.; Ryu, J.; Lee, J.S.; Jones, K.D.; Richeldi, L.; King, T.E.; et al. Idiopathic pulmonary fibrosis: CT and risk of death. *Radiol.* **2014**, *273*, 570–579. [CrossRef] [PubMed]

5

Retrospective Efficacy Analysis of Immune Checkpoint Inhibitor Rechallenge in Patients What Non-Small Cell Lung Cancer

Yuki Katayama [1,†], Takayuki Shimamoto [1,†], Tadaaki Yamada [1,*], Takayuki Takeda [2], Takahiro Yamada [3], Shinsuke Shiotsu [4], Yusuke Chihara [5], Osamu Hiranuma [6], Masahiro Iwasaku [1], Yoshiko Kaneko [1], Junji Uchino [1] and Koichi Takayama [1]

1 Department of Pulmonary Medicine, Graduate School of Medical Science, Kyoto Prefectural University of Medicine, Kyoto 602-8566, Japan; ktym2487@koto.kpu-m.ac.jp (Y.K.); m04035ts@koto.kpu-m.ac.jp (T.S.); miwasaku@koto.kpu-m.ac.jp (M.I.); kaneko-y@koto.kpu-m.ac.jp (Y.K.); uchino@koto.kpu-m.ac.jp (J.U.); takayama@koto.kpu-m.ac.jp (K.T.)

2 Department of Pulmonary Medicine, Japanese Red Cross Kyoto Daini Hospital, Kyoto 602-8026, Japan; dyckw344@yahoo.co.jp

3 Department of Pulmonary Medicine, Matsushita Memorial Hospital, Moriguchi 570-8540, Japan; t-yamada@koto.kpu-m.ac.jp

4 Department of Pulmonary Medicine, Japanese Red Cross Kyoto Daiichi Hospital, Kyoto 605-0981, Japan; sshiotsu@gmail.com

5 Department of Pulmonary Medicine, Uji-Tokushukai Medical Center, Uji 611-0041, Japan; c1981311@koto.kpu-m.ac.jp

6 Department of Pulmonary Medicine, Otsu City Hospital, Otsu 520-0804, Japan; osamu319@true.ocn.ne.jp

* Correspondence: tayamada@koto.kpu-m.ac.jp

† These authors contributed equally to this work and share first authorship.

Abstract: Little is known regarding the effectiveness and tolerability of immune checkpoint inhibitor (ICI) rechallenge after disease progression following initial ICI treatments. To identify eligible patients for ICI rechallenge, we retrospectively analyzed the relationship between clinical profiles and the effect of ICI rechallenge in patients with non-small cell lung cancer (NSCLC). We enrolled 35 NSCLC patients at six different institutions who were retreated with ICIs after discontinued initial ICI treatments due to disease progression. Cox proportional hazards models were used to assess the impact of clinical profiles on overall survival (OS) and progression-free survival (PFS). Median PFS and OS were 81 d (95% confidence interval, CI, 41–112 d) and 225 d (95% CI 106–361 d), respectively. The objective response rate was 2.9%, and the disease control rate was 42.9%. Multivariate analysis demonstrated that Eastern Cooperative Oncology Group Performance Score (ECOG-PS) ≥ 2 (hazard ratio, HR, 2.38; 95% CI 1.03–5.52; $p = 0.043$) and body mass index (BMI) > 20 (HR 0.43, 95% CI 0.19–0.95, $p = 0.036$) were significantly associated with PFS of ICI rechallenge. Our observations suggest that poor ECOG-PS and low BMI at intervention with ICI rechallenge may be negative predictors for ICI rechallenge treatment in patients with NSCLC.

Keywords: immunotherapy; rechallenge; non-small cell lung cancer; retrospective analysis

---

1. Introduction

Lung cancer is the leading cause of cancer death worldwide [1]. Current clinical studies have shown that some types of molecularly targeted therapies are able to successfully treat a subset of patients with advanced non-small cell lung cancer (NSCLC). In addition, cancer immunotherapies, such as programmed cell death protein 1 (PD-1)/programmed death ligand 1 (PD-L1) checkpoint inhibitors, are being developed as promising alternative strategies for treating patients with advanced NSCLC. Of the current immune checkpoint inhibitors (ICIs), nivolumab, pembrolizumab, atezolizumab, and durvalumab have been approved in the United States, Japan, and other countries for the treatment of patients with NSCLC based on phase III clinical trials [2–6]. However, the majority of patients with NSCLC ultimately acquire resistance to ICI treatments. After acquiring resistance to several therapeutic regimens, ICI rechallenge is considered to be one of the therapeutic options for patients with recurrent NSCLC. Unfortunately, ICI rechallenge treatment has been clinically effective in only a small number of NSCLC patients. Therefore, it is warranted to identify predictive clinical markers for the effectiveness of ICI rechallenge. Previous retrospective studies regarding ICI rechallenge have analyzed only limited numbers of NSCLC patients [7,8]. Hence, little is currently known regarding the effectiveness and tolerability of ICI rechallenge after disease progression following initial ICI treatments. In an effort to identify the patients eligible for ICI rechallenge treatment, we retrospectively analyzed the relationship between the clinical profiles and the effect of ICI rechallenge in patients with NSCLC.

2. Experimental Section

2.1. Patients

We enrolled 35 patients with NSCLC who were retreated with ICIs after their initial ICI treatments were discontinued due to disease progression. The patients were treated between April 2017 and November 2018 at one of six different institutions, which included University Hospital Kyoto Prefectural University of Medicine (Kyoto, Japan), Japanese Red Cross Kyoto Daiichi Hospital (Kyoto, Japan), Japanese Red Cross Kyoto Daini Hospital (Kyoto, Japan), Uji-Tokushukai Medical Center (Kyoto, Japan), Matsushita Memorial Hospital (Osaka, Japan), and Otsu City Hospital (Shiga, Japan). Patient clinical data were retrospectively obtained from their medical records, including age, sex, height, weight, body mass index (BMI) at the start of ICI rechallenge, histological subtype, PD-L1 expression level in tumors, epidermal growth factor receptor (EGFR) mutation status, disease staging, metastatic site, corticosteroid administration, Eastern Cooperative Oncology Group Performance Status (ECOG-PS), smoking status, laboratory findings at the time of ICI rechallenge, and overall survival (OS), progression-free survival (PFS), response rate, and disease control rate for the patients receiving ICI treatment based on the Response Evaluation Criteria in Solid Tumors (RECIST; version 1.1). The study protocol was approved by the ethics committee of each hospital. Tumor–node–metastasis (TNM) stage was classified using the TNM stage classification system, version 8. Six received 2.5 mg to 10 mg p.o. of corticosteroids administration due to improvement in the cachexia. We have added this information in the materials and methods section. This study is an exploratory trial.

2.2. Tumor PD-L1 Analysis

PD-L1 expression was analyzed by SRL, Inc. using a PD-L1 IHC 22C3 pharmDx assay (Agilent Technologies, Santa Clara, CA, USA). The PD-L1 tumor proportion score (TPS) was calculated as a percentage of at least 100 viable tumor cells with complete or partial membrane staining. Pathologists at SRL, Inc. interpreted the TPS results.

2.3. Statistical Analysis

Statistical analyses were performed using EZR statistical software, version 1.30 [9]. All statistical tests were two-sided, and p-values < 0.05 were regarded as statistically significant. The cutoff values for body mass index (BMI), albumin, lactate dehydrogenase (LDH), neutrophil to lymphocyte ratio (NLR), lymphocyte to monocyte ratio (LMR), platelet to lymphocyte ratio (PLR), and C-reactive protein (CRP) following prior therapy were determined according to previous reports [10–15]. The PFS and OS were calculated using the Kaplan–Meier method, and differences were compared using the log-rank test. The hazard ratios (HRs) and their 95% confidence intervals (CIs) were estimated using the Cox proportional hazards model in univariate analyses. The Cox proportional hazards model was also used for the multivariate analyses.

3. Results

3.1. Patient Characteristics

A total of 35 NSCLC patients treated with ICI rechallenge between April 2017 and November 2018 at six different institutions in Japan were enrolled. The median age was 70 years (range: 40–83 years), 24 patients (68.6%) were male, and 27 (77.1%) patients had a history of smoking. The histological subtypes were (23, i.e., 65.7%) adenocarcinoma and (10, i.e., 28.6%) squamous cell carcinoma. Metastatic disease was detected in the liver of five patients (14.3%) and in the brain of seven patients (20%). Of the patients, 10 (28.6%) had stage III disease, 19 (54.3%) had stage IV disease, and six (17.1%) had postoperative recurrence at the time of intervention with the initial ICI treatment. An EGFR mutation was detected in four patients (11.4%). There were no ALK-positive patients. ECOG-PS was 0–1 for 23 patients (65.7%) and 2–4 for 12 patients (34.3%). The PD-L1 TPS was ≥50% for 14 patients (50%), 1–49% for eight patients (7%), <0% for seven patients (29%), and not evaluated for six patients (17.1%). The BMI was ≥25 for 3 patients (8.6%), 20–25% for 16 patients (45.7%), and <20 for 16 patients (45.7%). Table 1 shows the baseline characteristics of patients.

Table 1. Patient characteristics at immune checkpoint inhibitor (ICI) rechallenge treatment.

Items	Group	*n* (%)
Age	Median (range)	70 (48–83)
Gender	Male	24 (68.6)
	Female	11 (31.4)
Eastern Cooperative Oncology Group Performance Score (ECOG-PS)	0–1	23 (65.7)
	2–4	12 (34.3)
Histology	Adenocarcinoma	23 (65.7)
	Squamous cell carcinoma	10 (28.6)
	Other	2 (5.7)
Smoking Status	Never smoker	8 (22.9)
	Current or former smoker	27 (77.1)
Staging	Stage III	10 (28.6)
	Stage IV	19 (54.3)
	Postoperative recurrence	6 (17.1)
Epidermal Growth Factor Receptor (EGFR) Mutations	Positive	4 (11.4)
	Negative	31 (88.6)
PD-L1 tumor proportion score (TPS)	≥50%	14 (40)
	1–49%	8 (22.9)
	<1%	7 (20)
	Not evaluated	6 (17.1)
Metastasis	Liver metastasis	5 (14.3)
	Brain metastasis	7 (20)
Body Mass Index (BMI)	BMI > 25	3 (8.6)
	25 ≥ BMI > 20	16 (45.8)
	BMI ≤ 20	16 (45.8)
Corticosteroid Administration	Yes	6 (17.1)
	No	29 (82.9)

Table 1. *Cont.*

Items	Group	*n* (%)
History of Treatment before ICI Rechallenge	Surgery Radiation therapy Chemotherapy (platinum) Chemotherapy (non-platinum)	6 (17.1) 12 (34.3) 30 (85.7) 25 (71.4)
First ICIs	Nivolumab Pembrolizumab Atezolizumab	19 (54.3) 12 (34.3) 4 (11.4)
Second ICIs	Nivolumab Pembrolizumab Atezolizumab	5 (14.3) 7 (20) 23 (65.7)
Line of First ICI	Median (range)	3 (1–15)
Line of Second ICI	Median (range)	4 (2–19)
Duration from the End of the First ICI to the Start of the Second ICI	Median (95% confidence interval; CI)	157 d (106–238)

3.2. Efficacy and Safety of ICI Treatments

The initial ICI treatment consisted of nivolumab for 19 (54.3%) patients, pembrolizumab for 12 (34.3%) patients, and atezolizumab for four (11.4%) patients. The rechallenge treatment consisted of nivolumab for five (14.3%) patients, pembrolizumab for 7 (20.0%) patients, and atezolizumab for 23 (65.7%) patients. The patients were treated with different regimens of ICIs between the initial and rechallenge treatments. In the initial ICI treatment, no patients experienced a complete response (0%), 12 experienced a partial response (34.3%), 12 experienced stable disease (34.3%), 10 experienced progressive disease (28.6%), and one was non-evaluable (2.9%). The objective response rate was 34.3%, and the disease control rate was 68.6% (Figure 1a). The PFS and OS of the initial ICI treatments were 120 d (95% CI 84–139 d) and 596 d (95% CI 455–864 d), respectively (Figure 2a,b). In the ICI rechallenge treatment, no patients experienced a complete response (0%), one experienced a partial response (2.9%), 14 experienced stable disease (40.0%), 18 experienced progressive disease (51.4%), and two were non-evaluable (5.7%). The objective response rate was 2.9% and the disease control rate was 45.7% (Figure 1b). The PFS and OS of the ICI rechallenge were 81 d (95% CI 41–112 d) and 225 d (95% CI 106–361 d), respectively (Figure 2c,d).

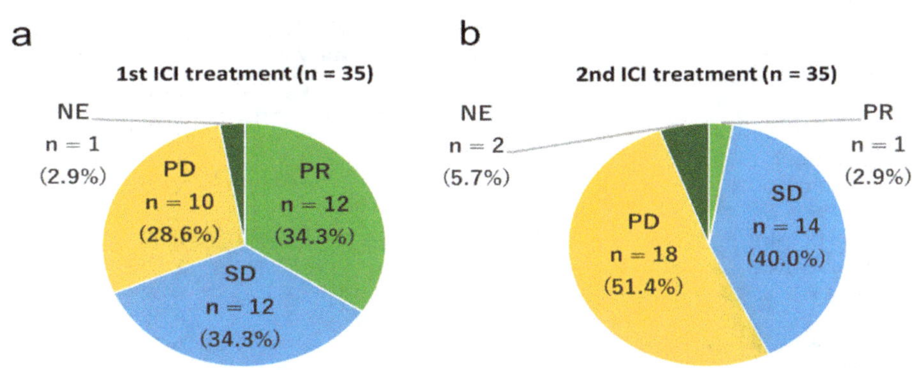

Figure 1. Frequency of the best overall response to immune checkpoint inhibitors (ICIs). (**a**) Frequency of the best overall response to first ICI treatment. (**b**) Frequency of the best overall response to ICI rechallenge treatment. PD, progressive disease; PR, partial response; SD, stable disease; NE, not evaluated.

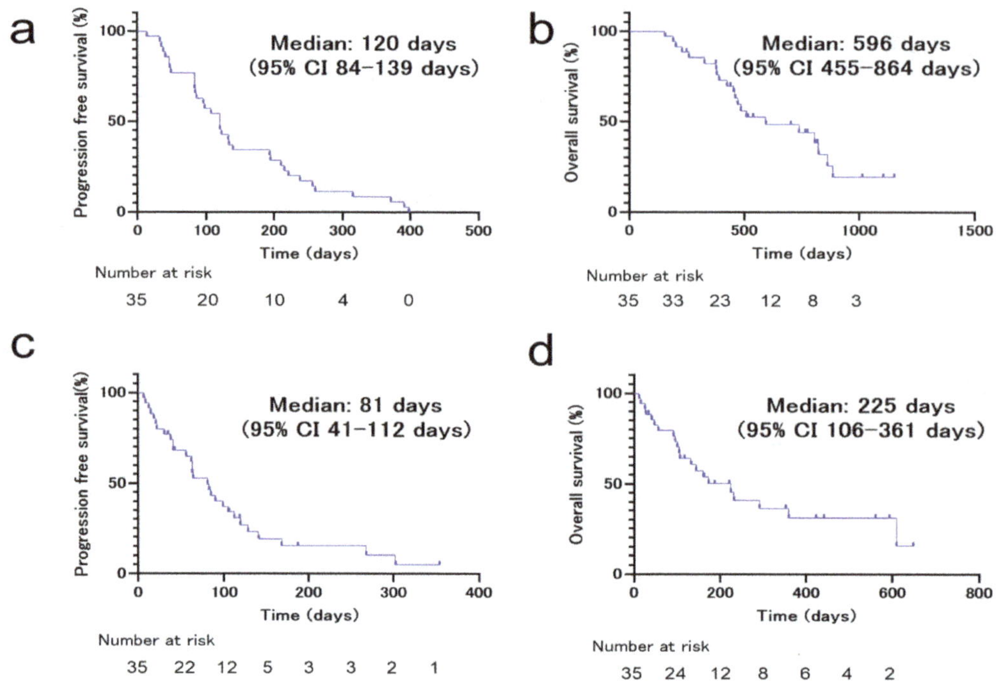

Figure 2. Kaplan–Meier survival curves of progression-free survival (PFS) and overall survival (OS) of patients who received immune checkpoint inhibitor (ICI) rechallenge treatment. (**a**) PFS of non-small cell lung cancer (NSCLC) patients (n = 35) on first ICI treatment. (**b**) OS of NSCLC patients (n = 35) on first ICI treatment. (**c**) PFS of NSCLC patients (n = 35) on ICI rechallenge treatment. (**d**) OS of NSCLC patients (n = 35) on ICI rechallenge treatment.

Univariate analyses of the patient data revealed that ECOG-PS ≥ 2 (HR 2.21, 95% CI 1.00–4.83, p = 0.048), BMI > 20 (HR 0.47, 95% CI 0.22–0.99, p = 0.047), NLR ≥ 5 (HR 2.22, 95% CI 1.02–4.84, p = 0.045), and LMR < 1.7 (HR 0.44, 95% CI 0.21–0.93, p = 0.032) were significantly associated with PFS of ICI rechallenge (Table 2). Moreover, multivariate analysis demonstrated that ECOG-PS ≥ 2 (HR 2.38, 95% CI 1.03–5.52, p = 0.043) and BMI > 20 (HR 0.43, 95% CI 0.19–0.95, p = 0.036) were significantly associated with PFS of ICI rechallenge (Table 3 and Figure 3).

Table 2. Cox proportional hazards and logistic regression models for progression-free survival (PFS) and overall survival (OS).

Items	PFS (Univariate Analysis)		OS (Univariate Analysis)	
	HR (95% CI)	p-Value	HR (95% CI)	p-Value
Age > 75 Years	0.81 (0.34–1.91)	0.63	1.45 (0.55–3.80)	0.45
Male Gender	1.47 (0.66–3.26)	0.35	2.39 (0.80–7.17)	0.12
Smoker	1.508 (0.63–3.59)	0.35	2.50 (0.73–8.58)	0.14
ECOG-PS ≥ 2	2.21 (1.00–4.83)	0.048	4.23 (1.65–10.89)	0.0028
Squamous Histology	1.08 (0.47–2.48)	0.86	0.67 (0.24–1.83)	0.43
EGFR Mutations Positive	0.83 (0.28–2.43)	0.73	1.17 (0.34–4.02)	0.80
BMI > 20	0.47 (0.22–0.99)	0.047	0.42 (0.17–1.02)	0.056
BMI > 25	0.54 (0.19–1.59)	0.27	0.92 (0.26–3.25)	0.90
Corticosteroids Administration	1.3 (0.49–3.52)	0.58	0.66 (0.19–2.27)	0.51
Alb > 3.5 g/dL	0.53 (0.25–1.11)	0.092	0.37 (0.15–0.90)	0.028
CRP > 1.0 mg/dL	1.44 (0.68–3.04)	0.34	2.92 (1.10–7.76)	0.032
LDH > 245 U/L	1.41 (0.67–2.99)	0.37	2.16 (0.89–5.24)	0.090
NLR > 5.0	2.22 (1.02–4.84)	0.045	1.98 (0.79–4.92)	0.14
LMR > 1.7	0.44 (0.21–0.93)	0.032	0.51 (0.21–1.23)	0.14
PLR > 262	2.23 (0.99–5.03)	0.054	2.80 (1.02–7.67)	0.045
Liver Metastasis	1.79 (0.61–5.28)	0.29	1.95 (0.55–6.886)	0.30

Table 2. *Cont.*

Items	PFS (Univariate Analysis)		OS (Univariate Analysis)	
	HR (95% CI)	*p*-Value	HR (95% CI)	*p*-Value
Brain Metastasis	1.17 (0.47–2.91)	0.73	0.58 (0.17–2.00)	0.39
PD-L1 TPS 1–49%	0.32 (0.096–1.05)	0.059	0.55 (0.16–1.89)	0.34
PD-L1 TPS > 50%	0.35 (0.12–1.05)	0.061	0.42 (0.12–1.49)	0.18
Lines between First and Second ICIs > 2	1.26 (0.55–2.87)	0.58	1.54 (0.59–4.04)	0.38
PFS of First ICI >120 d	1.06 (0.50–2.23)	0.89	1.30 (0.55–3.08)	0.54
Duration from the End of the First ICI to the Second ICI >157 d	0.97 (0.47–2.02)	0.94	0.77 (0.32–1.84)	0.55
Partial Response with First ICIs	0.58 (0.26–1.33)	0.20	0.99 (0.40–2.48)	0.98

Table 3. Cox proportional hazards and logistic regression models for progression-free survival (PFS) and overall survival (OS).

Items	PFS (Multivariate Analysis)		OS (Multivariate Analysis)	
	HR (95% CI)	*p*-Value	HR (95% CI)	*p*-Value
ECOG-PS ≥ 2	2.38(1.03–5.52)	0.043	3.01(1.10–8.24)	0.032
BMI > 20	0.43(0.19–0.95)	0.036		
Alb > 3.5 g/dL			0.48(0.18–1.28)	0.14
CRP > 1.0 mg/dL			1.51(0.48–4.75)	0.49
NLR > 5.0	1.08(0.22–5.18)	0.93		
LMR > 1.7	0.57(0.13–2.54)	0.46		
PLR > 262			1.93(0.68–5.43)	0.22

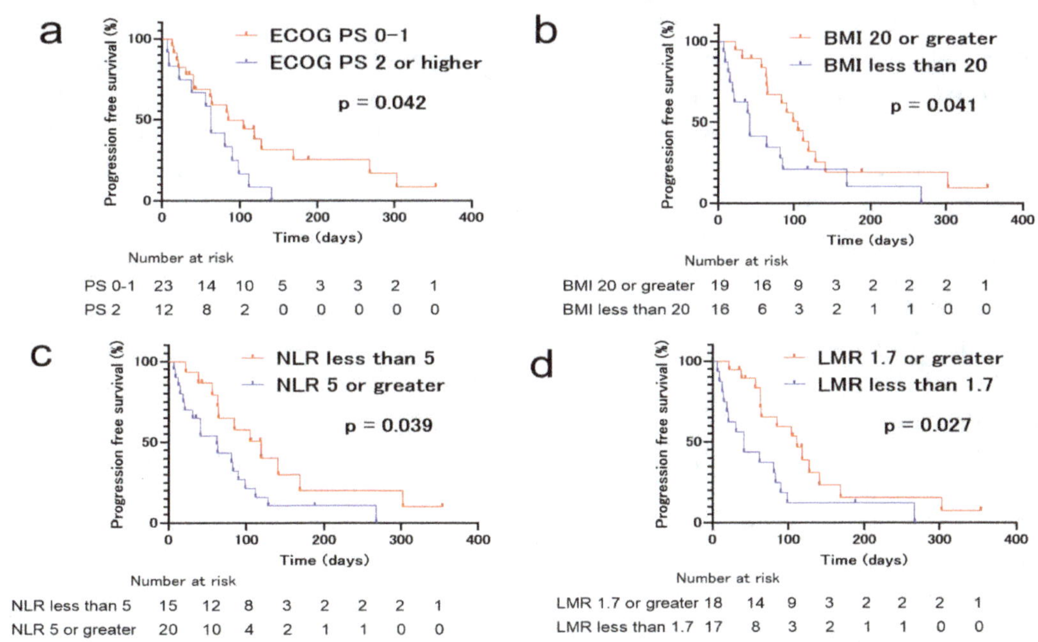

Figure 3. Kaplan–Meier survival curves for progression-free survival (PFS) of patients who received immune checkpoint inhibitor (ICI) rechallenge treatment. (**a**) Eastern Cooperative Oncology Group (ECOG-PS) ≥ 2, (**b**) body mass index (BMI) ≤ 20, (**c**) neutrophil-to-lymphocyte ratio (NLR) > 5, and (**d**) lymphocyte-to-monocyte ratio (LMR) ≤ 1.7 were significantly associated with inferior PFS.

Univariate analyses of the patient data revealed that ECOG-PS ≥ 2 (HR 4.23, 95% CI 1.65–10.89, $p = 0.0023$), CRP > 1.0 (HR 2.92, 95% CI 1.10–7.76, $p = 0.032$), albumin > 3.5 (HR 0.37, 95% CI 0.15–0.90, $p = 0.028$), and PLR > 262 (HR 2.80, 95% CI 1.02–7.67, $p = 0.045$) were significantly associated with OS of ICI rechallenge (Table 2). Multivariate analysis demonstrated that ECOG-PS ≥ 2 (HR 3.01, 95% CI 1.10–8.24, $p = 0.032$) was significantly associated with OS of ICI rechallenge (Table 3).

4. Discussion

PD-L1 expression in tumors has been used clinically as a positive predictive biomarker for the effective initial ICI treatment of patients with NSCLC [16]. However, clinically useful biomarkers have not yet been identified for predicting the efficacy of ICI rechallenge. Fujita et al. reported that objective response rate (ORR), disease control rate (DCR), and PFS values of pembrolizumab rechallenge after refractory nivolumab for 12 patients with NSCLC were 8.3%, 41.7%, and 3.1 months, respectively [8]. In addition, ORR, DCR, and PFS of atezolizumab rechallenge after refractory anti-PD-1 antibodies for 18 patients with NSCLC were 0%, 38.9%, and 2.9 months, respectively [17]. Another report showed that ORR, DCR, and PFS values of ICI rechallenge in 14 patients with ICI refractory tumors were 7.1%, 21.4%, and 1.6 months, respectively [7]. Our current observations showed that ORR, DCR, PFS, and OS values of ICI rechallenge in 35 patients with NSCLC were 2.9%, 42.9%, 2.7 months, and 7.5 months, respectively. These reproducible findings suggest that refractory NSCLC tumors for initial ICI treatments may exhibit poor responses to ICI rechallenge treatments, and the clinical benefits may be limited compared with those of the initial ICI treatment. However, a subset of patients with NSCLC demonstrate good outcomes with ICI rechallenge treatments. Therefore, there is a need for the elucidation of predictive clinical factors for re-treatment of ICI responders among patients with NSCLC.

Our multivariate analysis identified ECOG-PS and BMI as independent factors associated with poorer PFS of ICI rechallenge treatment in patients with NSCLC who were refractory to initial ICI treatment. This is the first report that identifies predictive clinical factors for the efficacy of ICI rechallenge in patients with NSCLC. The general and nutritional status of patients with NSCLC are closely related to the effects of ICI treatment. Several studies have demonstrated that poor ECOG-PS is a predictive negative factor related to clinical outcomes of initial ICI treatment in patients with NSCLC [10,13,18,19]. ECOG-PS is one of the factors that determines the tumor immune environment, and it has been reported that an imbalance of circulating T-lymphocyte subpopulations in patients with gastric cancer correlates with ECOG-PS [20]. BMI is widely used for relating weight to height, defining body size, and indicating nutritional status. In addition, a lower BMI is associated with increased mortality risk [21–24]. Our previous clinical study demonstrated that NSCLC patients with sarcopenia exhibit a significantly shorter median PFS following ICI treatment compared to that of non-sarcopenia patients [25]. Given these observations, a poor ECOG-PS and a low BMI at the time of ICI treatment intervention may be useful for predicting non-responders to initial ICI treatment, as well as ICI rechallenge treatment among patients with NSCLC. Recent clinical trials demonstrated that the ghrelin/growth hormone secretagogue receptor agonist anamorelin increases lean body mass and improves the performance status in NSCLC patients with cachexia [26,27]. Therefore, the administration of anamorelin may improve the effect of ICI rechallenge treatment.

The effectiveness of initial ICI treatments has been reported to be associated with PD-L1 expression in NSCLC tumors [28]. Our current observations show that the patients with PD-L1 expression tended to have longer PFS. This suggests that PD-L1 expression levels in pre-treatment tumors may be a factor to consider when with regard to ICI rechallenge treatment. Regardless, based on our observations, the values of blood NLR, LMR, and PLR at baseline may be useful tools for predicting responders to the ICI rechallenge treatment, which is consistent with the initial ICI treatment [10,13,15,29]. Thus, when considering ICI rechallenge treatment in patients with NSCLC, the inflammation markers, such as NLR, LMR, and PLR, may be useful to some extent for identifying responders to ICI rechallenge.

A previous report suggests that the response to initial ICI treatments correlates with the clinical response to ICI rechallenge treatment in patients with melanoma [30]. However, our results failed to indicate a relationship between clinical outcomes of initial ICI treatment and ICI rechallenge treatment in patients with NSCLC. This suggested that there may be differences between the immunological properties of NSCLC and melanoma.

The current study had several limitations. First, it consisted of a small retrospective sample. Therefore, a further large-cohort study is warranted to identify the predictive markers of ICI rechallenge treatment. Second, although the treatment was administered at multiple centers, there may have been bias in terms of the timing of evaluating the patients using CT scanning, even though it was performed every 1–3 months after treatment.

5. Conclusions

Our observations suggest that a poor ECOG-PS and a low BMI at the time of intervention with ICI rechallenge may be useful as negative predictors for ICI rechallenge treatment in patients with NSCLC. As this retrospective study was a relatively small-scale study, further experiments are needed to validate the observations.

Author Contributions: Conceptualization, Y.K. (Yuki Katayama), T.Y. (Tadaaki Yamada) and K.T.; methodology, Y.K. (Yuki Katayama); validation, Y.K. (Yuki Katayama), T.S. and T.Y.(Tadaaki Yamada); formal analysis, Y.K. (Yuki Katayama); investigation, Y.K. (Yuki Katayama); resources, T.S., T.Y. (Tadaaki Yamada), T.T., T.Y. (Takahiro Yamada), S.S., Y.C., O.H., M.I., Y.K. (Yoshiko Kaneko), J.U. and K.T.; writing—original draft preparation, Y.K. (Yuki Katayama), T.S. and T.Y. (Tadaaki Yamada); supervision, T.Y. (Tadaaki Yamada); project administration, T.Y. (Tadaaki Yamada). All authors have read and agreed to the published version of the manuscript.

Abbreviations

NSCLC, non-small cell lung cancer; PD-1, programmed cell death protein 1; PD-L1, programmed death-ligand 1; ICIs, immune checkpoint inhibitors; PFS, progression-free survival; OS, overall survival; BMI, body mass index; CRP, C-reaction protein; NLR, neutrophil to lymphocyte ratio; LMR, lymphocyte to monocyte ratio; PLR, platelet to lymphocyte ratio; RECIST, Response Evaluation Criteria in Solid Tumors; CR, complete response; PR, partial response; SD, stable disease; PD, progressive disease; NE, not evaluate; PS, Eastern Cooperative Oncology Group Performance Status; CI, confidence interval; HR, hazard ratio; TPS, tumor proportion score; EGFR, epidermal growth factor receptor.

References

1. Miller, K.D.; Goding Sauer, A.; Ortiz, A.P.; Fedewa, S.A.; Pinheiro, P.S.; Tortolero-Luna, G.; Martinez-Tyson, D.; Jemal, A.; Siegel, R.L. Cancer Statistics for Hispanics/Latinos, 2018. *CA Cancer J. Clin.* **2018**, *68*, 425–445. [CrossRef] [PubMed]
2. Borghaei, H.; Paz-Ares, L.; Horn, L.; Spigel, D.R.; Steins, M.; Ready, N.E.; Chow, L.Q.; Vokes, E.E.; Felip, E.; Holgado, E.; et al. Nivolumab versus Docetaxel in Advanced Nonsquamous Non-Small-Cell Lung Cancer. *N. Engl. J. Med.* **2015**, *373*, 1627–1639. [CrossRef] [PubMed]
3. Brahmer, J.; Reckamp, K.L.; Baas, P.; Crino, L.; Eberhardt, W.E.; Poddubskaya, E.; Antonia, S.; Pluzanski, A.; Vokes, E.E.; Holgado, E.; et al. Nivolumab versus Docetaxel in Advanced Squamous-Cell Non-Small-Cell Lung Cancer. *N. Engl. J. Med.* **2015**, *373*, 123–135. [CrossRef] [PubMed]
4. Herbst, R.S.; Baas, P.; Kim, D.W.; Felip, E.; Perez-Gracia, J.L.; Han, J.Y.; Molina, J.; Kim, J.-H.; Arvis, C.D.; Ahn, M.-J.; et al. Pembrolizumab versus docetaxel for previously treated, PD-L1-positive, advanced non-small-cell lung cancer (KEYNOTE-010): A Randomised Controlled Trial. *Lancet* **2016**, *387*, 1540–1550. [CrossRef]
5. Rittmeyer, A.; Barlesi, F.; Waterkamp, D.; Park, K.; Ciardiello, F.; von Pawel, J.; Gadgeel, S.M.; Hida, T.; Kowalski, D.M.; Dols, M.C.; et al. Atezolizumab versus docetaxel in patients with previously treated non-small-cell lung cancer (OAK): A phase 3, open-label, multicentre randomised controlled trial. *Lancet* **2017**, *389*, 255–265. [CrossRef]
6. Antonia, S.J.; Villegas, A.; Daniel, D.; Vicente, D.; Murakami, S.; Hui, R.; Yokoi, T.; Chiappori, A.; Lee, K.H.; Wit de, M.; et al. Durvalumab after Chemoradiotherapy in Stage III Non-Small-Cell Lung Cancer. *N. Engl. J. Med.* **2017**, *377*, 1919–1929. [CrossRef]
7. Watanabe, H.; Kubo, T.; Ninomiya, K.; Kudo, K.; Minami, D.; Murakami, E.; Ochi, N.; Ninomiya, T.; Harada, D.; Yasugi, M.; et al. The effect and safety of immune checkpoint inhibitor rechallenge in non-small cell lung cancer. *Jpn. J. Clin. Oncol.* **2019**, *49*, 762–765. [CrossRef]
8. Fujita, K.; Uchida, N.; Kanai, O.; Okamura, M.; Nakatani, K.; Mio, T. Retreatment with pembrolizumab in advanced non-small cell lung cancer patients previously treated with nivolumab: Emerging reports of 12 cases. *Cancer Chemother. Pharmacol.* **2018**, *81*, 1105–1109. [CrossRef]

9. Kanda, Y. Investigation of the freely available easy-to-use software 'EZR' for medical statistics. *Bone Marrow Transpl.* **2013**, *48*, 452–458. [CrossRef]
10. Bagley, S.J.; Kothari, S.; Aggarwal, C.; Bauml, J.M.; Alley, E.W.; Evans, T.L.; Kosteva, J.A.; Ciunci, C.A.; Gabriel, P.E.; Thompson, J.C.; et al. Pretreatment neutrophil-to-lymphocyte ratio as a marker of outcomes in nivolumab-treated patients with advanced non-small-cell lung cancer. *Lung Cancer* **2017**, *106*, 1–7. [CrossRef]
11. Kondo, T.; Nomura, M.; Otsuka, A.; Nonomura, Y.; Kaku, Y.; Matsumoto, S.; Muto, M. Predicting marker for early progression in unresectable melanoma treated with nivolumab. *Int. J. Clin. Oncol.* **2019**, *24*, 323–327. [CrossRef] [PubMed]
12. Inomata, M.; Hirai, T.; Seto, Z.; Tokui, K.; Taka, C.; Okazawa, S.; Kambara, K.; Ichikawa, T.; Imanishi, S.; Yamada, T.; et al. Clinical Parameters for Predicting the Survival in Patients with Squamous and Non-squamous-cell NSCLC Receiving PD-1 Inhibitor Therapy. *Pathol. Oncol. Res.* **2018**. [CrossRef] [PubMed]
13. Diem, S.; Schmid, S.; Krapf, M.; Flatz, L.; Born, D.; Jochum, W.; Templeton, A.J.; Fruh, M. Neutrophil-to-Lymphocyte ratio (NLR) and Platelet-to-Lymphocyte ratio (PLR) as prognostic markers in patients with non-small cell lung cancer (NSCLC) treated with nivolumab. *Lung Cancer* **2017**, *111*, 176–181. [CrossRef] [PubMed]
14. Liu, J.; Li, S.; Zhang, S.; Liu, Y.; Ma, L.; Zhu, J.; Xin, Y.; Wang, Y.; Yang, C.; Cheng, Y. Systemic immune-inflammation index, neutrophil-to-lymphocyte ratio, platelet-to-lymphocyte ratio can predict clinical outcomes in patients with metastatic non-small-cell lung cancer treated with nivolumab. *J. Clin. Lab. Anal.* **2019**, *33*, e22964. [CrossRef] [PubMed]
15. Failing, J.J.; Yan, Y.; Porrata, L.F.; Markovic, S.N. Lymphocyte-to-monocyte ratio is associated with survival in pembrolizumab-treated metastatic melanoma patients. *Melanoma Res.* **2017**, *27*, 596–600. [CrossRef] [PubMed]
16. Reck, M.; Rodriguez-Abreu, D.; Robinson, A.G.; Hui, R.; Csoszi, T.; Fulop, A.; Gottfried, M.; Peled, N.; Tafreshi, A.; Cuffe, S.; et al. Pembrolizumab versus Chemotherapy for PD-L1-Positive Non-Small-Cell Lung Cancer. *N. Engl. J. Med.* **2016**, *375*, 1823–1833. [CrossRef]
17. Fujita, K.; Uchida, N.; Yamamoto, Y.; Kanai, O.; Okamura, M.; Nakatani, K.; Sawai, S.; Mio, T. Retreatment With Anti-PD-L1 Antibody in Advanced Non-small Cell Lung Cancer Previously Treated With Anti-PD-1 Antibodies. *Anticancer Res.* **2019**, *39*, 3917–3921. [CrossRef]
18. Mezquita, L.; Auclin, E.; Ferrara, R.; Charrier, M.; Remon, J.; Planchard, D.; Ponce, S.; Ares, L.P.; Leroy, L.; Audigier-Valette, C.; et al. Association of the Lung Immune Prognostic Index With Immune Checkpoint Inhibitor Outcomes in Patients With Advanced Non-Small Cell Lung Cancer. *JAMA Oncol.* **2018**, *4*, 351–357. [CrossRef]
19. Katayama, Y.; Yamada, T.; Tanimura, K.; Yoshimura, A.; Takeda, T.; Chihara, Y.; Tamiya, N.; Kaneko, Y.; Uchino, J.; Takayama, K. Impact of bowel movement condition on immune checkpoint inhibitor efficacy in patients with advanced non-small cell lung cancer. *Thorac. Cancer* **2019**, *10*, 526–532. [CrossRef]
20. Wang, L.; Shen, Y. Imbalance of circulating T-lymphocyte subpopulation in gastric cancer patients correlated with performance status. *Clin. Lab.* **2013**, *59*, 429–433.
21. Naik, G.S.; Waikar, S.S.; Johnson, A.E.W.; Buchbinder, E.I.; Haq, R.; Hodi, F.S.; Schoenfeld, J.D.; Ott, P.A. Complex inter-relationship of body mass index, gender and serum creatinine on survival: Exploring the obesity paradox in melanoma patients treated with checkpoint inhibition. *J. Immunother. Cancer* **2019**, *7*, 89. [CrossRef] [PubMed]
22. Cortellini, A.; Bersanelli, M.; Buti, S.; Cannita, K.; Santini, D.; Perrone, F.; Giusti, R.; Tiseo, M.; Michiara, M.; Marino, P.D. A multicenter study of body mass index in cancer patients treated with anti-PD-1/PD-L1 immune checkpoint inhibitors: When overweight becomes favorable. *J. Immunother. Cancer* **2019**, *7*, 57. [CrossRef] [PubMed]
23. Xu, H.; Cao, D.; He, A.; Ge, W. The prognostic role of obesity is independent of sex in cancer patients treated with immune checkpoint inhibitors: A pooled analysis of 4090 cancer patients. *Int. Immunopharmacol.* **2019**, *74*, 105745. [CrossRef] [PubMed]
24. De Giorgi, U.; Procopio, G.; Giannarelli, D.; Sabbatini, R.; Bearz, A.; Buti, S.; Basso, U.; Mitterer, M.; Ortega, C.; Bidoli, P.; et al. Association of Systemic Inflammation Index and Body Mass Index with Survival in Patients with Renal Cell Cancer Treated with Nivolumab. *Clin. Cancer Res.* **2019**, *25*, 3839–3846. [CrossRef]

25. Nishioka, N.; Uchino, J.; Hirai, S.; Katayama, Y.; Yoshimura, A.; Okura, N.; Tanimura, K.; Hirai, S.; Imabayashi, T.; Chihara, Y.; et al. Association of Sarcopenia with and Efficacy of Anti-PD-1/PD-L1 Therapy in Non-Small-Cell Lung Cancer. *J. Clin. Med.* **2019**, *8*, 450. [CrossRef]
26. Katakami, N.; Uchino, J.; Yokoyama, T.; Naito, T.; Kondo, M.; Yamada, K.; Kitajima, H.; Yoshimori, K.; Sato, K.; Saito, H.; et al. Anamorelin (ONO-7643) for the treatment of patients with non-small cell lung cancer and cachexia: Results from a randomized, double-blind, placebo-controlled, multicenter study of Japanese patients (ONO-7643-04). *Cancer* **2018**, *124*, 606–616. [CrossRef]
27. Takayama, K.; Katakami, N.; Yokoyama, T.; Atagi, S.; Yoshimori, K.; Kagamu, H.; Saito, H.; Takiguchi, Y.; Aoe, K.; Koyama, A.; et al. Anamorelin (ONO-7643) in Japanese patients with non-small cell lung cancer and cachexia: Results of a randomized phase 2 trial. *Support Care Cancer* **2016**, *24*, 3495–3505. [CrossRef]
28. Grizzi, G.; Caccese, M.; Gkountakos, A.; Carbognin, L.; Tortora, G.; Bria, E.; Pilotto, S. Putative predictors of efficacy for immune checkpoint inhibitors in non-small-cell lung cancer: Facing the complexity of the immune system. *Expert Rev. Mol. Diagn.* **2017**, *17*, 1055–1069. [CrossRef]
29. Jiang, T.; Qiao, M.; Zhao, C.; Li, X.; Gao, G.; Su, C.; Ren, S.; Zhou, C. Pretreatment neutrophil-to-lymphocyte ratio is associated with outcome of advanced-stage cancer patients treated with immunotherapy: A meta-analysis. *Cancer Immunol. Immunother.* **2018**, *67*, 713–727. [CrossRef]
30. Nomura, M.; Otsuka, A.; Kondo, T.; Nagai, H.; Nonomura, Y.; Kaku, Y.; Matsumoto, S.; Muto, M. Efficacy and safety of retreatment with nivolumab in metastatic melanoma patients previously treated with nivolumab. *Cancer Chemother. Pharmacol.* **2017**, *80*, 999–1004. [CrossRef]

6

Final Results from a Phase II Trial of Osimertinib for Elderly Patients with Epidermal Growth Factor Receptor t790m-Positive Non-Small Cell Lung Cancer That Progressed during Previous Treatment

Akira Nakao [1,†], Osamu Hiranuma [2,†], Junji Uchino [3,*,†], Chikara Sakaguchi [4], Tomoyuki Araya [5], Noriya Hiraoka [6], Tamotsu Ishizuka [7], Takayuki Takeda [8], Masayuki Kawasaki [9], Yasuhiro Goto [10], Hisao Imai [11], Noboru Hattori [12], Keita Nakatomi [13], Hidetaka Uramoto [14], Kiyoaki Uryu [15], Minoru Fukuda [16], Yasuki Uchida [17], Toshihide Yokoyama [18], Masaya Akai [19], Tadashi Mio [20], Seiji Nagashima [21], Yusuke Chihara [3], Nobuyo Tamiya [3], Yoshiko Kaneko [3], Takako Mouri [3], Tadaaki Yamada [3], Kenichi Yoshimura [22], Masaki Fujita [1] and Koichi Takayama [3]

1 Department of Respiratory Medicine, Faculty of Medicine, Fukuoka University, Fukuoka 814-0180, Japan; akiran@fukuoka-u.ac.jp (A.N.); mfujita@fukuoka-u.ac.jp (M.F.)

2 Department of Respiratory Medicine, Otsu City Hospital, Shiga 520-0804, Japan; osamu319@true.ocn.ne.jp

3 Department of Pulmonary Medicine, Kyoto Prefectural University of Medicine, Kyoto 602-8566, Japan; c1981311@koto.kpu-m.ac.jp (Y.C.); koma@koto.kpu-m.ac.jp (N.T.); kaneko-y@koto.kpu-m.ac.jp (Y.K.); tmouri@koto.kpu-m.ac.jp (T.M.); tayamada@koto.kpu-m.ac.jp (T.Y.); takayama@koto.kpu-m.ac.jp (K.T.)

4 Department of Pulmonary Medicine, Rakuwakai Otowa Hospital, Kyoto 607-8062, Japan; rakuwadr1141@rakuwadr.com

5 Department of Respiratory Medicine, National Hospital Organization, Kanazawa Medical Center, Ishikawa 920-8650, Japan; komatsu_alone@yahoo.co.jp

6 Department of Respiratory Medicine, Japanese Red Cross Kyoto Daiichi Hospital, Kyoto 605-0981, Japan; noriya-hiraoka@kyoto1-jrc.org

7 Third Department of Internal Medicine, Faculty of Medical Sciences, University of Fukui, Fukui 910-1193, Japan; tamotsui@u-fukui.ac.jp

8 Department of Respiratory Medicine, Japanese Red Cross Society Kyoto Daini Hospital, Kyoto 602-8026, Japan; dyckw344@yahoo.co.jp

9 Department of Respiratory Medicine, National Hospital Organization, Omuta National Hospital, Fukuoka 837-0911, Japan; kawasaki.masayuki.hx@mail.hosp.go.jp

10 Department of Respiratory Medicine, Fujita Health University, Aichi 470-1192, Japan; gotoyasu@fujita-hu.ac.jp

11 Division of Respiratory Medicine, Gunma Prefectural Cancer Center, Gunma 373-8550, Japan; hi-imai@gunma-cc.jp

12 Department of Molecular and Internal Medicine, Graduate School of Biomedical & Health Sciences, Hiroshima University, Hiroshima 734-8553, Japan; nhattori@hiroshima-u.ac.jp

13 Department of Respiratory Medicine, Kyushu Central Hospital of the Mutual Aid Association of Public School Teachers, Fukuoka 815-8588, Japan; keita.nakatomi@icloud.com

14 Department of Thoracic Surgery, Kanazawa Medical University, Ishikawa 920-0293, Japan; hidetaka@kanazawa-med.ac.jp

15 Department of Respiratory Medicine, Yao Tokushukai General Hospital, Osaka 581-0011, Japan; kiyoaki.uryuu@tokushukai.jp

16 Second Department of Internal Medicine, Nagasaki University Hospital, Nagasaki 852-8523, Japan; mifukuda@nagasaki-u.ac.jp

17 Department of Respiratory Medicine, Shiga University of Medical Science Hospital, Shiga 520-2192, Japan; uchiy@belle.shiga-med.ac.jp

18 Department of Respiratory Medicine, Kurashiki Central Hospital, Okayama 710-8602, Japan; ty14401@kchnet.or.jp

19 Department of Respiratory Medicine, Japanese Red Cross Fukui Hospital, Fukui 918-8501, Japan; makai-0314@fukui-med.jrc.or.jp

[20] Division of Respiratory Medicine, Center for Respiratory Diseases, National Hospital Organization Kyoto Medical Center, Kyoto 612-8555, Japan; tmio.kmc@gmail.com
[21] Department of Respiratory Medicine, National Hospital Organization Nagasaki Medical Center, Nagasaki 856-0835, Japan; nagashima.seiji.kg@mail.hosp.go.jp
[22] Center for Integrated Medical Research, Hiroshima University Hospital, Hiroshima University, Hiroshima 734-8553, Japan; keyoshim@hiroshima-u.ac.jp
* Correspondence: uchino@koto.kpu-m.ac.jp
† Contributed equally.

Abstract: Epidermal growth factor receptor tyrosine kinase inhibitors (EGFR-TKIs) are used for treating EGFR-mutated lung cancer, and osimertinib is effective in cases that acquired T790M mutations after treatment with the first- and second-generation EGFR-TKIs. However, no study has evaluated its safety and efficacy in older patients. This phase II trial (jRCTs071180002) evaluated osimertinib in T790M mutation-positive Japanese patients who were ≥75 years old and had experienced relapse or progression after previous EGFR-TKI treatment. Our previous report that enrolled 36 patients showed the overall response rate (58.3%) and disease control rate (97.2%), while this report describes the results for the progression-free survival (PFS), overall survival (OS), and safety analyses. The median PFS was 11.9 months (95% confidence interval (CI): 7.9–17.5), and the median OS was 22.0 months (95% CI: 16.0 months–not reached). The most frequent adverse events were anemia/hypoalbuminemia (27 patients, 75.0%), thrombocytopenia (21 patients, 58.3%), and paronychia/anorexia/diarrhea/neutropenia (15 patients, 41.7%). Pneumonitis was observed in four patients (11.1%), including two patients (5.6%) with Grade 3–4 pneumonitis. These results suggest that osimertinib was relatively safe and effective for non-small cell lung cancer that acquired T790M mutations after previous EGFR-TKI treatment, even among patients who were ≥75 years old.

Keywords: non-small cell lung cancer; EGFR-TKI; T790M; osimertinib

1. Introduction

Treatment for epidermal growth factor receptor (EGFR)-mutated non-small cell lung cancer (NSCLC) typically involves EGFR tyrosine kinase inhibitors (EGFR-TKIs). Gefitinib and erlotinib are the first-generation EGFR-TKIs that provide significant survival benefits compared with platinum-based chemotherapy in clinical trials [1–6]. Afatinib and dacomitinib are the second-generation EGFR-TKIs that provide significantly longer progression-free survival (PFS) compared to that of platinum-based chemotherapy and first-generation EGFR-TKIs, although the second-generation EGFR-TKIs did not significantly improve overall survival (OS) [7–11]. In addition, these drugs are associated with more severe toxicity profiles, such as skin disorders, relative to the first-generation EGFR-TKIs.

Various mechanisms are responsible for resistance to the first-generation and second-generation EGFR-TKIs, with more than one-half of the cases involving the EGFR exon 20 T790M mutation [12]. Osimertinib is a third-generation EGFR-TKI that was developed to address this issue [12], and he AURA3 study revealed that it provided significantly longer PFS compared to platinum-based chemotherapy among patients with T790M-mutated lung cancer [13]. Moreover, the FLAURA trial conducted on first-line treatment revealed that osimertinib administered as an initial treatment for EGFR-mutated cases significantly prolonged PFS and OS compared with the first-generation EGFR-TKIs, with a median OS of >3 years [14,15]. Furthermore, osimertinib is expected to have good central nervous system translocation and a limited inhibition of the wild-type EGFR, which may make it less toxic, and therefore, the first choice for EGFR-mutated NSCLC [16–18]. Nevertheless, additional evidence is needed to support this application based on various patient populations. We have performed a phase II study to investigate the efficacy and safety of osimertinib in elderly Japanese patients (≥75 years old) with NSCLC containing the T790M mutation who progressed or experienced a relapse while receiving the first- and second- generations of EGFR-TKI treatment. In our previous report, the response rate was the primary endpoint, and the disease control rate was the secondary endpoint [19]. This report presents the results from our final analyses of PFS, OS, and safety events, which were the additional secondary endpoints in that trial.

2. Experimental Section

2.1. Patients

The study eligibility and exclusion criteria have been previously reported [19,20]. Patients were enrolled in this study between July 2016 and May 2018 if they met the following eligibility criteria: recurrence of NSCLC after achieving stable disease or better as their best overall response after treatment with the first- and second-generation of EGFR-TKIs; harboring an EGFR mutation (activating) and being T790M-positive; aged over 75 years; performance status of ≤1 based on the Eastern Cooperative Oncology Group (ECOG) scale; adequate bone marrow function (leukocyte count 3000–12,000/µL, platelet count ≥100,000/µL, and hemoglobin level ≥9.0 g/dL), adequate hepatic function (bilirubin level ≤1.5 mg/dL, aspartate aminotransferase of ≤100 IU/L, alanine aminotransferase of ≤100 IU/L), and adequate renal function (serum creatinine ≤2.0 mg/dL); a measurable lesion according to the Response Evaluation Criteria in Solid Tumors (RECIST) guidelines version 1.1; and provision of written informed consent. The exclusion criteria were pulmonary disorders; including idiopathic pulmonary fibrosis; interstitial pneumonia; pneumoconiosis; active radiation pneumonitis and drug-induced pneumonia, active infection; symptomatic brain metastasis; uncontrollable diabetes mellitus or severe comorbidities such as heart disease or renal disease; watery diarrhea; active concomitant malignancy; pregnancy or other medical problems that could prevent compliance with the protocol. The trial protocol was registered at Japan Registry of Clinical Trials (jRCTs071180002) and was approved by the ethical review board of Clinical Research Network Fukuoka Certified Review Board (CRB7180004). All patients provided written informed consent before enrollment.

2.2. Study Design, Treatments, and Endpoints

This single-arm-multicenter study involved daily oral administration of osimertinib (80 mg/day). Osimertinib had to be started at 80 mg/day, and if adverse events (AEs) occurred, dose reduction was performed according to the dose reduction criteria. Administration of osimertinib was continued until the patient met the discontinuation criteria or disease progression. Tumor assessments were performed at baseline, every 6 weeks (± 2 weeks) for 6 months, and then every 9 weeks (± 2 weeks) until disease progression. Baseline brain imaging was performed on a similar schedule. Among patients with T790M mutations, the objective response rate (ORR) was 62% (95% confidence interval [CI]: 54–68) in the AURA extension study (201 patients). In the AURA2 study (210 patients) the ORR was 70% (95% CI: 64–77) and the median PFS was 9.9 months (95% CI: 9.5–12.3) [21–23]. Docetaxel is the standard treatment for elderly patients based on the Japanese guidelines, as it provided an ORR of 22.7% in a study that compared docetaxel to vinorelbine [24]. Another recent study evaluated carboplatin plus pemetrexed for elderly Japanese patients and revealed an ORR of 41.2% [25]. Based on these findings, a required sample size of 31 patients was calculated according to the normal approximation method, with an expected response rate of 60%, a threshold response rate of 35%, two-sided alpha = 0.05, and 1 – beta = 0.8. However, the target sample size was increased to 35 patients to account for potential dropout cases. The primary endpoint for the trial was the overall response rate (ORR), while the secondary endpoints were PFS, OS, disease control rate (DCR), and safety events.

2.3. Statistical Methods

The ORR was calculated as the proportion of subjects with complete response or partial response as their best treatment responses. The DCR was calculated as the proportion of subjects who achieved stable disease (or better) as their best treatment response. The PFS interval was calculated from the date of enrollment to the first instance of disease progression, death from any cause, or the last follow-up without evidence of progression (for surviving patients with no evidence of progression). The OS interval was calculated from the date of enrollment to the date of death from any cause. Adverse events were evaluated from the first drug administration to 30 days after the last drug administration and were graded based on the Japanese JCOG translation of version 4.0 of the Common Terminology Criteria for Adverse Events.

The Wilson method was used to estimate the ORR and DCR with their two-sided 95% CIs. Statistical significance was considered present when the lower limit of the estimated 95% CI was above the threshold of 35% for ORR. The Kaplan–Meier method was used to evaluate the survival curves for PFS and OS, as well as the median and annual values. The Brookmeyer and Crowley method was used to estimate the CI values for median values, and Greenwood's formula was used to estimate the standard error for annual values.

3. Results

3.1. Patient Characteristics

The study enrolled 36 patients between July 2016 and May 2018, with 23 female patients (63.9%) with a median age of 80 years, and 19 patients (52.8%) who were ≥80 years old. The histological types were adenocarcinoma in 35 patients (97.2%) and a mixed type with small cell lung cancer in only 1 patient. Based on the 7th edition of the AJCC system for staging lung cancer, 25 cases (69.4%) were considered stage IV, 10 cases (27.8%) involved relapse after surgery, and 1 case (2.8%) was considered stage IIIB. Among the enrolled patients, 30.6% were former smokers. The EGFR gene mutations involved the exon 20 T790M mutation in all cases, as well as exon 19 deletion in 22 cases (61.1%) and the exon 21 L858R point mutation in 11 cases (30.6%). Brain metastasis was detected in 15 patients (41.7%) (Table 1).

Table 1. Patient characteristics.

		n (%)
Sex	Male	13 (36.1)
	Female	23 (63.9)
Age	Median (range)	80 (75–92)
	≥80 years	52.8 %
	>85 years	11.1 %
PS	0	8 (22.2)
	1	28 (77.8)
Histology	Adenocarcinoma	35 (97.2)
	Adenocarcinoma + SCLC	1 (2.8)
Stage	IIIB	1 (2.8)
	IV	25 (69.4)
	Relapse after surgery	10 (27.8)
EGFR mutation	T790M	36 (100.0)
	Exon 19 deletion	22 (61.1)
	L858R	11 (30.6)
	G719X	1 (2.8)
Smoking status	Ex-smoker	11(30.6)
Pre-treatment	Surgery	12 (33.3)

Table 1. *Cont.*

		n (%)
	Chemotherapy	13 (36.1)
	EGFR-TKI	36 (100.0)
	Afatinib	5 (13.9)
	Erlotinib	10 (27.8)
	Gefitinib	21 (58.3)
	Radiotherapy	10 (27.8)
	Thoracic drainage	4 (11.1)
Metastasis site	Lung	18 (50.0)
	Pleural dissemination	12 (33.3)
	Brain	15 (41.7)
	Bone	12 (33.3)
	Liver	8 (22.2)

PS: performance status, SCLC: small cell lung cancer.

3.2. *Efficacy*

The ORR from our previous report was 58.3% (95% CI: 42.2–72.9), which included a complete response rate of 2.8% and a partial response rate of 55.6%. The stable disease rate was 38.9%, and the DCR was 97.2%. The median response duration was 54.9 weeks (95% CI: 26.9–69.1), and a waterfall plot revealed that 33 patients (91.6%) experienced tumor shrinkage, which indicated favorable antitumor activity. Sixteen patients (44.4%) continued treatment beyond progression.

The median PFS was 11.9 months (95% CI: 7.9–17.5), with 1-year PFS rate of 50.0% and 2-year PFS rate of 18.3% (Figure 1). The median OS was 22.0 months (95% CI: 16.0–not reached), with 1-year OS rate of 77.8% and 2-year OS rate of 49.5% (Figure 2).

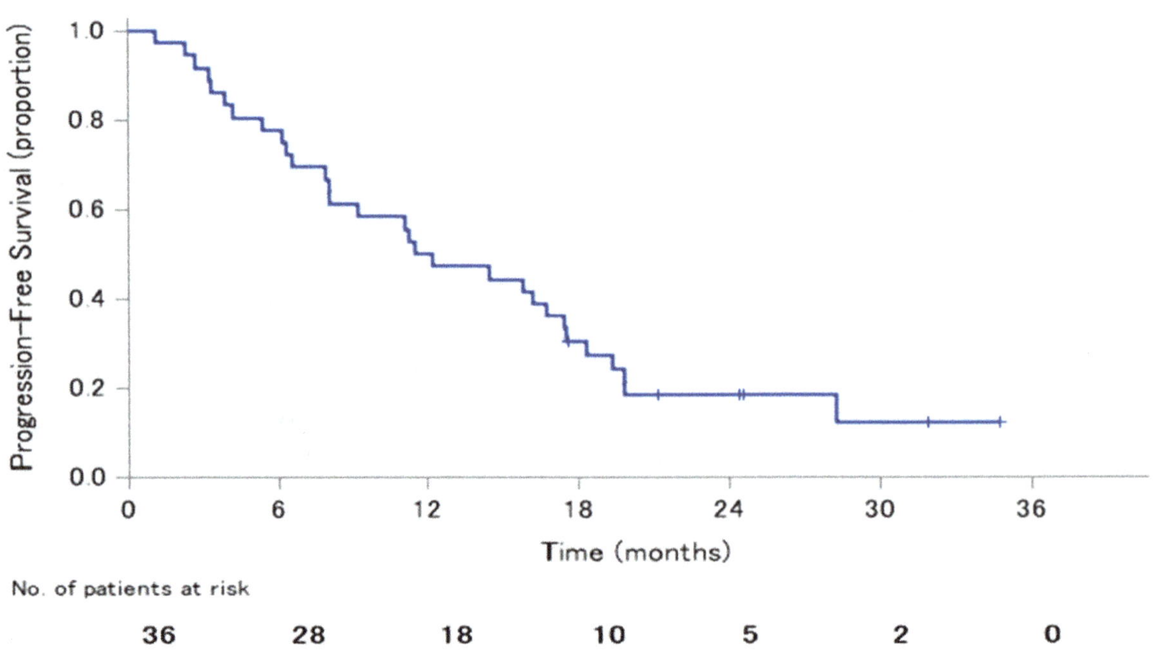

Figure 1. Progression-free survival.

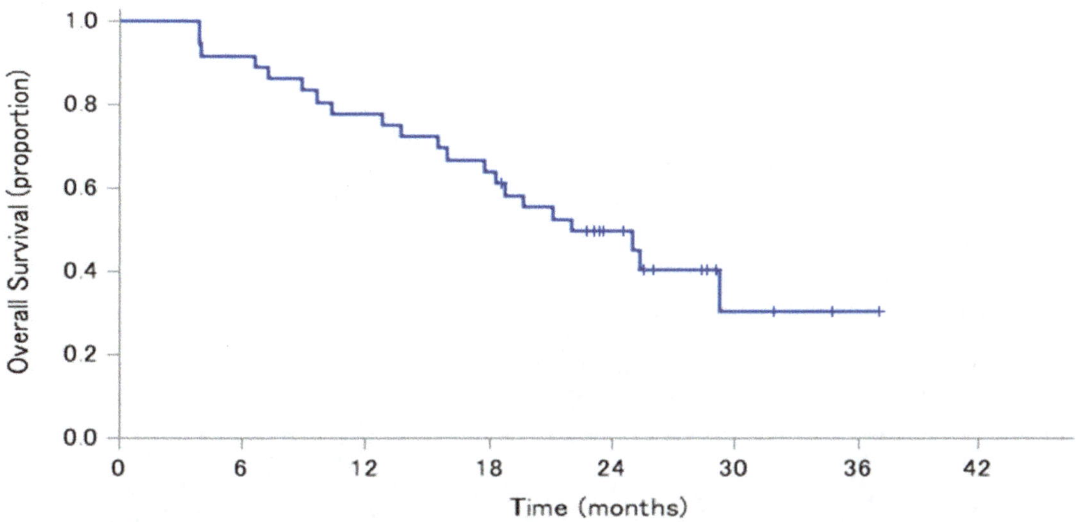

No. of patients at risk

36	33	28	23	12	3	1	0

Figure 2. Overall survival.

3.3. Safety

Adverse events occurred in 31 cases (86.1%), with Grade 3 or higher adverse events observed in 10 cases (27.8%). Seven patients (19.4%) required dose reductions, 10 patients (27.8%) discontinued treatment because of adverse events, and 1 patient died (2.8%). The adverse event leading to death was a pulmonary infection, although this was judged unlikely to have been caused by the osimertinib treatment. There were no death events caused by drug-induced lung injury. The most frequent adverse event was anemia/hypoalbuminemia (27 patients, 75.0%), which was followed by thrombocytopenia (21 patients, 58.3%), paronychia/anorexia/diarrhea/neutropenia (15 patients, 41.7%), leukopenia/aspartate aminotransferase increase (14 patients, 38.9%), fatigue/acneiform eruption (13 patients, 36.1%), and alanine aminotransferase increase/alkaline phosphatase increase/creatinine increase (11 patients, 30.6%). The Grade 3–4 adverse events included fatigue, anorexia, diarrhea, cardiac ejection fraction decreased, prolonged QT, leukopenia, neutropenia, and aspartate aminotransferase increase. The cases of cardiac ejection fraction were decreased and the cases of prolonged QT were different cases, and delirium and hallucinations were observed in the same patient. Pneumonitis was observed in four patients (11.1%), including two patients (5.6%) with Grade 3–4 pneumonitis (Table 2).

Table 2. Adverse events.

	Any Grade	Grade 3–4
All adverse events > 15%, *n* (%)		
Anemia	27 (75.0)	0 (0.0)
Hypoalbuminemia	27 (75.0)	0 (0.0)
Platelet count decreased	21 (58.3)	0 (0.0)
Neutrophil count decreased	15 (41.7)	1 (2.8)
Paronychia	15 (41.7)	0 (0.0)
Decreased appetite	15 (41.7)	4 (11.1)
Diarrhea	15 (41.7)	1 (2.8)
White blood cell decreased	14 (38.9)	1 (2.8)
Aspartate aminotransferase increased	14 (38.9)	2 (5.6)

Table 2. *Cont.*

	Any Grade	Grade 3–4
Fatigue	13 (36.1)	3 (8.3)
Dermatitis acneiform	13 (36.1)	0 (0.0)
Alanine aminotransferase increased	11 (30.6)	0 (0.0)
Alkaline phosphatase increased	11 (30.6)	2 (5.6)
Creatinine increased	11 (30.6)	0 (0.0)
Pruritus	8 (22.2)	0 (0.0)
Mucositis oral	8 (22.2)	0 (0.0)
Grade 3–4 adverse events, *n* (%)		
Pneumonitis	4 (11.1)	2 (5.6)
Left ventricular systolic dysfunction	1 (2.8)	1 (2.8)
Electrocardiogram QT prolongation	1 (2.8)	1 (2.8)
Delirium	1 (2.8)	1 (2.8)
Hallucination	1 (2.8)	1 (2.8)
Dyspnea	1 (2.8)	1 (2.8)
Dehydration	1 (2.8)	1 (2.8)
Lung infection	2 (5.6)	1 (2.8)
Sinusitis	1 (2.8)	1 (2.8)

4. Discussion

Treatment of NSCLC has advanced dramatically after the introduction of molecularly targeted drugs, such as EGFR-TKIs for EGFR-mutated cases. The first- and second-generation of EGFR-TKIs proved to be highly effective in several studies, although the effects tended to only last for approximately 1 year [1–11]. Approximately one-half of the resistant cases involved a gatekeeper mutation in exon 20 (T790M), and osimertinib was developed and approved for the treatment of these cases [12,13]. The results of the FLAURA trials positioned osimertinib as a standard treatment option, and even as an initial treatment option [14,15]. However, many cases still involve treatment in the second line or later, as the T790M mutation was identified via re-biopsy in patients who received first-generation or second-generation EGFR-TKIs as their initial treatment. When the T790M mutation was identified in these cases, patients typically received osimertinib.

Aging populations are becoming increasingly common worldwide, and many lung cancer cases involve older patients [26,27]. There are concerns that older patients have a higher risk of developing adverse events, which may necessitate dose reduction or treatment discontinuation, and subsequently result in decreased efficacy. Thus, this phase II study aimed to evaluate the safety and efficacy of osimertinib in elderly patients with EGFR-mutated lung cancer involving the T790M mutation. The primary endpoint was the ORR, and our previous report found that the ORR was 58.3% (95% CI: 42.2–72.9), which fulfilled the efficacy criterion (the lower limit of the CI exceeded the threshold response rate of 35%) [19]. This report describes the secondary endpoints, which include the DCR (97.2%), median PFS (11.9 months), and median OS (22.0 months). In terms of efficacy, the pooled results from the AURA expansion and AURA2 studies revealed an ORR of 66%, a DCR of 91%, a median PFS of 9.9 months, and a median OS of 26.8 months [23]. In addition, phase 3 AURA3 studies revealed an ORR of 70.6%, a DCR of 93.2%, a median PFS of 10.1 months, and a median OS of 26.8 months [13,28]. Thus, while our ORR was lower than that shown in the previous studies, it agrees with the slightly lower ORR (61.1%) that was retrospectively observed in another sample of elderly Japanese patients [29]. Furthermore, our findings regarding PFS and OS do not appear inferior to the results from previous studies, thereby suggesting that osimertinib was effective in elderly Japanese patients. Regarding the effects based on the PS, the ORR of PS0 and PS1 was 75% and 53.6%, respectively, and the PFS was 13.7 months and 11.9 months, respectively. Since there were few cases, it was impossible to discuss the significant differences, but the PS0 group tended to be superior.

It is also important to compare the results from osimertinib treatment to those from cytotoxic anticancer drugs, which are the alternative options if osimertinib is not used for T790M-positive cases. For example, the control group for the AURA3 study received platinum plus pemetrexed, which provided an ORR of 31%, a DCR of 74%, a median PFS of 4.4 months, and a median OS of 22.5 months [13,28]. A subgroup analysis of ≥70-year-old Japanese patients from the JACAL study evaluated carboplatin plus pemetrexed and revealed an ORR of 24%, a DCR of 68%, a median PFS of 5.2 months, and a median OS of 16.8 months [30,31]. Thus, our OS findings may be comparable to the results from the entire AURA3 population, although our ORR, DCR, and PFS outcomes are comparable or even slightly better. Interestingly, 71% of the patients in the group that received platinum plus pemetrexed subsequently received additional treatment, with 60% experiencing a greater effect after crossing over to osimertinib treatment. Therefore, while the JACAL study had only included EGFR-mutated cases and did not specifically consider older patients, we believe that osimertinib may provide good outcomes among older patients with EGFR-mutated (T790M) NSCLC.

Safety is also an important consideration in this setting, given the concerns regarding the potentially higher risk of adverse events among older patients. In the AURA3 study, it appears that Japanese patients had a higher risk of paronychia, diarrhea, and skin pruritus, although no clear increase was observed among elderly patients. However, elderly patients had a clearly increased frequency of myelosuppression events, such as anemia (75% in this study vs. 8% in AURA3 study), leukopenia (38.9% in this study vs. 8% in AURA3 study), neutropenia (41.7% in this study vs. 8% in AURA3 study), and thrombocytopenia (58.3% in this study vs. 10% in AURA3 study), although the frequencies of Grade 3–4 adverse events were generally comparable. Osimertinib has also been reported to be more frequently myelosuppressed than in other EGFR-TKI in a pivotal study [13,14]. In addition, myelosuppression was reported to be stronger in the analysis of the Japanese population [32]. Although the obvious mechanism was unclear, it was suggested that racial differences might be involved. Since myelosuppression was observed more frequently in the present study than in the aforementioned analysis of the Japanese population, caution should be exercised in the elderly Japanese. Fiala et al. reported that pre-treatment hypoalbuminemia correlated with poor prognosis in advanced NSCLC patients treated with erlotinib [33]. The present study also revealed that anorexia and exhaustion were common (30–40% of cases vs. 16-18% of cases in AURA3 study, including some Grade 3–4 cases), as well as hypoalbuminemia (75% of cases vs. N/A in AURA3 study). Therefore, careful follow-up is needed for elderly patients who are receiving osimertinib. Elevated alkaline phosphatase and creatinine values were also observed, albeit not serious cases, and related follow-up testing is also important. Cardiac adverse events, such as decreased left heart ejection fraction and QT prolongation, were observed in some cases, although only one patient experienced a Grade 3–4 cardiac adverse event. Central nervous system events, such as delirium and hallucination, may be explained by the large proportion of cases with brain metastasis (41.7%), although caution should be exercised if these events present in conjunction with sinusitis and pulmonary infection. Regarding AE by PS, no clear difference was observed between PS0 and PS1.

All-grade pneumonitis was observed in 11.1% of cases, and Grade 3–4 pneumonitis was observed in 5.6% of cases. The rates after conventional EGFR-TKI treatment were 4% in the AURA3 study and 7.3% in the Japanese subset of patients, which suggests that Japanese patients may have a higher rate of pneumonitis [13,34]. The difference between our findings and the previous findings may be related to differences in the proportions of patients with a history of smoking (69.4% for the present study, 32.2% for the AURA3 study, and 31.7% for the Japanese subset of the AURA3 population). In addition, the Japanese subset of the FLAURA study population had a higher frequency of pulmonary disorders (all grades: 12%, Grade 3 or higher: 2%); it should be noted that this is a first-line trial. Other reports have also suggested that osimertinib may be associated with an increased incidence of pulmonary disorders relative to other EGFR-TKIs [32]. Nevertheless, the odds ratio for pulmonary disorders after gefitinib treatment was 1.92-fold higher among Japanese patients who were ≥55 years old, which suggests that careful follow-up is required for patients who are ≥75 years old [35].

The present study revealed all-grade AEs in 86.1%, Grade 3 or worse AEs in 27.8%, and fatal AEs in 2.8% of the patients. These rates did not appear to be substantially elevated among elderly patients, based on results from the AURA3 study and its Japanese subgroup (all-grade: 97.8% and 100%, Grade 3 or higher: 22.6% and 31.7%, and fatal AEs: 1.4% and 0%). However, AEs leading to treatment discontinuation occurred in 12 patients (33.3%) in our study, which was more common than the rates of 6.8% in the AURA3 study and 7.3% in the Japanese subgroup. For example, we observed drug-induced lung injury in four patients (11.1%), and these patients needed to stop treatment. In addition, three patients (8.3%) discontinued treatment because of Grade 4 AEs (pulmonary infection, hallucinations, and hepatic dysfunction), although those events were judged unlikely to be associated with their treatment. One patient (2.8%) required a two-step dose reduction, and two patients (5.6%) were unable to continue the treatment protocol because of a ≥4-week treatment disruption. Treatment was also stopped in one case involving Grade 3 aspiration pneumonia, one case at the attending physician's discretion, and one case because the patient refused to continue treatment. Thus, although the safety of osimertinib outside the study protocol has not been evaluated, most of these AEs and treatment discontinuations were likely not to have been caused by a drug-induced pulmonary injury.

Most all-grade adverse events involved anorexia, fatigue, myelosuppression, and gastrointestinal symptoms. These complications were generally not serious and could be addressed using conventional management strategies. However, it is important to note that the frequency of drug-induced lung injury may increase, which highlights the importance of a careful follow-up in this population. Despite the potential need for a careful follow-up and the small sample size, which was the limitation in this study, it appears that osimertinib can be a standard treatment even for the elderly patients harboring T790M mutation.

While the present study provided encouraging data, we are conducting an additional phase II study (SPIRAL-0) to confirm the safety and efficacy of osimertinib in ≥75-year-old patients with untreated NSCLC harboring EGFR-activating mutations [36]. This may provide further information to guide the increasing use of osimertinib treatment in this setting.

Author Contributions: Conceptualization, J.U.; validation, J.U., A.N., and K.T.; formal analysis, K.Y.; investigation, O.H., C.S., T.A., N.H., T.I., T.T., M.K., Y.G., H.I., N.H., K.N., H.U., K.U., M.F. (Minoru Fukuda), Y.U., T.Y. (Toshihide Yokoyama), M.A., T.M. (Tadashi Mio), S.N., Y.C., N.T., Y.K., T.M. (Takako Mouri), T.Y. (Tadaaki Yamada) and M.F. (Masaki Fujita); data curation, K.Y.; writing—original draft preparation, A.N.; writing—review and editing, J.U.; supervision, K.T.; project administration, J.U.; funding acquisition, J.U. All authors have read and agreed to the published version of the manuscript.

Acknowledgments: We thank all of the patients who participated in this study, as well as their families. We also thank the Clinical Research Support Center Kyushu for managing the study.

References

1. Mok, T.S.; Wu, Y.L.; Thongprasert, S.; Yang, C.H.; Chu, D.T.; Saijo, N.; Sunpaweravong, P.; Han, B.; Margono, B.; Ichinose, Y.; et al. Gefitinib or carboplatin-paclitaxel in pulmonary adenocarcinoma. *N. Engl. J. Med.* **2009**, *361*, 947–957. [CrossRef] [PubMed]
2. Maemondo, M.; Inoue, A.; Kobayashi, K.; Sugawara, S.; Oizumi, S.; Isobe, H.; Gemma, A.; Harada, M.; Yoshizawa, H.; Kinoshita, I.; et al. Gefitinib or chemotherapy for non-small-cell lung cancer with mutated EGFR. *N. Engl. J. Med.* **2010**, *362*, 2380–2388. [CrossRef] [PubMed]
3. Mitsudomi, T.; Morita, S.; Yatabe, Y.; Negoro, S.; Okamoto, I.; Tsurutani, J.; Seto, T.; Satouchi, M.; Tada, H.; Hirashima, T.; et al. Gefitinib versus cisplatin plus docetaxel in patients with non-small-cell lung cancer harbouring mutations of the epidermal growth factor receptor (WJTOG3405): An open label, randomised phase 3 trial. *Lancet Oncol.* **2010**, *11*, 121–128. [CrossRef]

4. Zhou, C.; Wu, Y.L.; Chen, G.; Feng, J.; Liu, X.Q.; Wang, C.; Zhang, S.; Wang, J.; Zhou, S.; Ren, S.; et al. Erlotinib versus chemotherapy as first-line treatment for patients with advanced EGFR mutation-positive non-small-cell lung cancer (OPTIMAL, CTONG-0802): A multicentre, open-label, randomised, phase 3 study. *Lancet Oncol.* **2011**, *12*, 735–742. [CrossRef]
5. Rosell, R.; Carcereny, E.; Gervais, R.; Vergnenegre, A.; Massuti, B.; Felip, E.; Palmero, R.; Garcia-Gomez, R.; Pallares, C.; Sanchez, J.M.; et al. Erlotinib versus standard chemotherapy as first-line treatment for European patients with advanced EGFR mutation-positive non-small-cell lung cancer (EURTAC): A multicentre, open-label, randomised phase 3 trial. *Lancet Oncol.* **2012**, *13*, 239–246. [CrossRef]
6. Wu, Y.L.; Zhou, C.; Liam, C.K.; Wu, G.; Liu, X.; Zhong, Z.; Lu, S.; Cheng, Y.; Han, B.; Chen, L.; et al. First-Line erlotinib versus gemcitabine/cisplatin in patients with advanced EGFR mutation-positive non-small-cell lung cancer: Analyses from the phase III, randomized, open-label, ENSURE study. *Ann. Oncol.* **2015**, *26*, 1883–1889. [CrossRef] [PubMed]
7. Sequist, L.V.; Yang, J.C.; Yamamoto, N.; O'Byrne, K.; Hirsh, V.; Mok, T.; Geater, S.L.; Orlov, S.; Tsai, C.M.; Boyer, M.; et al. Phase III study of afatinib or cisplatin plus pemetrexed in patients with metastatic lung adenocarcinoma with EGFR mutations. *J. Clin. Oncol.* **2013**, *31*, 3327–3334. [CrossRef]
8. Wu, Y.L.; Zhou, C.; Hu, C.P.; Feng, J.; Lu, S.; Huang, Y.; Li, W.; Hou, M.; Shi, J.H.; Lee, K.; et al. Afatinib versus cisplatin plus gemcitabine for first-line treatment of Asian patients with advanced non-small-cell lung cancer harbouring EGFR mutations (LUX-Lung 6): An open-label, randomised phase 3 trial. *Lancet Oncol.* **2014**, *15*, 213–222. [CrossRef]
9. Park, K.; Tan, E.H.; O'Byme, K.; Zhang, L.; Boyer, M.; Mok, T.; Hirsh, V.; Yang, J.C.; Lee, K.H.; Lu, S.; et al. Afatinib versus gefitinib as first-line treatment of patients with EGFR mutation-positive non-small-cell lung cancer (LUX-Lung 7): A phase 2B, open-label, randomised controlled trial. *Lancet Oncol.* **2016**, *17*, 577–589. [CrossRef]
10. Paz-Ares, L.; Tan, E.H.; O'Byme, K.; O'Byrne, K.; Zhang, L.; Hirsh, V.; Boyer, M.; Yang, J.C.; Mok, T.; Lee, K.H.; et al. Afatinib versus gefitinib in patients with EGFR mutation-positive advanced non-small-cell lung cancer: Overall survival data from the phase IIb LUX-Lung 7 trial. *Ann. Oncol.* **2017**, *28*, 270–277. [CrossRef]
11. Wu, Y.L.; Cheng, Y.; Zhou, X.; Lee, K.H.; Nakagawa, K.; Niho, S.; Tsuji, F.; Linke, R.; Rosell, R.; Corral, J.; et al. Dacomitinib versus gefitinib as first-line treatment for patients with EGFR-mutation-positive non-small-cell lung cancer (ARCHER 1050): A randomised, open-label, phase 3 trial. *Lancet Oncol.* **2017**, *18*, 1454–1466. [CrossRef]
12. Yu, H.A.; Arcila, M.E.; Rekhtman, N.; Sima, C.S.; Zakowski, M.F.; Pao, W.; Kris, M.G.; Miller, V.A.; Ladanyi, M.; Riely, G.J. Analysis of tumor specimens at the time of acquired resistance to EGFR-TKI therapy in 155 patients with EGFR-mutant lung cancers. *Clin. Cancer Res.* **2013**, *19*, 2240–2247. [CrossRef] [PubMed]
13. Mok, T.S.; Wu, Y.L.; Ahn, M.J.; Garassino, M.C.; Kim, H.R.; Ramalingam, S.S.; Shepherd, F.A.; He, Y.; Akamatsu, H.; Theelen, W.S.; et al. Osimertinib or platinum-pemetrexed in EGFR T790M-positive lung cancer. *N. Engl. J. Med.* **2017**, *376*, 629–640. [CrossRef] [PubMed]
14. Soria, J.C.; Ohe, Y.; Vansteenkiste, J.; Reungwetwattana, T.; Chewaskulyong, B.; Lee, K.H.; Dechaphunkul, A.; Imamura, F.; Nogami, N.; Kurata, T.; et al. Osimertinib in untreated EGFR-mutated advanced non-small-cell lung cancer. *N. Engl. J. Med.* **2018**, *378*, 113–125. [CrossRef]
15. Ramalingam, S.S.; Vanteenkiste, J.; Planchard, D.; Cho, B.C.; Gray, J.E.; Ohe, Y.; Zhou, C.; Reungwetwattana, T.; Cheng, Y.; Chewaskulyong, B.; et al. Overall survival with Osimertinib in untreated, EGFR-mutated advanced NSCLC. *N. Engl. J. Med.* **2020**, *382*, 41–50. [CrossRef]
16. Nanjo, S.; Ebi, H.; Takeuchi, S.; Takeuchi, S.; Yamada, T.; Mochizuki, S.; Okada, Y.; Nakada, M.; Murakami, T.; Yano, S. High efficacy of third generation EGFR inhibitor AZD9291 in a leptomeningeal carcinomatosis model with EGFR-mutant lung cancer cells. *Oncotarget* **2016**, *7*, 3847–3856. [CrossRef]
17. Nanjo, S.; Hata, A.; Okuda, C.; Kaji, R.; Okada, H.; Tamura, D.; Irie, K.; Okada, H.; Fukushima, S.; Katakami, N. Standard-Dose osimertinib for refractory leptomeningeal metastases in T790M-positive EGFR-mutant non-small cell lung cancer. *Br. J. Cancer* **2018**, *118*, 32–37. [CrossRef]
18. Cross, D.A.; Ashton, S.E.; Ghiorghlu, S.; Eberlein, C.; Nebhan, C.A.; Spitzler, P.J.; Orme, J.P.; Finlay, M.R.; Ward, R.A.; Mellor, M.J.; et al. AZD9291, an irreversible EGFR TKI, overcomes T790M-mediated resistance to EGFR inhibitors in lung cancer. *Cancer Discov.* **2014**, *4*, 1046–1061. [CrossRef]

19. Nakao, A.; Hiranuma, O.; Uchino, J.; Sakaguchi, C.; Kita, T.; Hiraoka, N.; Ishizuka, T.; Kubota, Y.; Kawasaki, M.; Goto, Y.; et al. Osimertinib in elderly patients with epidermal growth factor receptor T790M-positive non-small-cell lung cancer who progressed during prior treatment: A phase II trial. *Oncologist* **2019**, *24*, 593-e170. [CrossRef]

20. Uchino, J.; Nakao, A.; Tamiya, N.; Kaneko, Y.; Yamada, T.; Yoshimura, K.; Fujita, M.; Takayama, K. Treatment rationale and design of the SPIRAL study: A phase II trial of osimertinib in elderly epidermal growth factor receptor T790M-positive nonsmall-cell lung cancer patients who progressed during prior EGFR-TKI treatment. *Medicine* **2018**, *97*, e11081. [CrossRef]

21. Yang, J.C.; Ahn, M.J.; Kim, D.W.; Ramalingam, S.S.; Sequist, L.V.; Su, W.C.; Kim, S.W.; Kim, J.H.; Planchard, D.; Felip, E.; et al. Osimertinib in pretreated T790M-positive advanced non-small-cell lung cancer: AURA study phase II extension component. *J. Clin. Oncol.* **2017**, *35*, 1288–1296. [CrossRef] [PubMed]

22. Goss, G.; Tsai, C.M.; Shepherd, F.A.; Bazhenova, L.; Lee, J.S.; Chang, G.C.; Crino, L.; Satouchi, M.; Chu, Q.; Hida, T.; et al. Osimertinib for pretreated EGFR Thr790Met-positive advanced non-small-cell lung cancer (AURA2): A multicentre, open-label, single-arm, phase 2 study. *Lancet Oncol.* **2016**, *17*, 1643–1652. [CrossRef]

23. Ahn, M.J.; Tsai, C.M.; Shepherd, F.A.; Bazhenova, L.; Sequist, L.V.; Hida, T.; Yang, J.; Ramalingam, S.S.; Mitsudomi, T.; Jänne, P.A.; et al. Osimertinib in patients with T790M mutation-positive, advanced non-small cell lung cancer: Long-term follow-up from a pooled analysis of 2 phase 2 studies. *Cancer* **2019**, *125*, 892–901. [CrossRef] [PubMed]

24. Kudoh, S.; Takeda, K.; Nakagawa, K.; Takada, M.; Katakami, N.; Matsui, K.; Shinkai, T.; Sawa, T.; Goto, I.; Semba, H.; et al. Phase III study of docetaxel compared with vinorelbine in elderly patients with advanced non-small-cell lung cancer: Results of the West Japan Thoracic Oncology Group Trial (WJTOG 9904). *J. Clin. Oncol.* **2006**, *24*, 3657–3663. [CrossRef]

25. Tamiya, M.; Tamiya, A.; Kaneda, H.; Nakagawa, K.; Yoh, K.; Goto, K.; Okamoto, H.; Shimokawa, T.; Abe, T.; Tanaka, H.; et al. A phase II study of pemetrexed plus carboplatin followed by maintenance pemetrexed as first-line chemotherapy for elderly patients with advanced non-squamous non-small cell lung cancer. *Med. Oncol.* **2016**, *33*, 2. [CrossRef]

26. Barta, J.A.; Zinner, R.G.; Unger, M. Lung cancer in the older patient. *Clin. Geriatr. Med.* **2017**, *33*, 563–577. [CrossRef]

27. Torre, L.A.; Siegel, R.L.; Ward, E.M.; Jemal, A. Global cancer incidence and mortality rates and trends—An update. *Cancer Epidemiol. Biomark. Prev.* **2016**, *25*, 16–27. [CrossRef]

28. Wu, Y.L.; Mok, T.S.; Han, J.; Ahn, M.J.; Delmonte, A.; Ramalingam, S.S.; Kim, S.; Shepherd, F.A.; Laskin, J.; He, Y.; et al. Overall Survival (OS) from the AURA3 phase III study: Osimertinib vs Platinum-Pemetrexed (PLT-PEM) in Patients (PTS) with EGFR T790M advanced Non-Small Cell Lung Cancer (NSCLC) and progression on a prior EGFR-tyrosine kinase inhibitor (TKI). *Ann. Oncol.* **2019**, *20* (Suppl. 9), ix157–ix181.

29. Furuta, H.; Uemura, T.; Yoshida, T.; Kobara, M.; Yamaguchi, T.; Watanabe, N.; Shimizu, J.; Horio, Y.; Kuroda, H.; Sakao, Y.; et al. Efficacy and safety data of Osimertinib in elderly patients with NSCLC who harbor the EGFR T790M mutation after failure of initial EGFR-TKI treatment. *Anticancer Res.* **2018**, *38*, 5231–5237. [CrossRef]

30. Okamoto, I.; Aoe, K.; Kato, T.; Hosomi, Y.; Yokoyama, A.; Imamura, F.; Kiura, K.; Hirashima, T.; Nishio, M.; Nogami, N.; et al. Pemetrexed and carboplatin followed by pemetrexed maintenance therapy in chemo-naïve patients with advanced nonsquamous non-small-cell lung cancer. *Investig. New Drugs* **2013**, *31*, 1275–1282. [CrossRef]

31. Nogami, N.; Nishio, M.; Okamoto, I.; Enatsu, S.; Suzukawa, K.; Takai, H.; Nakagawa, K.; Tamura, T. Pemetrexed and carboplatin combination therapy followed by pemetrexed maintenance in Japanese patients with non-squamous non-small cell lung cancer: A subgroup analysis of elderly patients. *Respir. Investig.* **2019**, *57*, 27–33. [CrossRef] [PubMed]

32. Ohe, Y.; Imamura, F.; Nogami, N.; Okamoto, I.; Kurata, T.; Kato, T.; Sugawara, S.; Ramalingam, S.S.; Uchida, H.; Hodge, R.; et al. Osimertinib versus standard-of-care EGFR-TKI as first-line treatment for EGFRm advanced NSCLC: FLAURA Japanese subset. *Jpn. J. Clin. Oncol.* **2019**, *49*, 29–36. [CrossRef] [PubMed]

33. Fiala, O.; Pesek, M.; Finek, J.; Racek, J.; Minarik, M.; Benesova, L.; Bortlicek, Z.; Sorejs, O.; Kucera, R.; Topolcan, O. Serum albumin is a strong predictor of survival in patients with advanced-stage non-small cell lung cancer treated with erlotinib. *Neoplasma* **2016**, *63*, 471–476. [CrossRef] [PubMed]
34. Akamatsu, H.; Katakami, N.; Okamoto, I.; Kato, T.; Kim, Y.H.; Imamura, F.; Shinkai, M.; Hodge, R.A.; Uchida, H.; Hida, T. Osimertinib in Japanese patients with EGFR T790M mutation-positive advanced non-small-cell lung cancer: AURA3 trial. *Cancer Sci.* **2018**, *109*, 1930–1938. [CrossRef] [PubMed]
35. Kudoh, S.; Kato, H.; Nishiwaki, Y.; Fukuoka, M.; Nakata, K.; Ichinose, Y.; Tsuboi, M.; Yokota, S.; Nakagawa, K.; Suga, M. Interstitial lung disease in Japanese patients with lung cancer: A cohort and nested case-control study. *Am. J. Respir. Crit. Care Med.* **2008**, *177*, 1348–1357. [CrossRef]
36. Chihara, Y.; Yamada, T.; Uchino, J.; Tamiya, N.; Kaneko, Y.; Kishimoto, J.; Takayama, K. Rationale and design of a phase II trial of osimertinib as first-line treatment for elderly patients with epidermal growth factor receptor mutation-positive advanced non-small cell lung cancer (SPIRAL-0 study). *Transl. Lung Cancer Res.* **2019**, *8*, 1086–1090. [CrossRef]

7

Negative Effect of Reduced NME1 Expression on Recurrence-Free Survival in Early Stage Non-Small Cell Lung Cancer

Dohun Kim [1], Yujin Kim [2], Bo Bin Lee [2], Dongho Kim [2], Ok-Jun Lee [3], Pildu Jeong [4], Wun-Jae Kim [4], Eun Yoon Cho [5], Joungho Han [5], Young Mog Shim [6] and Duk-Hwan Kim [2,*]

1 Department of Thoracic and Cardiovascular Surgery, Chungbuk National University Hospital, College of Medicine, Chungbuk National University, Cheongju 28644, Korea; mwille@naver.com
2 Department of Molecular Cell Biology, Sungkyunkwan University School of Medicine, Suwon 16419, Korea; yujin0328@hanmail.net (Y.K.); whitebini@hanmail.net (B.B.L.); jindonghao2001@hotmail.com (D.K.)
3 Department of Pathology, College of Medicine, Chungbuk National University, Cheongju 28644, Korea; ojlee@chungbuk.ac.kr
4 Department of Urology, College of Medicine, Chungbuk National University, Cheongju 28644, Korea; leo24fly@chungbuk.ac.kr (P.J.); wjkim@chungbuk.ac.kr (W.-J.K.)
5 Department of Pathology, Samsung Medical Center, Sungkyunkwan University School of Medicine, Seoul 06351, Korea; eunyoon.cho@samsung.com (E.Y.C.); joungho.han@samsung.com (J.H.)
6 Department of Thoracic and Cardiovascular Surgery, Samsung Medical Center, Sungkyunkwan University, School of Medicine, Seoul 06351, Korea; youngmog.shim@samsung.com
* Correspondence: dukhwan.kim@samsung.com

Abstract: This study aimed to understand whether the effect of non-metastatic cells 1 (NME1) on recurrence-free survival (RFS) in early stage non-small cell lung cancer (NSCLC) can be modified by β-catenin overexpression and cisplatin-based adjuvant chemotherapy. Expression levels of NME1 and β-catenin were analyzed using immunohistochemistry in formalin-fixed paraffin-embedded tissues from 425 early stage NSCLC patients. Reduced NME1 expression was found in 39% of samples. The median duration of follow-up was 56 months, and recurrence was found in 186 (44%) of 425 patients. The negative effect of reduced NME1 expression on RFS was worsened by cisplatin-based adjuvant chemotherapy (adjusted hazard ratio = 3.26, 95% CI = 1.16–9.17, p = 0.03). β-catenin overexpression exacerbated the effect of reduced NME1 expression on RFS and the negative effect was greater when receiving cisplatin-based adjuvant chemotherapy: among patients treated with cisplatin-based adjuvant chemotherapy, hazard ratios of patients with reduced NME1 expression increased from 5.59 (95% confidence interval (CI) = 0.62–50.91, p = 0.13) to 15.52 (95% CI = 2.94–82.38, p = 0.001) by β-catenin overexpression, after adjusting for confounding factors. In conclusion, the present study suggests that cisplatin-based adjuvant chemotherapy needs to be carefully applied to early stage NSCLC patients with overexpressed β-catenin in combination with reduced NME1 expression.

Keywords: adjuvant chemotherapy; β-catenin; lung neoplasms; nucleotide-diphosphate kinase; recurrence

---

1. Introduction

Lung cancer is one of the most common causes of cancer-related deaths in the world. Despite recent advances in the early detection and treatment of lung cancer, the prognosis is very poor, partly because of a high rate of recurrence even after curative resection. Approximately half of the patients diagnosed with non-small cell lung cancer (NSCLC) develop recurrence and die of the disease even after curative resection. Adjuvant chemotherapy plays an important role in preventing recurrence following curative resection of lung cancer. A survival benefit of platinum-based adjuvant chemotherapy in NSCLC was confirmed by phase III trials and the Lung Adjuvant Cisplatin Evaluation (LACE) meta-analysis [1,2]. However, some NSCLC patients receiving such adjuvant chemotherapy show no progress in survival. Accordingly, it is critically important to identify biomarkers that can select patients who will not respond well to adjuvant therapy so that an appropriate treatment plan can be provided to patients. Given that occult micro-metastatic cancer cells might be present systemically at the time of surgery, altered expression of metastasis-related genes might be useful as molecular biomarkers to distinguish patients at high risk of recurrence after surgery.

Non-metastatic cells 1 (NME1), also known as NM23-H1, was the first metastasis suppressor discovered by its reduced mRNA transcript levels in a murine melanoma cell line exhibiting high metastatic activity [3]. In addition to its known function as a nucleotide-diphosphate kinase that converts nucleoside diphosphates to nucleoside triphosphates at the expense of adenosine triphosphate (ATP), NME1 is involved in several pathological processes such as motility and metastasis of tumor cells [4]. An inverse relationship between metastatic potential and NME1 expression has been reported in several types of cancers, including non-small cell lung cancer [5,6], melanoma [7], breast cancer [8], hepatocellular carcinoma [9], gastric cancer [10], and colorectal cancer [11]. Transfection of the *NME1* gene into different types of cancer cells has resulted in the inhibition of metastatic properties, including migration, invasion, and colonization [12–16]. *NME1* silencing is known to upregulate β-catenin-dependent TCF/LEF-1 (T-cell factor/lymphoid enhancer-binding factor) transactivation through glycogen synthase kinase (GSK)-3β-independent mechanisms by promoting nuclear translocation of β-catenin [17].

Activation of the canonical Wnt signaling pathway inhibits axin-mediated β-catenin phosphorylation and degradation and allows β-catenin to accumulate in the cytoplasm and then translocate into the nucleus. Nuclear β-catenin forms a stable complex with members of the TCF/LEF transcription factor family and induces the expression of target genes such as *c-MYC* and *CCND1*, and influences the metastatic cascade by regulating the expression of genes such as *AXIN2*, *SNAIL*, *ZEB1*, *COX2*, and *S100A4* [18]. It has been reported that the Wnt/β-catenin signaling pathway is involved in the invasion and metastasis of tumor cells in patients with NSCLC [19–22]. In addition to the nuclear translocation of β-catenin by *NME1* silencing, Wnt/β-catenin-mediated resistance to cisplatin has been demonstrated in human cancers [23,24]. Based on these reports, we hypothesized that NME1 and the Wnt signal may cooperatively affect patient prognosis and cisplatin treatment.

In this study, we analyzed whether the effect of NME1 on recurrence-free survival (RFS) can be modified by cisplatin-based adjuvant chemotherapy and β-catenin overexpression in early stage NSCLC.

2. Materials and Method

2.1. Study Population

This was a retrospective study. Formalin-fixed paraffin-embedded (FFPE) tissue specimens stored at room temperature were obtained from 425 patients with pathologic stage I–IIIA NSCLC who had undergone anatomical lung resection with mediastinal lymph node dissection between November 1994 and April 2004 at Samsung Medical Center in Seoul, Korea. Patients with incomplete resection of lung tissue (e.g., positive malignant cell in resection margin) or history of neoadjuvant therapy were excluded from this study. Postoperative follow-up was performed according to a previously described protocol [25]. Information including recurrence, death, and platinum-based adjuvant chemotherapy was obtained from our hospital's electronic medical records (EMRs) and outside medical records as of 31 July 2018. Thirty-two (7.5%) patients received postoperative adjuvant chemotherapy comprising cisplatin combined with vinorelbine, vinblastine, etoposide, fluorouracil, gemcitabine, pemetrexed, or docetaxel. The chemotherapy regimens were selected by medical oncologists responsible for treatment decisions. This study was approved by the Institutional Review Board of the Samsung Medical Center (2018-04-153), and pre-operative informed consent for the use of samples was obtained from all patients. Pathologic stage was determined according to the guideline of the 7th edition of the tumor-node-metastasis (TNM) staging system maintained by the American Joint Committee on Cancer [26]. Supporting data for this study are available from the corresponding author upon request.

2.2. Immunohistochemistry

Tissue microarrays (TMAs) were constructed from paraffin blocks prepared from 425 NSCLC samples. Expression levels of β-catenin and NME1 proteins were analyzed using immunohistochemistry. In brief, serial sections of 4 μM in thickness were cut from TMA blocks, deparaffinized in xylene, and rehydrated through a series of decreasing concentrations of alcohols. Antigens were recovered by heating these sections in 10 mM (pH 6) citrate buffer for 10 min using a pressure cooker. These sections were then incubated with primary antibody β-catenin clone 17C2 (Leica Biosystems, Buffalo Grove, IL, USA) or NME1 clone 4B2 (GeneTex, Irvine, CA, USA) at 4 °C overnight. Immunoreactivity of each primary antibody was detected with Envision™ + peroxidase (Dako, Carpinteria, CA, USA). Antibody-bound peroxidase activity was visualized after incubating with chromogen 3,3′-diaminobenzidine (DAB) at room temperature for 1–5 min. Normal bronchial epithelial cells were used for positive control of staining, and primary antibody was replaced by immunoglobin for negative control. All sections were counterstained with Mayer's hematoxylin.

2.3. Interpretation of Immunohistochemical Staining

Immunohistochemical staining was interpreted by consensus between two authors (O.-J.L. and D.-H.K.) in a double-blinded fashion to minimize inter-rater variability. Samples with a Cohen's kappa coefficient of less than 0.20 were removed from further analysis. Although immunoreactivity for β-catenin was found in the membrane, cytoplasm, and nucleus, only cytoplasmic staining was assessed for scoring. The expression of NME1 protein in tumor cells was evaluated based on cytoplasmic staining. Cytoplasmic staining of both proteins was semi-quantitatively evaluated using a score calculated by multiplying the intensity score (0, none; 1, weak; 2, moderate; 3, strong) with the proportion score of positive cells (0, absent; 1, 0–10%; 2, 10–50%; 3, 50–80%; 4, >80%). For NME1, its expression was defined as reduced if a composite score was less than two in a tumor. β-catenin expression was considered to be overexpressed in a tumor with a composite score greater than or equal to two. Staining was performed in triplicate and average values of scores were used to determine the expression levels. Cutoff values for the abnormal expression of NME1 and β-catenin were determined considering an internal control consisting of 23 normal lung cores. Representative positive stainings for β-catenin and NME1 expression are shown in adenocarcinoma and squamous cell carcinoma (Figure 1A). Details of the immunohistochemical staining procedure and interpretation for Ki-67 (MKI67) proteins were reported previously [27].

2.4. Study Design

Patients were randomly selected without stratification or matching by age. The median duration of follow-up was 56 months. The clinical endpoint of the study was recurrence-free survival (RFS), which was defined as the time from the date of the diagnosis to the first recurrence. Variables such as age, sex, histology, pathologic stage, NME1 expression, and adjuvant chemotherapy were initially considered for the analysis of RFS. FFPE tissue samples were obtained from 425 patients because at least 365 patients were needed for analysis of the effect of NME1 expression on RFS under 2-sided $\alpha = 0.05$ and $\beta = 0.1$ (i.e., 90% power).

2.5. Statistical Analyses

To find factors associated with NME1 reduction in NSCLC, chi-square test (or Fisher's exact test) and Student's t-test (or one-way ANOVA) were used for univariate analyses of continuous and categorical variables, respectively. A linear relationship between two continuous variables was analyzed using Pearson's correlation coefficient. The prognostic significance of NME1 on RFS was evaluated by Kaplan–Meier survival curves. The difference between two survival curves was assessed using the log-rank test. Variables with $P \leq 0.25$ in the univariate analysis were included in the multivariate model. Hazard ratios of predictor variables for survival were estimated using the Cox proportional hazards model after controlling for potential confounding factors. The effect of β-catenin expression and adjuvant chemotherapy on NME1 function was analyzed using a stratified Cox proportional hazards model. No replacement was made for missing values. All statistical analyses were two-sided with a type I error of 5%.

3. Results

3.1. Clinicopathological Characteristics

A total of 425 patients with early stage NSCLC were included in the data analysis without dropout. The mean age of the patients at diagnosis was 61 years (range, 37–82 years), and men accounted for 74% of the cases. Adenocarcinoma and squamous cell carcinoma comprised 46% and 47% of the cases, respectively. Patients at I, II, and IIIA stages accounted for 56%, 43%, and 5%, respectively. The relationship between NME1 expression and clinicopathological characteristics is summarized in Supplementary Table S1. NME1 expression was found to be reduced in 165 (39%) of 425 patients. Reduced NME1 expression was not associated with patient's age, sex, tumor size, or exposure to tobacco smoke. However, reduced NME1 expression was found to have a significantly higher prevalence in squamous cell carcinoma (46%) than in adenocarcinoma (34%), and the difference was statistically significant ($p = 0.01$; Figure 1B).

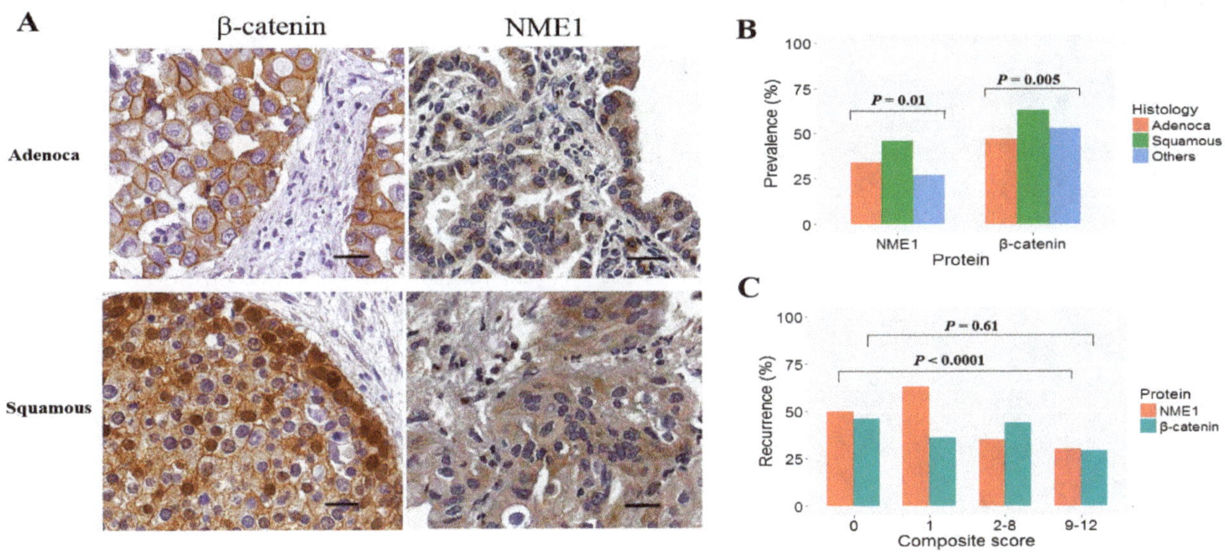

Figure 1. Immunohistochemical staining for non-metastatic cells 1 (NME1) and β-catenin expression in non-small cell lung cancer. (**A**) Expression levels of NME1 and β-catenin were analyzed using immunohistochemical staining (scale bar = 100 μm). Representative images of positive staining are shown in adenocarcinoma (upper) and squamous cell carcinoma (lower) at magnification of ×200. Cytoplasmic staining was considered positive for NME1 and β-catenin expression. (**B**) Prevalence of reduced NME1 expression and β-catenin overexpression was compared according to histologic subtypes. *p*-values were based on Pearson's chi-square test. (**C**) Association between recurrence and the expression levels of NME1 or β-catenin was analyzed in 425 participants.

Postoperative recurrence occurred in 186 (44%) of 425 patients. Patients with reduced NME1 expression had a higher recurrence rate than those without (62% vs. 32%, $p < 0.0001$). β-catenin was overexpressed in 55% of patients, with a higher prevalence in squamous cell carcinoma than that in adenocarcinoma ($p = 0.005$; Figure 1B). Recurrence was found at a high prevalence in patients with reduced NME1 expression but not β-catenin overexpression irrespective of histologic subtypes (Figure 1C).

3.2. Reduced NME1 Expression Is Significantly Associated with Poor RFS Irrespective of Histology or Pathologic Stage

Univariate analysis was performed to discover prognostic factors that affect RFS in early stage NSCLC. RFS was negatively associated with reduced NME1 expression but not with β-catenin overexpression and cisplatin-based adjuvant chemotherapy (Supplementary Table S2). Patients were stratified according to histology and pathologic stage to analyze whether the relationship between RFS and NME1 expression was modified by histology or pathologic stage. RFS was compared between patients with and without reduced NME1 expression in histologic subtypes. Reduced NME1 expression was significantly associated with RFS ($p < 0.0001$; Supplementary Figure S1A): Five-year RFS rate after surgery was 38% for those with reduced NME1 expression and 68% for those without reduced NME1 expression. Reduced NME1 expression had a negative effect on RFS in adenocarcinoma ($p < 0.0001$; Supplementary Figure S1B) and in squamous cell carcinoma ($p < 0.0001$; Supplementary Figure S1C).

The effect of reduced NME1 expression on RFS was further analyzed based on pathologic stage (Figure 2). The number of patients with stage IIIA NSCLC was five, which was too small to analyze RFS. Therefore, patients with stage IIIA NSCLC were combined with those who had stage IIB NSCLC to analyze RFS. Reduced NME1 expression was significantly associated with poor RFS in stage IA ($p = 0.0005$; Figure 2A), stage IB ($p = 0.001$; Figure 2B), and stage IIA ($p = 0.01$; Figure 2C). It was marginally associated with poor RFS in stage IIB–IIIA ($p = 0.08$; Figure 2D). The relationship between β-catenin overexpression and RFS was also analyzed based on pathologic stage and histology. However, no association was found between them.

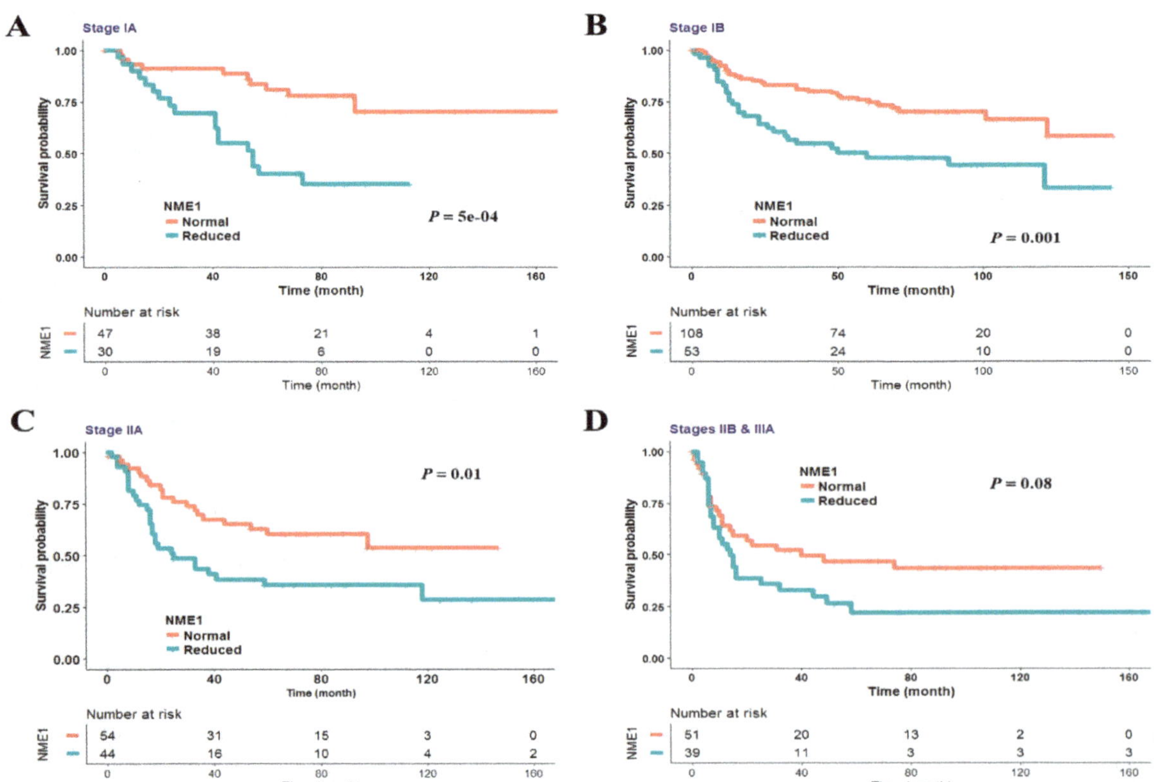

Figure 2. Impact of NME1 on recurrence-free survival (RFS) according to pathologic stages. The effect of reduced NME1 expression on RFS was estimated using the Kaplan–Meier survival curve in 77 patients with stage IA (**A**), 161 with stage IB (**B**), 98 with stage IIA (**C**), and 89 stage IIB–IIIA (**D**). Statistical difference between two survival curves was calculated using the log-rank test.

3.3. Negative Effect of Reduced NME1 Expression on RFS in Patients with Cisplatin-Based Adjuvant Chemotherapy and β-Catenin Overexpression

Cisplatin-based adjuvant chemotherapy was not associated with RFS irrespective of histologic subtypes in univariate analysis. The effect of NME1 or β-catenin on RFS was further analyzed considering cisplatin-based adjuvant chemotherapy. The negative effect of reduced NME1 expression on RFS was worse in patients treated with (Figure 3A) cisplatin-based adjuvant chemotherapy than in those treated without (Figure 3B). Reduced NME1 expression was not associated with β-catenin overexpression in this study. However, it is known that there is a complex interplay between NME1 and β-catenin in a variety of cancers. Therefore, data were further stratified according to β-catenin overexpression. The negative effect of reduced NME1 expression on RFS was much greater in patients with overexpression of β-catenin (Figure 3C) than in those without (Figure 3D).

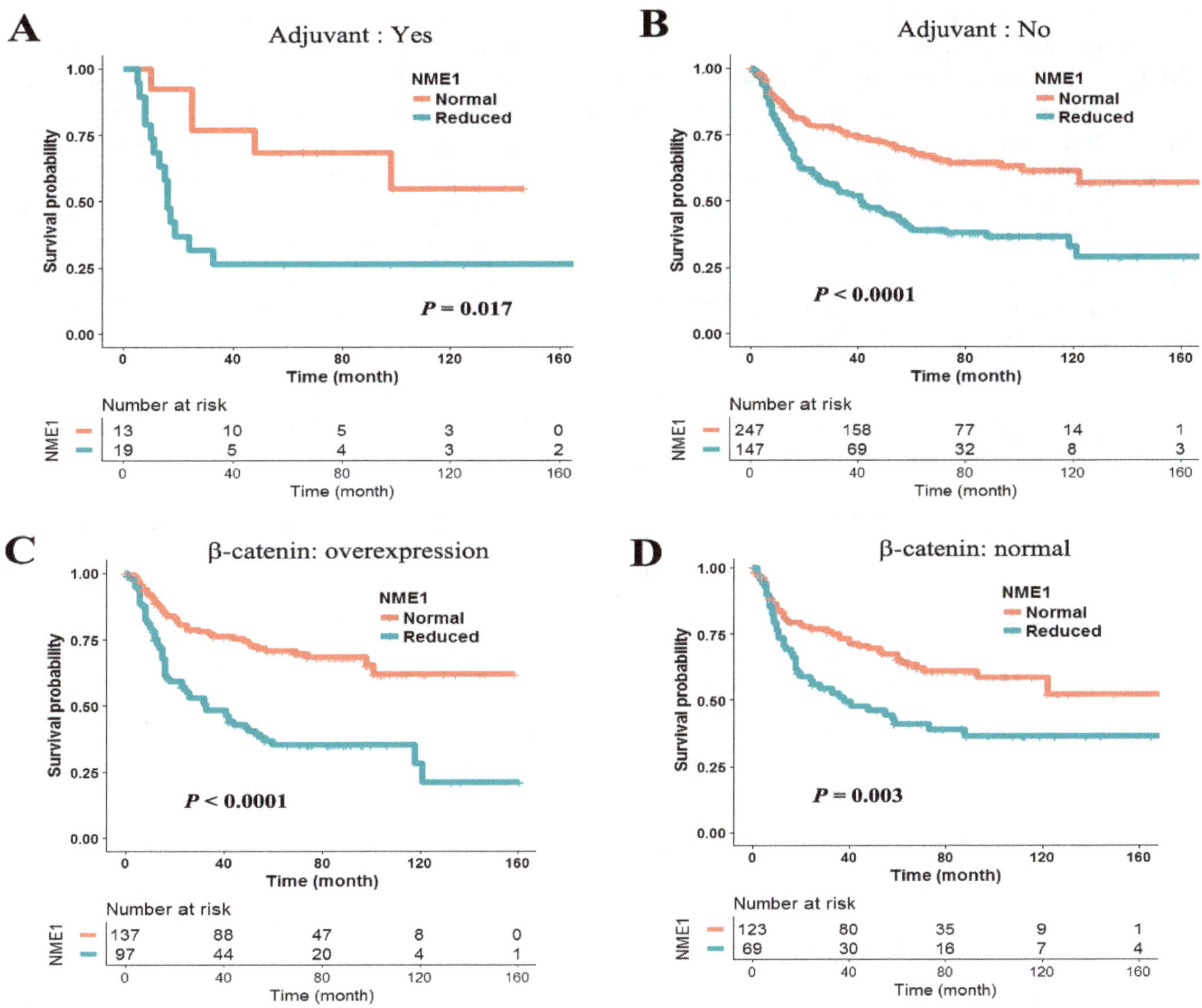

Figure 3. Effect of NME1 on recurrence-free survival, stratified by β-catenin expression and cisplatin-based adjuvant chemotherapy. To understand whether the effect of NME1 on RFS was confounded by β-catenin expression or cisplatin-based adjuvant chemotherapy, data were stratified by β-catenin overexpression (**A**,**B**) or cisplatin-based adjuvant chemotherapy (**C**,**D**) and then the survival curves were compared according to NME1. The survival was compared using the log-rank test in 425 non-small cell lung cancers (NSCLCs).

3.4. *Multivariate Cox Proportional Hazards Analysis*

Multivariate Cox proportional hazards analysis was conducted to measure the effect of reduced NME1 expression on RFS in early stage NSCLC, after adjusting for potential confounding effects of variables. Considering the pathological stage, hazard ratios for RFS ranged from 1.64 to 3.93, after adjusting for patient age, sex, β-catenin expression, adjuvant chemotherapy, and histology (Supplementary Table S3). The hazard ratio for RFS in a total of 425 patients was 2.27 (95% CI = 1.70–3.03, $p < 0.0001$) times worse in patients with reduced NME1 expression than in those without (Supplementary Table S4). However, the hazard ratio was not associated with age (HR = 1.01, 95% CI = 0.99–1.03, $p = 0.18$), sex (HR = 1.02, 95% CI = 0.71–1.47, $p = 0.93$), adjuvant chemotherapy (HR = 1.03, 95% CI = 0.86–2.23, $p = 0.89$), and β-catenin expression (HR = 0.99, 95% CI = 0.75–1.34, $p = 0.99$).

To test our hypothesis that the effect of NME1 expression on RFS may be affected by Wnt signal and cisplatin treatment, we stratified patients according to adjuvant chemotherapy and β-catenin expression. The negative effect of reduced NME1 expression on RFS was exacerbated by cisplatin-based adjuvant chemotherapy (adjusted hazard ratio = 3.26, 95% CI = 1.16–9.17, $p = 0.03$; Supplementary Table S5). For patients who did not receive cisplatin-based adjuvant chemotherapy, the hazard ratio of reduced NME1 expression was increased from 1.89 (95% confidence interval (CI) = 1.21–2.95, $p = 0.005$) to 2.54 (95% CI = 1.66–3.89, $p < 0.0001$; Table 1) by β-catenin overexpression after adjusting for patient age, sex, histology, and pathologic stage. Among patients with β-catenin overexpression who received cisplatin-based adjuvant chemotherapy, patients with reduced NME1 expression were determined to have 15.52 (95% CI = 2.94–82.38, $p = 0.001$; Table 1) times poorer RFS than those without. These results suggest that the negative effect of reduced NME1 expression on RFS may be worsen by cisplatin-based adjuvant chemotherapy and β-catenin overexpression in early stage NSCLC.

Table 1. Cox proportional hazards analysis [a] of RFS according to NME1 in early stage NSCLC stratified by cisplatin-based adjuvant chemotherapy and β-catenin overexpression

<table>
<tr><th>Adjuvant Chemotherapy</th><th>β-Catenin Overexpression</th><th>Reduced NME1 Expression</th><th>HR</th><th>95% CI</th><th>p-Value</th></tr>
<tr><td rowspan="4">No</td><td rowspan="2">No (N = 176)</td><td>No</td><td>1</td><td></td><td></td></tr>
<tr><td>Yes</td><td>1.89</td><td>1.21–2.95</td><td>0.005</td></tr>
<tr><td rowspan="2">Yes (N = 217)</td><td>No</td><td>1</td><td></td><td></td></tr>
<tr><td>Yes</td><td>2.54</td><td>1.66–3.89</td><td><0.0001</td></tr>
<tr><td rowspan="4">Yes</td><td rowspan="2">No (N = 16)</td><td>No</td><td>1</td><td></td><td></td></tr>
<tr><td>Yes</td><td>5.59</td><td>0.62–50.91</td><td>0.13</td></tr>
<tr><td rowspan="2">Yes (N = 16)</td><td>No</td><td>1</td><td></td><td></td></tr>
<tr><td>Yes</td><td>15.52</td><td>2.94–82.38</td><td>0.001</td></tr>
</table>

[a] Adjusted for age, sex, histology, and pathologic stage. Abbreviations: HR, hazard ratio; CI, confidence interval.

3.5. *Relationship between Ki-67 Labeling Index and Expression of NME1 and β-Catenin*

Ki-67 proliferation index was analyzed to investigate whether the effect of NME1 and β-catenin on cisplatin-resistance might be confounded by different cell proliferation activity. Ki-67 proliferation was not significantly different according to abnormal expression of NME1 or β-catenin irrespective of histology (Figure 4A) and cisplatin-based adjuvant chemotherapy (Figure 4B). These observations suggest that NME1 and β-catenin may affect cisplatin-based adjuvant chemotherapy through other mechanisms rather than through any changes in cell proliferation.

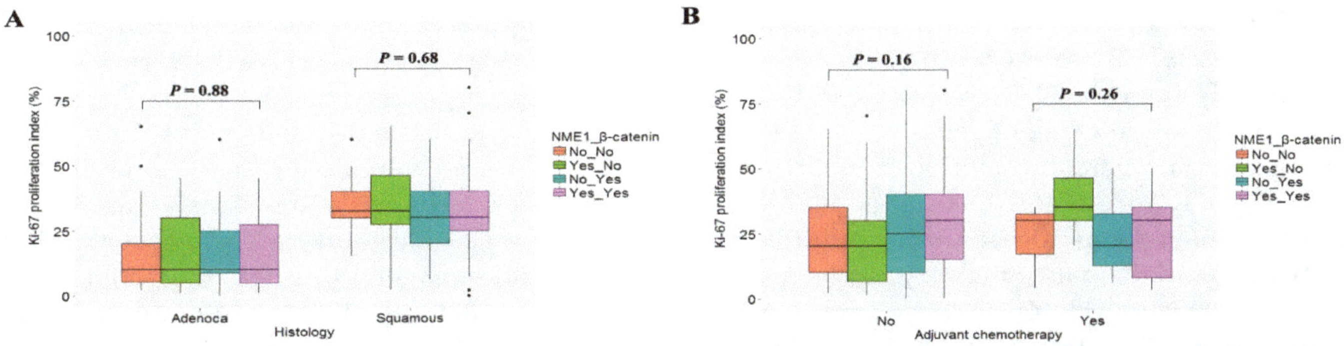

Figure 4. Ki-67 (MKI67) proliferation index according to altered expression of NME1 and β-catenin. Ki-67 proliferation was compared according to expression statuses of NME1 and β-catenin, stratified by histology (**A**) and adjuvant chemotherapy (**B**). "Adenoca" and "Squamous" represent adenocarcinoma and squamous cell carcinoma, respectively. "No" and "Yes" indicate the absence and presence of altered expression, respectively. p-values were calculated using one-way ANOVA.

3.6. The Relationship between NME1 and Nuclear β-Catenin Expression

NME1 silencing is known to induce a redistribution of β-catenin from the cell surface into the cytoplasm and nucleus by activating the Wnt pathway [17]. To understand whether NME1 expression affects the nuclear translocation of β-catenin, we analyzed the levels of nuclear β-catenin expression (Figure 5A) according to NME1 expression. The levels of nuclear β-catenin expression showed a linear relationship with those of cytoplasmic β-catenin expression (Pearson's correlation coefficient $\gamma = 0.74$, $p = 0.002$; Figure 5B) but not to those of NME1 expression ($\gamma = -0.03$, $p = 0.80$; Figure 5C).

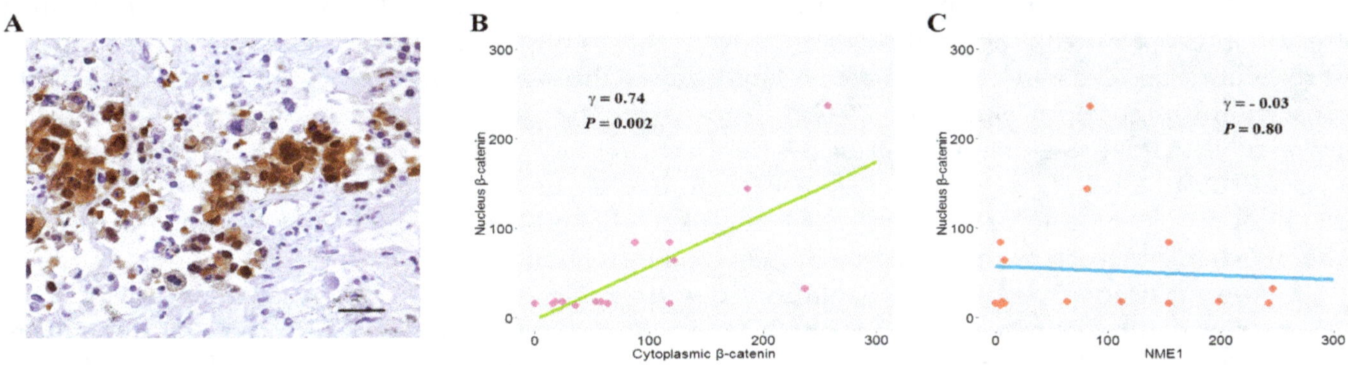

Figure 5. The relationship between NME1 and nuclear β-catenin expression. (**A**) β-catenin expression (scale bar, 100 μm) are shown in nucleus. (**B**,**C**) X- and Y-axis scores were obtained by multiplying the intensity score of staining with the proportion of positive stained cells. The linear relationship between two variables was calculated using Pearson's correlation coefficient.

4. Discussion

The epithelial–mesenchymal transition (EMT) plays a crucial role in promoting metastasis of carcinoma derived from epithelial cells. Tumor cells lose their epithelial characteristics such as cell polarity and gain mesenchymal features such as increased migratory and invasive potentials during EMT. Our data did not show an association of NME1 expression with tumor growth (Figure 4), consistent with a previous study showing that *NME1* silencing does not provide epithelial cancer cells with a selective growth advantage [17]. A number of groups have reported the relationship between NME1 expression and patient prognosis in NSCLC with different results. Some groups have reported no association between NME1 expression and overall survival [28,29]. In contrast, reduced NME1 expression has been found to be associated with bone metastasis and poor survival in patients with pulmonary adenocarcinoma [30]. Ohta et al. [31] have also reported that NME1 expression is inversely correlated with the microdissemination of tumor cells in stage I NSCLC. In addition, stage

I NSCLC patients with NME1-negative expression show a significantly poorer survival than those without [32,33]. The present study also showed the negative effect of reduced NME1 expression on RFS in early stage NSCLC, consistent with findings from previous groups [30–33].

The negative effect of reduced NME1 expression on RFS in this study was worse in patients with β-catenin overexpression than in those without. How does β-catenin overexpression influence the effect of reduced NME1 expression on RFS? Mechanisms underlying the metastasis suppression of NME1 have been addressed in multiple types of cancer cells. Early efforts have revealed that NME1 may mediate its inhibitory effects on cellular motility and invasion through interactions with signaling cascades [16,34–36]. For example, NME1 negatively regulates Rac1 (Rac family small GTPase 1) and Cdc42 (Cell division cycle 42) GTPase by interacting with Rac1-specific nucleotide exchange factors, TIAM Rac1 associated GEF1 (Tiam1) and TGF_BETA_2 domain-containing protein (Dbl-1), respectively [36]. A splicing variant of *NME1* inhibits the metastasis of lung cancer cells by interacting with Inhibitor of nuclear factor Kappa-B Kinase subunit beta (IKKβ) in an isotype-specific fashion and regulating tumor necrosis factor alpha (TNFα)-stimulated Nuclear Factor kappa-light-chain-enhancer of activated B cells (NF-κB) signaling negatively [16]. In addition, NME1 inhibits the liver metastasis of colon cancer cells by regulating the phosphorylation of myosin light chains in nude mice [35]. *NME1* silencing induces the nuclear translocation of β-catenin by disrupting adherence junction complexes mediated by E-cadherin and promotes extracellular matrix invasion by increasing invadopodia formation and pericellular matrix metalloproteinase (MMP) activity [17].

In addition to its effect on signaling pathways, NME1 is also known to regulate gene transcription by binding to single-stranded DNA. A promoter region between –922 to –846 of Kangai 1 (KAI1) is known to suppress metastasis through the inhibition of cell movement. It responds to NME1 in high-metastatic lung cancer cell line L9981 [37]. NME1 suppresses motile and invasive phenotypes of melanoma cells by inducing the transcription of integrin beta-3 (*ITGβ3*) gene through direct physical interaction with the promoter [38]. NME1 also plays a role as a co-regulator of transcription by regulating expression of metastasis-related genes through direct or indirect interactions with transcription-regulatory elements [39–42]. However, the present study showed no relationship between NME1 expression and nuclear β-catenin expression (Figure 5), suggesting that the adverse effect of NME1 on RFS exacerbated by β-catenin overexpression might not be due to the nuclear translocation of β-catenin by reduced NME1. It is likely that NME1 may interact with β-catenin through other mechanisms such as upregulation of many genes related to cell cycle, apoptosis, and metastasis.

Platinum derivatives such as cisplatin are widely used chemotherapeutic agents for NSCLC. However, cisplatin resistance is a major challenge in the use of these drugs. The molecular mechanism of cisplatin resistance in lung cancer cells is not fully understood. Therefore, there are few efficient strategies to overcome such resistance. Cisplatin-based adjuvant chemotherapy in the present study did not affect RFS in univariate analysis. However, it worsened the RFS in patients with reduced NME1 expression (Supplementary Table S5). A functional link between NME1 expression and responsiveness to cisplatin-based adjuvant chemotherapy has been reported by several groups. Cisplatin increases interstrand DNA cross-links and inhibits pulmonary metastatic colonization in *NME1*-transfected breast cancer cells [43]. NME1 has 3′-5′ exonuclease activity potentially involved in DNA proofreading [44]. Thus, reduced expression of NME1 may contribute to chemoresistance by allowing metastatic cells to escape from apoptosis. Knockdown of *NME1* by shRNA transfection in head and neck squamous carcinoma cells attenuates the chemosensitivity of cells to cisplatin by downregulating cyclins E and A and reducing cisplatin-induced S-phase accumulation [45]. These lines of evidence suggest that reduced NME1 expression might be involved in cisplatin resistance through various mechanisms. Therefore, restoring NME1 expression might be a therapeutic intervention strategy to surmount cisplatin resistance.

Previous studies have demonstrated Wnt/β-catenin-mediated resistance to cisplatin in various types of cancers [23,24]. Transient interference of cytoplasmic GSK-3β increases cisplatin resistance by activating Wnt/β-catenin signaling in cisplatin-resistant A549 cells [23]. Recently, Zhang and colleagues [24] have reported that the interference of β-catenin expression by siRNA can decrease mRNA and protein levels of anti-apoptotic gene *Bcl-xl* and increase cisplatin sensitivity in A549 wild-type cells. Despite these associations of β-catenin overexpression and cisplatin resistance in various types of cancer cells, β-catenin overexpression alone was not associated with cisplatin resistance in the present study. However, β-catenin overexpression aggravated RFS when patients with reduced NME1 received cisplatin-based adjuvant chemotherapy (Table 1). Further studies are needed to better understand the combined effect of β-catenin and NME1 on RFS of patients receiving platinum-based adjuvant chemotherapy in early stage NSCLC.

This study was limited by several factors. First, this was a retrospective study that was prone to selection and surveillance biases. Second, it is necessary to investigate combined effects of β-catenin and NME1 on apoptosis, migration, invasion, or metastasis in different cell types of lung cancer to clearly understand the molecular mechanisms underlying the effect of β-catenin and NME1 on poor RFS. Third, the lack of a negative effect of β-catenin in the univariate analysis (Supplementary Table S2) in this study might be due to the small sample size and short duration of follow-up. Fourth, *EcoR1* (rs34214448-G/T) polymorphism in *NME1* gene is associated with increased susceptibility to NSCLC [46] and could potentially affect the results of the current analysis, which is based only on expression levels. Fifth, the relationship between the Th1 (T helper cell type 1) and Th 2 (T helper cell type 2) ratio and β-catenin levels were not analyzed in this study. The balance between Th1 and Th2 in the tumor microenvironment is regulated by several factors, and β-catenin may affect the tumor microenvironment. Thus, for the understanding of their relationship and the analysis of β-catenin levels, it may be informative to know the Th1/Th2 ratio of patients. Sixth, the number of patients receiving adjuvant chemotherapy was too small. Accordingly, prospective large-scale studies are needed to validate the effect of β-catenin and cisplatin-based adjuvant chemotherapy on NME1-related RFS in early stage NSCLC.

In conclusion, the present study suggests that the adverse effect of reduced NME1 expression on RFS may be exacerbated by cisplatin-based adjuvant chemotherapy and β-catenin overexpression through other mechanisms rather than through the nuclear translocation of β-catenin in early stage NSCLC. Accordingly, it is recommended that cisplatin-based adjuvant chemotherapy in patients with completely resected stage I–IIIA NSCLC be carefully applied after examining the expression levels of β-catenin and NME1.

Supplementary Materials:
Table S1: Relationship between NME1 expression and clinicopathological characteristics (N = 425). Table S2: Univariate analysis of RFS (N = 425). Table S3: Cox proportional hazards analysis of RFS according to NME1 in early stage NSCLC (N = 425), stratified by pathologic stages. Table S4: Cox proportional hazards analysis[†] for RFS in early stage NSCLCs (N = 425). Table S5: Cox proportional hazards analysis[†] for RFS according to NME1 expression in 425 early stage NSCLCs treated with and without cisplatin-based adjuvant chemotherapy. Figure S1: Kaplan–Meier plot of recurrence-free survival according to NME1 expression in histologic subtypes: (A) Total, (B) Adenocarcinoma, (C) Squamous cell carcinoma.

Author Contributions: Conceptualization D.K. (Dohun Kim) and D.-H.K.; data curation, Y.K. and W.-J.K.; formal analysis, Y.K., B.B.L., and D.K. (Dongho Kim); methodology, O.-J.L. and P.J.; resources, E.Y.C., J.H., and Y.M.S.; supervision, D.-H.K.; writing—original draft preparation, D.K. (Dohun Kim) and D-H.K.; writing—review and editing, D.K. (Dohun Kim), Y.K., B.B.L., D.K. (Dongho Kim), O.-J.L., P.J., W.-J.K., E.Y.C., J.H., Y.M.S., and D.-H.K.; funding acquisition, D.-H.K. All authors have read and agreed to the published version of the manuscript.

Acknowledgments: The authors thank Eunkyung Kim and Jin-Hee Lee for data collection and management, and Hoon Suh for sample collection.

References

1. Pignon, J.-P.; Tribodet, H.; Scagliotti, G.V.; Douillard, J.-Y.; Shepherd, F.A.; Stephens, R.J.; Dunant, A.; Torri, V.; Rosell, R.; Seymour, L.; et al. Lung Adjuvant Cisplatin Evaluation: A Pooled Analysis by the LACE Collaborative Group. *J. Clin. Oncol.* **2008**, *26*, 3552–3559. [CrossRef] [PubMed]

2. Arriagada, R.; Dunant, A.; Pignon, J.-P.; Bergman, B.; Chabowski, M.; Grunenwald, D.; Kozlowski, M.; Le Péchoux, C.; Pirker, R.; Pinel, M.-I.S.; et al. Long-Term Results of the International Adjuvant Lung Cancer Trial Evaluating Adjuvant Cisplatin-Based Chemotherapy in Resected Lung Cancer. *J. Clin. Oncol.* **2010**, *28*, 35–42. [CrossRef] [PubMed]
3. Steeg, P.S.; Bevilacqua, G.; Kopper, L.; Thorgeirsson, U.P.; Talmadge, J.E.; Liotta, L.A.; Sobel, M.E. Evidence for a Novel Gene Associated with Low Tumor Metastatic Potential. *J. Natl. Cancer Inst.* **1988**, *80*, 200–204. [CrossRef]
4. Boissan, M.; Dabernat, S.; Peuchant, E.; Schlattner, U.; Lascu, I.; Lacombe, M.-L. The mammalian Nm23/NDPK family: From metastasis control to cilia movement. *Mol. Cell. Biochem.* **2009**, *329*, 51–62. [CrossRef]
5. Goncharuk, V.N.; Del-Rosario, A.; Kren, L.; Anwar, S.; E Sheehan, C.; Carlson, J.A.; Ross, J.S. Co-downregulation of PTEN, KAI-1, and nm23-H1 tumor/metastasis suppressor proteins in non-small cell lung cancer. *Ann. Diagn. Pathol.* **2004**, *8*, 6–16. [CrossRef] [PubMed]
6. Ayabe, T.; Tomita, M.; Matsuzaki, Y.; Ninomiya, H.; Hara, M.; Shimizu, T.; Edagawa, M.; Onitsuka, T.; Hamada, M. Micrometastasis and expression of nm23 messenger RNA of lymph nodes from lung cancer and the postoperative clinical outcome. *Ann. Thorac. Cardiovasc. Surg.* **2004**, *10*, 152–159.
7. Sarris, M.; Scolyer, R.A.; Konopka, M.; Thompson, J.F.; Harper, C.G.; Lee, C.S. Cytoplasmic expression of nm23 predicts the potential for cerebral metastasis in patients with primary cutaneous melanoma. *Melanoma Res.* **2004**, *14*, 23–27. [CrossRef]
8. Khan, I.; Gril, B.; Steeg, P.S. Metastasis Suppressors NME1 and NME2 Promote Dynamin 2 Oligomerization and Regulate Tumor Cell Endocytosis, Motility, and Metastasis. *Cancer Res.* **2019**, *79*, 4689–4702. [CrossRef]
9. Khera, L.; Paul, C.; Kaul, R. Hepatitis C Virus E1 protein promotes cell migration and invasion by modulating cellular metastasis suppressor Nm23-H1. *Virology* **2017**, *506*, 110–120. [CrossRef]
10. Guan-Zhen, Y.; Ying, C.; Can-Rong, N.; Guo-Dong, W.; Jian-Xin, Q.; Jie-Jun, W. Reduced protein expression of metastasis-related genes (nm23, KISS1, KAI1 and p53) in lymph node and liver metastases of gastric cancer. *Int. J. Exp. Pathol.* **2007**, *88*, 175–183. [CrossRef]
11. Yang, T.; Chen, B.Z.; Li, D.F.; Wang, H.M.; Lin, X.S.; Wei, H.F.; Zeng, Y.M. Reduced NM23 Protein Level Correlates with Worse Clinicopathologic Features in Colorectal Cancers: A Meta-Analysis of Pooled Data. *Medicine (Baltimore)* **2016**, *95*, e2589. [PubMed]
12. Rasool, R.U.; Nayak, D.; Chakraborty, S.; Jamwal, V.L.; Mahajan, V.; Katoch, A.; Faheem, M.M.; Iqra, Z.; Amin, H.; Gandhi, S.G.; et al. Differential regulation of NM23-H1 under hypoxic and serum starvation conditions in metastatic cancer cells and its implication in EMT. *Eur. J. Cell Boil.* **2017**, *96*, 164–171. [CrossRef] [PubMed]
13. Horak, C.; Mendoza, A.; Vega-Valle, E.; Albaugh, M.; Graff-Cherry, C.; McDermott, W.G.; Hua, E.; Merino, M.J.; Steinberg, S.M.; Khanna, C.; et al. Nm23-H1 Suppresses Metastasis by Inhibiting Expression of the Lysophosphatidic Acid Receptor EDG2. *Cancer Res.* **2007**, *67*, 11751–11759. [CrossRef] [PubMed]
14. Khan, I.; Steeg, P.S. The relationship of NM23 (NME) metastasis suppressor histidine phosphorylation to its nucleotide diphosphate kinase, histidine protein kinase and motility suppression activities. *Oncotarget* **2017**, *9*, 10185–10202. [CrossRef]
15. Che, G.; Chen, J.; Liu, L.; Wang, Y.; Li, L.; Qin, Y.; Zhou, Q. Transfection of nm23-H1 increased expression of beta-Catenin, E-Cadherin and TIMP-1 and decreased the expression of MMP-2, CD44v6 and VEGF and inhibited the metastatic potential of human non-small cell lung cancer cell line L9981. *Neoplasma* **2006**, *53*, 530–537.
16. You, D.-J.; Park, C.R.; Lee, H.B.; Moon, M.J.; Kang, J.-H.; Lee, C.; Oh, S.-H.; Ahn, C.; Seong, J.Y.; Hwang, J.-I. A Splicing Variant of NME1 Negatively Regulates NF-κB Signaling and Inhibits Cancer Metastasis by Interacting with IKKβ. *J. Boil. Chem.* **2014**, *289*, 17709–17720. [CrossRef]
17. Boissan, M.; De Wever, O.; Lizarraga, F.; Wendum, D.; Poincloux, R.; Chignard, N.; Desbois-Mouthon, C.; Dufour, S.; Nawrocki-Raby, B.; Birembaut, P.; et al. Implication of Metastasis Suppressor NM23-H1 in Maintaining Adherens Junctions and Limiting the Invasive Potential of Human Cancer Cells. *Cancer Res.* **2010**, *70*, 7710–7722. [CrossRef]
18. Hansen, M.T.; Forst, B.; Cremers, N.; Quagliata, L.; Ambartsumian, N.; Grum-Schwensen, B.; Klingelhöfer, J.; Abdul-Al, A.; Herrmann, P.; Osterland, M.; et al. A link between inflammation and metastasis: Serum amyloid A1 and A3 induce metastasis, and are targets of metastasis-inducing S100A4. *Oncogene* **2014**, *34*, 424–435. [CrossRef]

19. He, W.; He, S.; Wang, Z.; Shen, H.; Fang, W.; Zhang, Y.; Qian, W.; Lin, M.; Yuan, J.; Wang, J.; et al. Astrocyte elevated gene-1(AEG-1) induces epithelial-mesenchymal transition in lung cancer through activating Wnt/β-catenin signaling. *BMC Cancer* **2015**, *15*, 107. [CrossRef]
20. Shukla, S.; Sinha, S.; Khan, S.; Kumar, S.; Singh, K.; Mitra, K.; Maurya, R.; Meeran, S.M. Cucurbitacin B inhibits the stemness and metastatic abilities of NSCLC via downregulation of canonical Wnt/β-catenin signaling axis. *Sci. Rep.* **2016**, *6*, 21860. [CrossRef]
21. Lu, J.; Du, C.; Yao, J.; Wu, B.; Duan, Y.; Zhou, L.; Xu, N.; Zhou, F.; Gu, L.; Zhou, H.; et al. C/EBPα Suppresses Lung Adenocarcinoma Cell Invasion and Migration by Inhibiting β-Catenin. *Cell. Physiol. Biochem.* **2017**, *42*, 1779–1788. [CrossRef] [PubMed]
22. Yang, S.; Liu, Y.; Li, M.-Y.; Ng, C.S.H.; Yang, S.-L.; Wang, S.S.; Zou, C.; Dong, Y.; Du, J.; Long, X.; et al. FOXP3 promotes tumor growth and metastasis by activating Wnt/β-catenin signaling pathway and EMT in non-small cell lung cancer. *Mol. Cancer* **2017**, *16*, 124. [CrossRef]
23. Gao, Y.; Liu, Z.; Zhang, X.; He, J.; Pan, Y.; Hao, F.; Xie, L.; Li, Q.; Qiu, X.; Wang, E. Inhibition of cytoplasmic GSK 3β increases cisplatin resistance through activation of Wnt/β catenin signaling in A549/DDP cells. *Cancer Lett.* **2013**, *336*, 231–239. [CrossRef] [PubMed]
24. Zhang, J.; Liu, J.; Li, H.; Wang, J. β-Catenin signaling pathway regulates cisplatin resistance in lung adenocarcinoma cells by upregulating Bcl-xl. *Mol. Med. Rep.* **2016**, *13*, 2543–2551. [CrossRef] [PubMed]
25. Kim, J.S.; Kim, J.-W.; Han, J.; Shim, Y.M.; Park, J.; Kim, D.-H. Cohypermethylation of p16 and FHIT Promoters as a Prognostic Factor of Recurrence in Surgically Resected Stage I Non–Small Cell Lung Cancer. *Cancer Res.* **2006**, *66*, 4049–4054. [CrossRef]
26. Edge, S.B.; Byrd, D.R.; Compton, C.C.; Fritz, A.G.; Greene, F.L.; Troth, A. American Joint Committee on Cancer. In *AJCC Cancer Staging Manual*, 7th ed.; Springer: New York, NY, USA, 2010; pp. 253–270.
27. Kim, J.S.; Han, J.; Shim, Y.M.; Park, J.; Kim, D.H. Aberrant methylation of H-cadherin (CDH13) promoter is associated with tumor progression in primary nonsmall cell lung cancer. *Cancer* **2005**, *104*, 1825–1833.
28. MacKinnon, M. p53, c-erbB-2 and nm23 expression have no prognostic significance in primary pulmonary adenocarcinoma. *Eur. J. Cardio-Thoracic Surg.* **1997**, *11*, 838–842. [CrossRef]
29. Tomita, M.; Ayabe, T.; Matsuzaki, Y.; Onitsuka, T. Immunohistochemical analysis of nm23-H1 gene product in node-positive lung cancer and lymph nodes. *Lung Cancer* **1999**, *24*, 11–16. [CrossRef]
30. Yang, M.; Sun, Y.; Sun, J.; Wang, Z.; Zhou, Y.; Yao, G.; Gu, Y.; Zhang, H.; Zhao, H. Differentially expressed and survival-related proteins of lung adenocarcinoma with bone metastasis. *Cancer Med.* **2018**, *7*, 1081–1092. [CrossRef]
31. Ohta, Y.; Nozawa, H.; Tanaka, Y.; Oda, M.; Watanabe, Y. Increased vascular endothelial growth factor and vascular endothelial growth factor–c and decreased nm23 expression associated with microdissemination in the lymph nodes in stage i non–small cell lung cancer. *J. Thorac. Cardiovasc. Surg.* **2000**, *119*, 804–813. [CrossRef]
32. Katakura, H.; Tanaka, F.; Oyanagi, H.; Miyahara, R.; Yanagihara, K.; Otake, Y.; Wada, H. Clinical significance of nm23 expression in resected pathologic-stage I, non-small cell lung cancer. *Ann. Thorac. Surg.* **2002**, *73*, 1060–1064. [CrossRef]
33. Liu, C.; Liu, J.; Wang, X.; Mao, W.; Jiang, L.; Ni, H.; Mo, M.; Wang, W. Prognostic impact of nm23-H1 and PCNA expression in pathologic stage I non-small cell lung cancer. *J. Surg. Oncol.* **2011**, *104*, 181–186. [CrossRef] [PubMed]
34. Otsuki, Y.; Tanaka, M.; Yoshii, S.; Kawazoe, N.; Nakaya, K.; Sugimura, H. Tumor metastasis suppressor nm23H1 regulates Rac1 GTPase by interaction with Tiam1. *Proc. Natl. Acad. Sci. USA* **2001**, *98*, 4385–4390. [CrossRef] [PubMed]
35. Suzuki, E.; Ota, T.; Tsukuda, K.; Okita, A.; Matsuoka, K.; Murakami, M.; Doihara, H.; Shimizu, N. nm23-H1 reduces in vitro cell migration and the liver metastatic potential of colon cancer cells by regulating myosin light chain phosphorylation. *Int. J. Cancer* **2004**, *108*, 207–211. [CrossRef] [PubMed]
36. Murakami, M.; Meneses, P.I.; Lan, K.; Robertson, E.S. The suppressor of metastasis Nm23-H1 interacts with the Cdc42 Rho family member and the pleckstrin homology domain of oncoprotein Dbl-1 to suppress cell migration. *Cancer Boil. Ther.* **2008**, *7*, 677–688. [CrossRef]
37. You, J.; Chang, R.; Liu, B.; Zu, L.; Zhou, Q. Nm23-H1 was involved in regulation of KAI1 expression in high-metastatic lung cancer cells L9981. *J. Thorac. Dis.* **2016**, *8*, 1217–1226. [CrossRef]

38. Leonard, M.K.; Novak, M.; Snyder, D.; Snow, G.; Pamidimukkala, N.; McCorkle, J.R.; Yang, X.H.; Kaetzel, D. The metastasis suppressor NME1 inhibits melanoma cell motility via direct transcriptional induction of the integrin beta-3 gene. *Exp. Cell Res.* **2019**, *374*, 85–93. [CrossRef]
39. Subramanian, C.; Robertson, E.S. The Metastatic Suppressor Nm23-H1 Interacts with EBNA3C at Sequences Located between the Glutamine- and Proline-Rich Domains and Can Cooperate in Activation of Transcription. *J. Virol.* **2002**, *76*, 8702–8709. [CrossRef]
40. Curtis, C.D.; Likhite, V.S.; McLeod, I.X.; Yates, J.R.; Nardulli, A.M. Interaction of the Tumor Metastasis Suppressor Nonmetastatic Protein 23 Homologue H1 and Estrogen Receptor Alters Estrogen-Responsive Gene Expression. *Cancer Res.* **2007**, *67*, 10600–10607. [CrossRef]
41. Horak, C.; Lee, J.H.; Elkahloun, A.G.; Boissan, M.; Dumont, S.; Maga, T.K.; Arnaud-Dabernat, S.; Palmieri, D.; Stetler-Stevenson, W.G.; Lacombe, M.-L.; et al. Nm23-H1 Suppresses Tumor Cell Motility by Down-regulating the Lysophosphatidic Acid Receptor EDG2. *Cancer Res.* **2007**, *67*, 7238–7246. [CrossRef]
42. Choudhuri, T.; Murakami, M.; Kaul, R.; Sahu, S.K.; Mohanty, S.; Verma, S.; Kumar, P.; Robertson, E.S. Nm23-H1 can induce cell cycle arrest and apoptosis in B cells. *Cancer Boil. Ther.* **2010**, *9*, 1065–1078. [CrossRef]
43. Ferguson, A.W.; Flatow, U.; Macdonald, N.J.; Larminat, F.; A Bohr, V.; Steeg, P.S. Increased sensitivity to cisplatin by nm23-transfected tumor cell lines. *Cancer Res.* **1996**, *56*, 2931–2935.
44. Ma, D.; McCorkle, J.R.; Kaetzel, D. The Metastasis Suppressor NM23-H1 Possesses 3′-5′ Exonuclease Activity. *J. Boil. Chem.* **2004**, *279*, 18073–18084. [CrossRef] [PubMed]
45. Wang, Y.-F.; Chang, C.-J.; Chiu, J.-H.; Lin, C.-P.; Li, W.-Y.; Chang, S.-Y.; Chu, P.-Y.; Tai, S.-K.; Chen, Y.-J. NM23-H1 expression of head and neck squamous cell carcinoma in association with the response to cisplatin treatment. *Oncotarget* **2014**, *5*, 7392–7405. [CrossRef] [PubMed]
46. Shi, X.; Jin, H.; Peng, M.; Li, B.; She, M.; Zhu, T.; Wen, S.; Qin, D.-C. Association between NME1 polymorphisms and cancer susceptibility: A meta-analysis based on 1644 cases and 2038 controls. *Pathol. Res. Pract.* **2018**, *214*, 467–474. [CrossRef] [PubMed]

8

Identification of Clonality through Genomic Profile Analysis in Multiple Lung Cancers

Rumi Higuchi [1,†], Takahiro Nakagomi [1,2,†], Taichiro Goto [1,2,*], Yosuke Hirotsu [3,†], Daichi Shikata [1], Yujiro Yokoyama [1,2], Sotaro Otake [1], Kenji Amemiya [3], Toshio Oyama [4], Hitoshi Mochizuki [3] and Masao Omata [3,5]

1. Lung Cancer and Respiratory Disease Center, Yamanashi Central Hospital, Yamanashi 400-8506, Japan; lumi.hgc.236@gmail.com (R.H.); nakagomi.takahiro@gmail.com (T.N.); shikarupd@yahoo.co.jp (D.S.); dooogooodooo@me.com (Y.Y.); sotaro.otake@gmail.com (S.O.)
2. Department of Surgery, School of Medicine, Keio University, Tokyo 160-8582, Japan
3. Genome Analysis Center, Yamanashi Central Hospital, Yamanashi 400-8506, Japan; hirotsu-bdyu@ych.pref.yamanashi.jp (Y.H.); amemiya-bdcd@ych.pref.yamanashi.jp (K.A.); h-mochiduki2a@ych.pref.yamanashi.jp (H.M.); m-omata0901@ych.pref.yamanashi.jp (M.O.)
4. Department of Pathology, Yamanashi Central Hospital, Yamanashi 400-8506, Japan; t-oyama@ych.pref.yamanashi.jp
5. Department of Gastroenterology, The University of Tokyo Hospital, Tokyo 113-8655, Japan

* Correspondence: taichiro@1997.jukuin.keio.ac.jp

† These authors contributed equally to this work.

Abstract: In cases of multiple lung cancers, individual tumors may represent either a primary lung cancer or both primary and metastatic lung cancers. In this study, we investigated the differences between clinical/histopathological and genomic diagnoses to determine whether they are primary or metastatic. 37 patients with multiple lung cancers were enrolled in this study. Tumor cells were selected from tissue samples using laser capture microdissection. DNA was extracted from those cells and subjected to targeted deep sequencing. In multicentric primary lung cancers, the driver mutation profile was mutually exclusive among the individual tumors, while it was consistent between metastasized tumors and the primary lesion. In 11 patients (29.7%), discrepancies were observed between genomic and clinical/histopathological diagnoses. For the lymph node metastatic lesions, the mutation profile was consistent with only one of the two primary lesions. In three of five cases with lymph node metastases, the lymph node metastatic route detected by genomic diagnosis differed from the clinical and/or pathological diagnoses. In conclusion, in patients with multiple primary lung cancers, cancer-specific mutations can serve as clonal markers, affording a more accurate understanding of the pathology of multiple lung cancers and their lymphatic metastases and thus improving both the treatment selection and outcome.

Keywords: lung cancer; multiple cancers; metastasis; sequencing; mutation; genomic diagnosis

1. Introduction

In patients with synchronous or metachronous multiple cancers, individual tumors may appear as either a primary lung cancer or both primary and metastatic lung cancers. The selection of treatment in such cases is dependent on the resulting characteristics. In patients with multiple lung cancers, the nature of a tumor (i.e., whether it is metastatic or primary) can usually be judged on the basis of diagnostic imaging findings, clinical course, and/or pathology. If individual tumors composing multiple lung cancers are histologically inconsistent in terms of histological morphology and/or cellular atypism, the multiple onset of primary cancers is highly likely. However, there are no specific radiological, clinical or histological features that can be utilized to unambiguously distinguish intrapulmonary metastases from multiple primary cancers and the cut diagnosis can be perplexing in the clinical setting. The differing biological activities of tumors allow for prognostic distinctions to be drawn and patients with intrapulmonary metastasis are supposed to have a poorer prognosis. Therefore, it is critically important to develop improved methods for the identification of tumors by exploring new, practical techniques and markers. We have previously demonstrated that as a more precise and clinically applicable method, a comparison of the driver mutation profiles enables elucidation of the clonal origin of tumors and thus facilitates an accurate discrimination between primary and metastatic tumors [1]. However, this finding was based on only 12 multiple lung cancer cases; hence, validation through a study involving a larger number of such cases was needed. Moreover, the significance of these findings in the clinical setting remained to be determined. In view of this, we extended the case accrual period to 5 years and included 37 patients with multiple lung cancers in the present study. In addition, we analyzed the clinical course in individual patients in detail to examine the use of mutation data for the diagnosis of multiple lung cancers in clinical practice and to determine the actual contribution of this approach to an improvement of clinical practice. Furthermore, we analyzed gene mutations in primary lung cancers as well as metastatic lymph nodes and genetically examined the pathology of the metastatic lymph nodes to accurately understand the pathology of lymphatic metastasis and thus enhance the postoperative treatment outcome.

2. Methods

2.1. Patients and Sample Preparation

The study enrolled 37 patients who had undergone surgery for multiple lung cancers in our department between January 2015 and July 2019. Written informed consent for genetic research was obtained from all patients, which was performed in accordance with protocols approved by the institutional review board in our hospital. Histological typing was performed according to the World Health Organisation (WHO) classification (3rd edition) [2] and clinical staging was performed according to the International Union Against Cancer Tumor-Node-Metastasis (TNM) classification (8th edition) [3].

A serial section from formalin-fixed, paraffin-embedded (FFPE) tissue was stained with hematoxylin-eosin and subsequently microdissected using an ArcturusXT laser capture microdissection system (Thermo Fisher Scientific, Tokyo, Japan). DNA was extracted using the QIAamp DNA FFPE Tissue Kit (Qiagen, Tokyo, Japan). FFPE DNA quality was verified using primers for the ribonuclease P locus. Peripheral blood was drawn from each patient immediately before surgery. A buffy coat was isolated by centrifugation and DNA was extracted from these cells using the QIAamp DNA Blood Mini Kit (Qiagen).

2.2. Targeted Deep Sequencing and Data Analysis

A panel covering the exons of 53 lung cancer-related genes (see Supplementary Table S1) was designed in-house to perform targeted sequencing. These genes were selected after a literature search based on the following criteria: (a) genes involved in lung cancer according to The Cancer Genome Atlas [4,5] and other, similar projects [6–10] or (b) genes frequently mutated in lung cancer according to the Catalogue Of Somatic Mutations In Cancer (COSMIC) database [11]. Ion AmpliSeq designer software (Thermo Fisher Scientific) was utilized for the primer composition, as previously reported [1,12,13]. An Ion AmpliSeq Library kit (Thermo Fisher Scientific) was utilized for the preparation of sequencing libraries. The library samples were bar-coded with an Ion Xpress Barcode Adapters kit (Thermo Fisher Scientific), purified using Agencourt AMPure XP reagent (Beckman Coulter, Tokyo, Japan) and subsequently quantified using an Ion Library Quantitation Kit (Thermo Fisher Scientific). The libraries were templated with an Ion PI Template OT2 200 Kit v3 (Thermo

Fisher Scientific). Sequencing was performed on Ion Proton (Ion Torrent) with an Ion PI Sequencing 200 Kit v3.

The sequence data were processed on standard Ion Torrent Suite Software. Raw signal data were measured using the Torrent Suite version 4.0. The pipeline consisted of signaling processing, base calling, quality score assignment, read alignment to the human genome 19 reference (hg19), mapping quality control and coverage analysis. After the data analysis, the annotation of single-nucleotide variants and indels (insertions and deletions) was performed on the Ion Reporter Server System (Thermo Fisher Scientific). Blood cell DNA extracted from the peripheral blood was used as a normal control to detect variants (Tumor-Normal pair analysis). Sequencing data were visually analyzed using an Integrative Genomics Viewer.

3. Results

3.1. Patient Characteristics

The 37 patients recruited in this study (age range, 54–85 years; mean age, 70.5 ± 7.5 years) were divided into different groups according to the following characteristics (Supplementary Table S2): 31 males, 6 females; 30 smokers, 7 non-smokers; and pathological stage IA (n = 10), IB (n = 15), IIA (n = 2), IIB (n = 4), IIIA (n = 5) and IIIB (n = 1). The maximum tumor diameter ranged from 2 mm to 80 mm (mean tumor diameter, 24.5 ± 15.9 mm).

Twenty nine patients were diagnosed with double or triple primary lung cancers on the basis of histopathological characteristics, including 15 patients with adenocarcinoma–adenocarcinoma, 3 patients with squamous cell carcinoma–squamous cell carcinoma, 5 patients with adenocarcinoma–squamous cell carcinoma and 6 patients with other combinations. In terms of tumor development, tumors developed synchronously and metachronously in 26 and 11 patients, respectively. In patients with metachronous tumors, the tumors were designated as tumor 1 (T1), T2 and T3 in chronological order from the earliest to the latest. In those with synchronous tumors, this designation was based on the order of size from the largest to the smallest.

3.2. Targeted Sequencing Identified Somatic Mutations in the Lung Cancers

Targeted sequencing was performed on 76 surgically resected tumors and 8 lymph nodes obtained from 37 patients, with their blood cell samples utilized as normal controls. The mean coverage depth was 1411-fold for cancer samples (range, 106- to 5096-fold) and 1387-fold for blood cell samples (range, 76- to 6960-fold). Sequence analyses detected 314 somatic mutations with an allele fraction ≥1% from 84 cancer lesions (1–54 mutations per tumor) (Supplementary Table S3). Among these mutations, 137 mutations (44%) were present at an allele fraction ≥20% (Supplementary Table S3).

In 29 patients, the gene, amino-acid substitution and nucleotide changes that were caused by these somatic mutations within individual tumors composing the multiple lung cancers lacked consistency (Figure 1, Supplementary Table S3). Thus, there were no shared or overlapping mutations among the individual lung cancers detected in these patients. This finding demonstrated that the multiple lung cancers in these cases were independently developed primary lung cancers (Figure 1). Meanwhile, in 8 patients, the gene mutation profile was consistent among the individual tumors, suggesting the presence of intrapulmonary metastasis (Figure 2). Importantly, in these cases, nucleotide position and mutation variance were entirely consistent across the tumors (Supplementary Table S3).

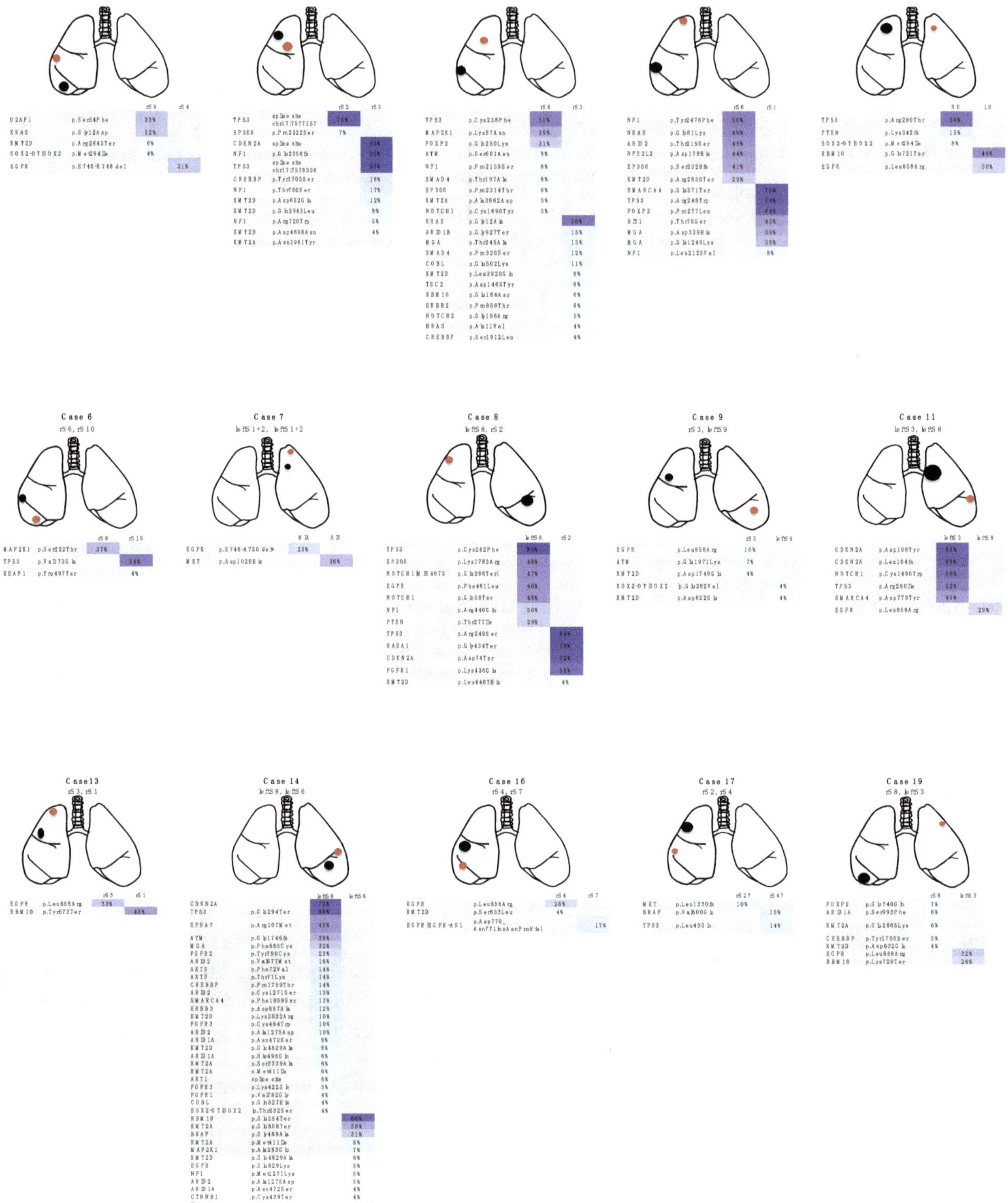

Figure 1. *Cont.*

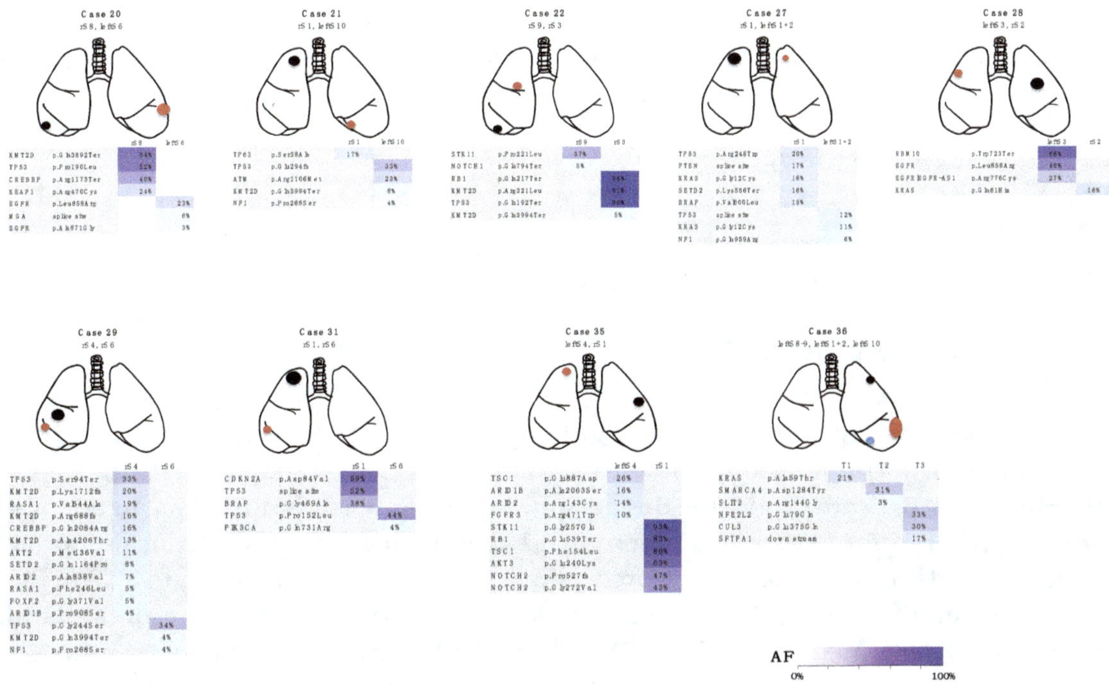

Figure 1. Heatmap of gene mutations in patients with double or triple primary lung cancers. These maps visualize the gene mutations in each cancer. Two or three lung cancers in each patient were characterized by different mutation profiles and all patients were diagnosed with double or triple primary lung cancers. Case 21, 22 and 28 were metachronous cancers, while the other cases in this figure were synchronous cancers. The remaining 5 cases of double primary lung cancers (cases 12, 18, 24, 26 and 34 in Table 1 and Table S2) that are not shown in this figure are described in detail in the Case presentation section. Black, red and blue indicate tumor 1 (T1), T2 and T3, respectively. r, right; S, segment; AF, allele fraction; MIA, microinvasive adenocarcinoma; AIS, adenocarcinoma in situ.

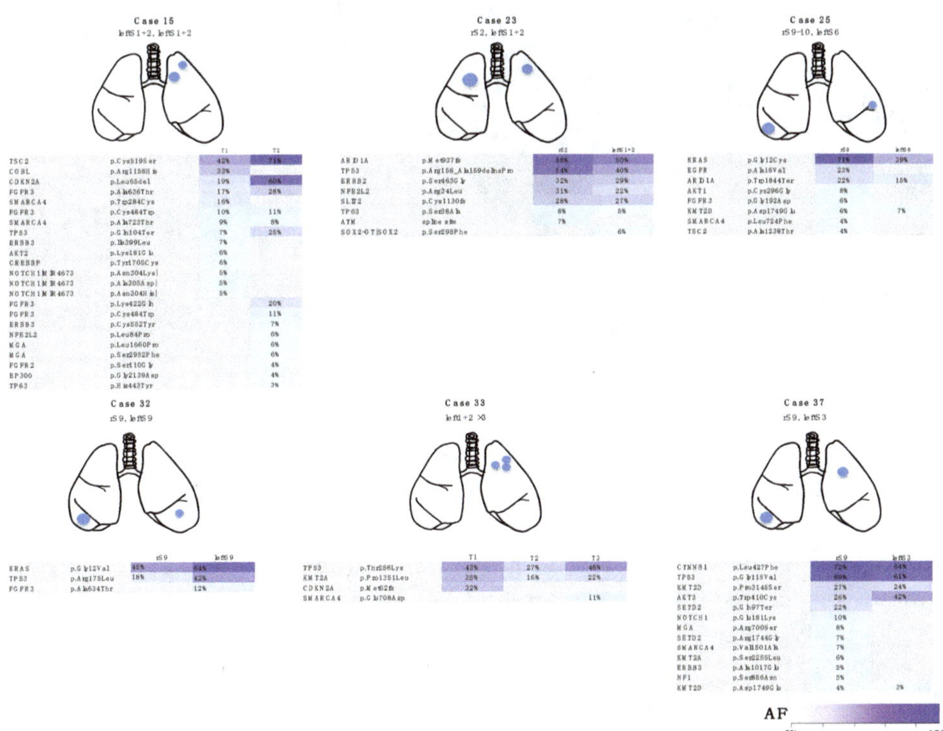

Figure 2. Heatmap of gene mutations in patients with metastatic lung cancers. The mutation profiles were consistent between the individual tumors in each case and the tumors were identified as

intrapulmonary metastasis. Case 33 was synchronous cancers, while the other cases in this figure were metachronous cancers. The remaining 2 cases of metastatic lung cancers (cases 10 and 30 in Table 1 and Table S2) that are not shown in this figure are described in detail in the Case presentation section. r, right; S, segment; AF, allele fraction.

3.3. *Case Presentations*

Three Representative Cases are Described in Detail Below

Case A (Case 30 in Table 1 and Table S2)

A 74-year-old man had two tumors in the right upper lobe that were resected through right upper lobectomy. Both tumors morphologically had an irregular surface; thus, they were diagnosed as primary lung cancers (Figure 3A,B). Pathologically, the peripheral lesion was identified as an adenosquamous carcinoma comprised of squamous cell carcinoma and acinar-predominant adenocarcinoma, whereas the central lesion was identified as papillary-predominant adenocarcinoma (Figure 3C,D). On the basis of the histopathological differences, the tumors were judged as double primary tumors. Pathologically, the cancer stage was determined to be pT1cN2M0, stage IIIA. However, the genetic mutation profiles were completely consistent between these two tumors, suggesting they are metastases (Figure 3E). Moreover, their mutation profiles were also consistent with the mutation profile of the metastatic lymph node. (Figure 3E). Based on the genetic diagnosis, the cancer stage was ultimately upgraded to T3N2M0, stage IIIB. At the patient's request, he was placed on follow-up without any postoperative adjuvant chemotherapy. The patient has remained alive for 2 years postoperatively without any recurrence.

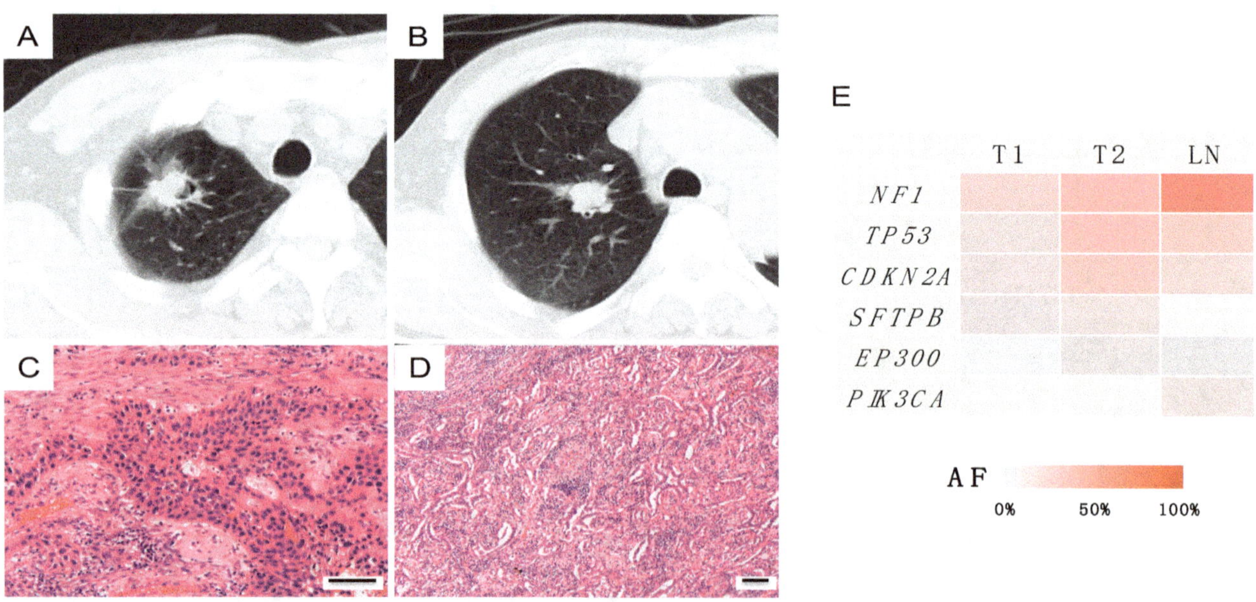

Figure 3. Radiological, histopathological and genomic findings in case A. (**A**,**B**) Right upper lobe nodules: one tumor was located in the peripheral region, whereas the other was located in the central region. (**C**) Histologically, the peripheral tumor (T1) was identified as an adenosquamous carcinoma. (**D**) The central tumor (T2) was histologically identified as an adenocarcinoma. Each scale bar indicates 100 μm. (**E**) The heatmap revealed that the same mutation profiles were shared by the two tumors and the lymph node metastasis. AF, allele fraction; LN, lymph node

Case B (Case 10 in Table 1 and Table S2)

A 59-year-old woman presented with 0.7-cm nodules in the right lower lobe 1.5 years after undergoing right upper lobectomy for cancer. The tumors were round and had a smooth surface. Because of their morphology, they were suspected of being metastatic lesions. After 4 months of follow-up, there was no increase in the number of lung lesions, suggesting solitary intrapulmonary metastasis. Subsequently, wedge resection was performed. Although both tumors were pathologically papillary-predominant adenocarcinoma (Figure 4C,D), a lepidic pattern was observed in the periphery of the smaller nodule (Figure 4E), leading to a diagnosis of double primary lung cancers. However, the genetic mutation profile was consistent between the two tumors, suggesting them to be metastases (Figure 4F). The patient was positive for a mutation in the epidermal growth factor receptor (EGFR) gene (exon 19 deletion); hence, oral administration of an EGFR-tyrosine kinase inhibitor (gefitinib) was continued. The patient has remained alive without recurrence for 4 years after the second surgery.

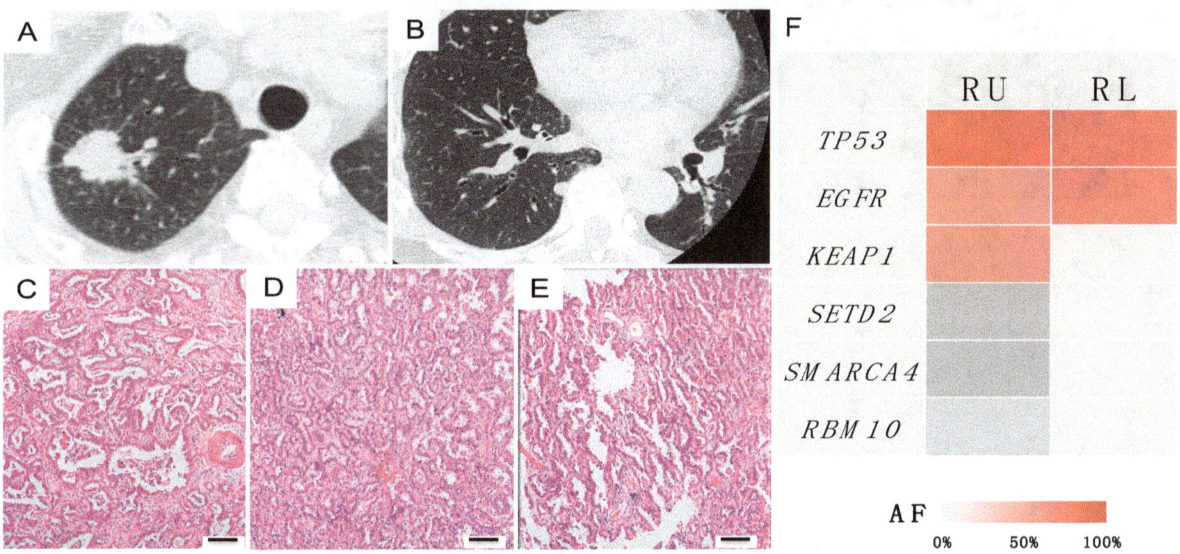

Figure 4. Radiological, histopathological and genomic findings in case B. (**A**) Lung cancer in the right upper lobe. (**B**) A small nodule in the right lower lobe. (**C**) Histology of the lung cancer in the right upper lobe. (**D**,**E**) Histology of the nodule in the right lower lobe. A lepidic pattern was observed in the periphery of the small nodule. Each scale bar indicates 100 μm. (**F**) Heatmap of the gene mutations of the two lung tumors. The significant mutations identified in the right upper lobe tumor were homologous with those detected in the right lower lobe tumor. RU, right upper lobe; RL, right lower lobe; AF, allele fraction

Case C (Case 18 in Table 1 and Table S2)

A 74-year-old man presented with tumors measuring 4.0 cm and 1.8 cm in the left upper lobe, so left upper lobectomy was performed (Figure 5A,B). As both tumors were closely located and pathologically similar squamous cell carcinomas, they were assumed to be single origin pulmonary metastases (Figure 5C,D). However, the mutation profile was completely different between the two tumors genetically, suggesting double primary cancers (Figure 5E).

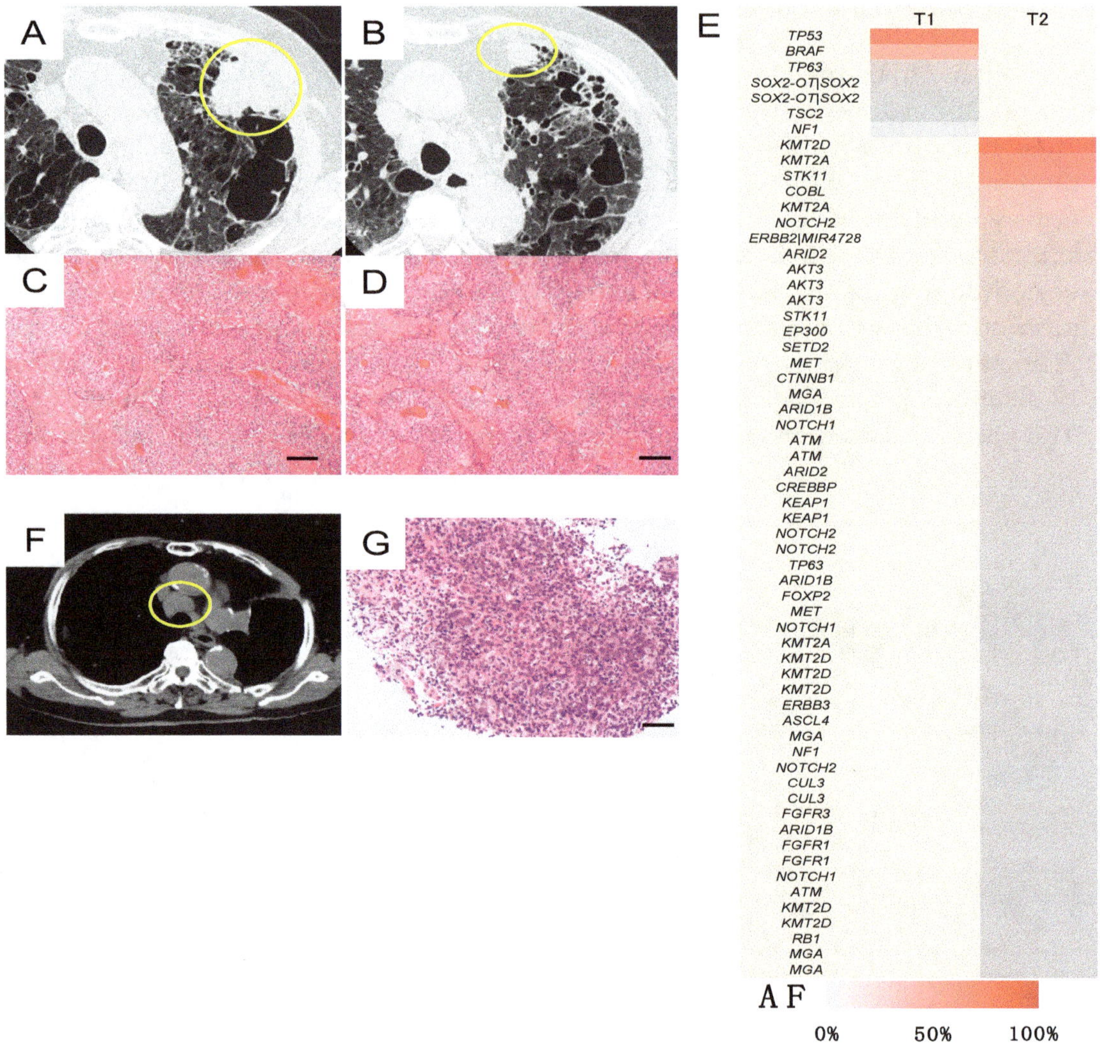

Figure 5. Radiological, histopathological and genomic findings in case C. (**A**,**B**) Two tumors, a large one (T1) and a small one (T2), were located in the left upper lobe in proximity to each other. (**C**,**D**) The tumors exhibited a similar histology of squamous cell carcinoma. Each scale bar indicates 100 µm. (**E**) Heatmap of the gene mutations of the two lung tumors. The mutation profiles of T1 and T2 were completely different. (**F**,**G**) Postoperatively, tracheobronchial lymph node enlargement was observed and the tumor was identified as a squamous cell carcinoma. Each scale bar indicates 100 µm. AF, allele fraction.

3.4. Investigation of the Discrepancies between the Clinical and/or Histopathological Diagnoses and Genetic Diagnosis

Table 1 shows the discrepancies between and among the clinical, pathological and genetic diagnoses of the primary or metastatic lesions in all 37 patients. The clinical diagnoses were comprehensively determined, mainly on the basis of imaging findings and clinical course by the cancer board of the hospital (comprised of thoracic surgeons, pulmonologists, pathologists and radiologists). The pathological diagnoses were determined on the basis of the postoperative pathological findings, especially the differences in the tissue morphology and cellular atypia detected by pathologists. The genetic diagnoses were determined on the basis of digital and statistical analyses of overlaps in the mutation profiles of individual tumors. Discrepancies between the genetic diagnosis and clinical and/or histopathological diagnoses were observed in 11 patients (29.7%). In the patients with synchronous tumors, primary and metastatic tumors were eventually diagnosed on the basis of genetic diagnosis in 24 and 2 patients, respectively. In the 11 patients with metachronous tumors, primary and metastatic tumors were diagnosed in 5 and 6 patients, respectively, in the same manner. The distribution of primary and metastatic tumors between synchronous and metachronous tumors was significantly different; thus synchronous multiple lung tumors were deemed likely to be primary lesions.

Table 1. Mutation analysis of the multiple lung cancers.

Case	Occurrence of Tumors	Interval between the 1st and 2nd Tumors	Clinical Dx	Pathological Dx	Genomic Dx
1	Synchronous	-	Double	Double	Double
2	Synchronous	-	Double	Double	Double
3	Synchronous	-	Double	Double	Double
4	Synchronous	-	Metastasis	Metastasis	Double *
5	Synchronous	-	Double	Double	Double
6	Synchronous	-	Double	Double	Double
7	Synchronous	-	Double	Double	Double
8	Synchronous	-	Double	Double	Double
9	Synchronous	-	Double	Double	Double
10	Metachronous	14 months	Metastasis	Double	Metastasis *
11	Synchronous	-	Double	Double	Double
12	Synchronous	-	Metastasis	Double	Double *
13	Synchronous	-	Double	Double	Double
14	Synchronous	-	Double	Double	Double
15	Metachronous	15 months	Double	Metastasis	Metastasis *
16	Synchronous	-	Double	Double	Double
17	Synchronous	-	Double	Double	Double
18	Synchronous	-	Metastasis	Metastasis	Double *
19	Synchronous	-	Double	Double	Double
20	Synchronous	-	Double	Double	Double
21	Metachronous	17 months	Double	Double	Double
22	Metachronous	28 months	Double	Double	Double
23	Metachronous	23 months	Double	Metastasis	Metastasis *
24	Metachronous	37 months	Double	Double	Double
25	Metachronous	37 months	Double	Double	Metastasis *
26	Synchronous	-	Double	Double	Double
27	Synchronous	-	Double	Double	Double
28	Metachronous	41 months	Double	Double	Double
29	Synchronous	-	Double	Double	Double
30	Synchronous	-	Double	Double	Metastasis *
31	Synchronous	-	Double	Double	Double
32	Metachronous	16 months	Double	Metastasis	Metastasis *
33	Synchronous	-	Double	Metastasis	Metastasis *
34	Metachronous	13 months	Double	Double	Double
35	Synchronous	-	Double	Double	Double
36	Synchronous	-	triple	triple	triple
37	Metachronous	46 months	Double	Double	Metastasis *

The cases in which the diagnoses were inconsistent in the clinicopathological and genetic examinations are indicated by *.

3.5. Genetic Diagnosis of Lymph Node Metastasis in Patients with Multiple Lung Cancers

Lymph node metastasis was detected in five patients with double primary lung cancers (Table 2). It occurred approximately at the time of surgery in three patients and was identified as postoperative lymph node recurrence in two patients (Table 2). In some patients, the route of lymph node metastasis was apparent from the timing of the metastasis as well as the location and pathological findings of the metastatic lesions (cases 4 and 5 in Table 2). In contrast, it was difficult to identify the clonal origin of lymph node metastasis on the basis of the clinical and pathological findings in the other patients, especially in those in whom the primary lesions were both squamous cell carcinomas (cases 1–3 in Table 2). However, even in these patients, a comparison of the mutation profiles of the primary and lymph node metastatic lesions revealed the route of lymph node metastasis (Figure 6).

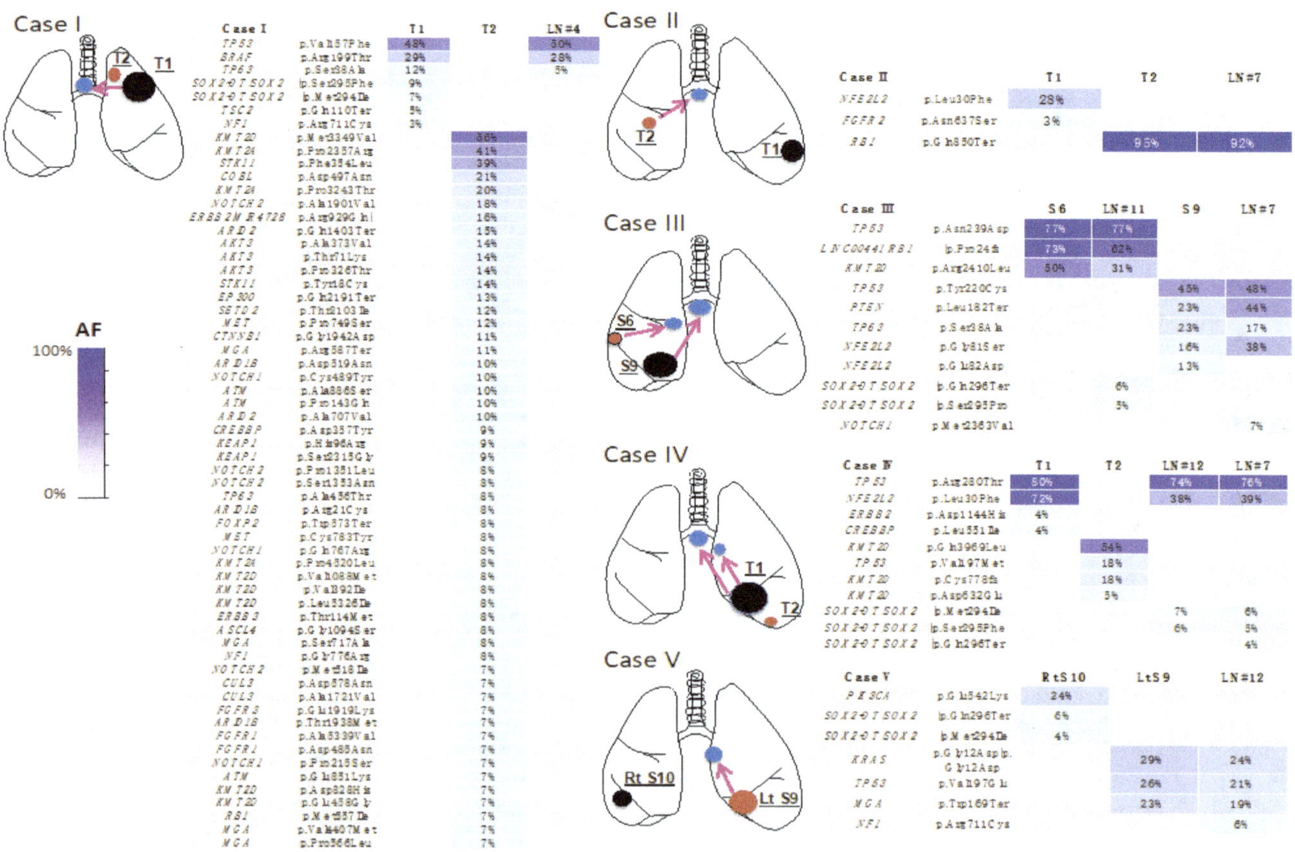

Figure 6. Schema of lymphatic metastasis and mutation profiles in multiple lung cancers. On the basis of the coincidence and differences in the mutation profiles, the clonality of each tumor and the pathway of lymphatic progression are clearly elucidated in each case. The arrows indicate the lymphatic routes of the cancer invasion. Tumor 1 is shown in black, tumor 2 in red and lymph node metastasis in blue. #4, tracheobronchial lymph node; #7, subcarinal lymph node; #11, interlobar lymph node; and #12, hilar lymph node. S, segment; LN, lymph node; AF, allele fraction

Table 2. LN metastasis in patients with multiple lung cancers.

Case	Case No. in Table 1	Location and Histology of T1	Location and Histology of T2	Location and Histology of LN	LN Biopsy Method	Occurrence of LN Metastasis	Inconsistency between Clinical and Genomic Diagnoses
I	18	Left upper, Sq	Left upper, Sq	Right tracheobronchial, Sq	EBUS-TBNA	Postoperative	+
II	34	Left lower, Sq	Middle, Sq	Subcarinal, Sq	EBUS-TBNA	Postoperative	+
III	26	Right S9, Sq	Right S6, Sq	Interlobar and subcarinal, Sq	Surgery	Simultaneous	+
IV	12	Left S6, Sq	Left S10, small	Subcarinal, Sq	Surgery	Simultaneous	–
V	24	Right lower, acinar Ad	Left lower, solid Ad	Left lobar, solid Ad	Surgery	Simultaneous	–

S, segment; LN, lymph node; Sq, squamous cell carcinoma; Ad, adenocarcinoma; small, small cell carcinoma; EBUS-TBNA, endobronchial ultrasound-guided transbronchial needle aspiration.

3.6. Case Presentations

Three Representative Cases are Described in Detail Below

Case D (Case I in Table 2 and Figure 6)

A 74-year-old man, described as case C in the previous section, presented with paratracheal and mediastinal lymph node metastases 1 year after left upper lobectomy (Figure 5F). Although it was not possible to pathologically identify the metastasizing primary lesion (Figure 5G), the mutation profile of the metastatic lymph node was genetically consistent with that of the larger cancer. The genetic diagnosis was lymph node metastasis of the larger cancer (Figure 6).

Case E (Case II in Table 2 and Figure 6)

A 77-year-old man with lung cancer underwent left lower lobectomy (Figure 7A). One year later, a nodule appeared in the middle lobe (Figure 7B). Middle lobectomy was performed based on the assumption that the lesion was a double primary tumor. However, after 1 year, subcarinal lymph node metastasis occurred (Figure 7C). Pathologically, all three lesions were of squamous cell carcinoma type and it was impossible to determine which primary lesion had metastasized (Figure 7D–F). Given the tumor size, the tumor in the left lobe was clinically more likely to have metastasized. However, mutation analysis revealed that the two lung lesions had different mutation profiles; therefore, they were diagnosed as double primary lung cancers. Furthermore, the mutation profiles were consistent between the middle lobe lung cancer and the metastatic lymph node. Thus, lymph node metastasis of the middle lobe lung cancer was determined (Figure 6). Programmed death-ligand 1 (PD-L1) staining of tumor cells was 0% and 90% in the left lower lobe and middle lobe tumors, respectively. Treatment with an anti-PD-1 antibody (nivolumab) was administered and a complete response has been maintained for 1 year since the recurrence in the lymph node.

Case F (Case III in Table 2 and Figure 6)

A 72-year-old man presented with two tumors in the right lower lobe. Imaging findings suggested double primary lung cancers and right lower lobectomy was performed (Figure 7G,H). Postoperative pathological examination revealed metastases in the interlobar and subcarinal lymph nodes. All four lesions, including the double primary lesions and two metastatic lymph nodes, were pathologically similar squamous cell carcinomas. Therefore, it was impossible to determine which primary lesion had metastasized to the lymph nodes (Figure 7I–L). Clinically, the larger segment 9 tumor was likely to have metastasized to the two lymph nodes. However, both segment 6 and 9 tumors, which had different mutation profiles, were genetically identified as double primary lung cancers. In addition, it was found that the larger segment 9 tumor had metastasized to the interlobar lymph node, whereas the smaller segment 6 tumor had metastasized to the subcarinal lymph node (Figure 6). PD-L1 staining of tumor cells was 0% and 70% in the segment 9 and segment 6 tumors, respectively. Despite the administration of an anti-PD-1 antibody (nivolumab), the patient did not respond to the treatment and died of progression of the cancer at 17 months postoperatively.

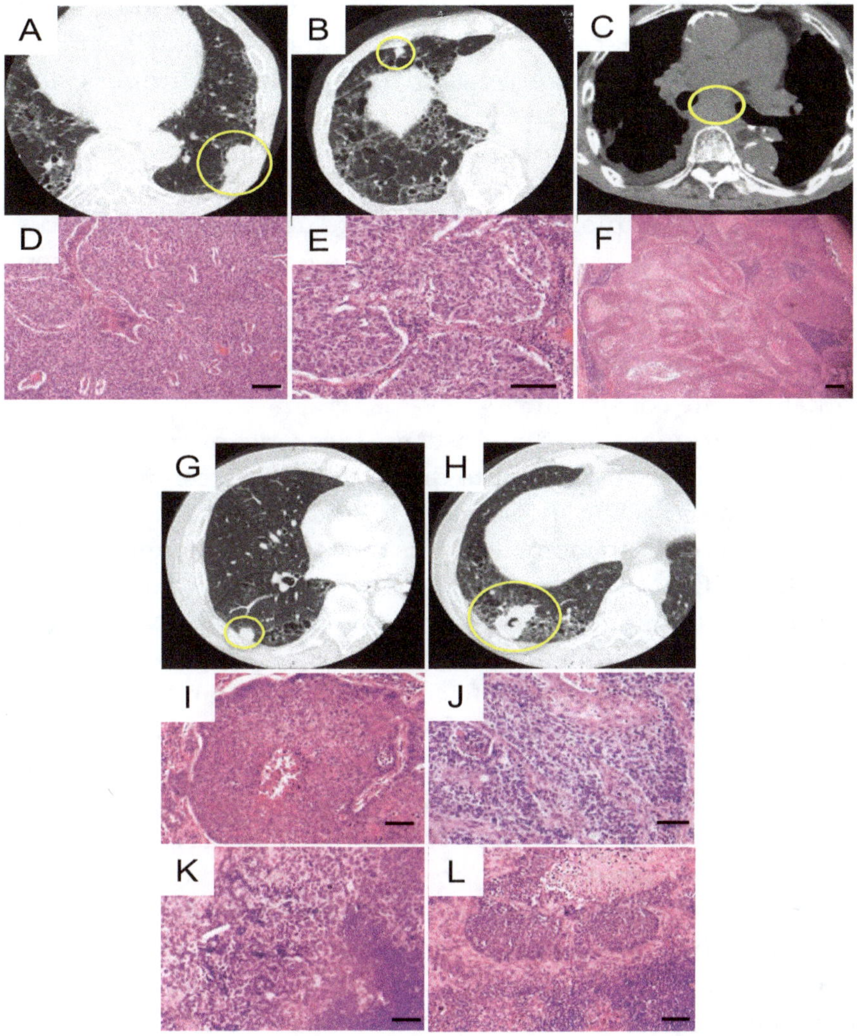

Figure 7. Radiological and histopathological findings in cases E and F. (**A–F**) Findings in case E. (**A**) Primary lesion in the left lower lobe. (**B**) Primary lesion in the middle lobe. (**C**) Subcarinal lymph node metastasis. (**D–F**) The three lesions displayed a similar histology of squamous cell carcinoma. (**G–L**) Findings in case F. (**G**) Primary lesion in right segment 6. (**H**) Primary lesion in right segment 9. (**I**) Histology of the primary lesion in segment 6. (**J**) Histology of the primary lesion in segment 9. (**K**) Histology of the subcarinal lymph node. (**L**) Histology of the interlobar lymph node. Histologically, the four lesions displayed a similar histology of squamous cell carcinoma. Each scale bar indicates 100 μm.

4. Discussion

In cases of multiple lung cancers, clinical differentiation between primary and metastatic tumors can be difficult, rendering treatment selection challenging. Furthermore, in patients with multiple lung cancers metastasized to the lymph nodes or distal sites, the focus of treatment varies depending on the cancer that has metastasized. Thus, determining the origin of the metastasizing cancer is clinically important. Therefore, we performed lung cancer mutation analysis through targeted deep sequencing and demonstrated that mutations of individual lung cancers are able to provide clonal markers, enabling discrimination of the clonal origin of multiple lung cancers and their metastases.

The consistency of mutations across multiple sites, with complete concordance in the position and patterns of base-pair substitutions or indels, cannot be a coincidental phenomenon. Although discordance between two tumors was noted in mutations with an allele fraction <20%, this can be interpreted as tumor heterogeneity [14]. In general, cancers comprise populations of cells with various molecular and phenotypic features, a phenomenon termed intratumor heterogeneity [14,15]. This may bolster tumor adaptation, cancer progression and metastasis, and/or therapeutic failure through negative selection [14,16]. Conversely, a driver mutation triggers clonal expansion and is retained ubiquitously within the tumors of the same clone [16,17]. These theories can be interpreted as the "trunk and branch" mutation models; early somatic events that drive tumor progress in early clonal founders are represented by the "trunk" of the tumor [18,19]. Such trunk somatic mutations to be found at the early stages of tumor development are ubiquitous events occurring at all sites of disease. Meanwhile, later somatic events that occur in the wake of branched separation of subclones represent heterogeneity. Such subclonal heterogeneity may be spatially divided among regions of the same tumor or its metastatic sites [18–20]. In this context, clonally dominant mutations are important clonal markers. Primary and metastatic tumors can be differentiated by determining whether such ubiquitous driver mutations are consistent.

It is relatively straightforward to diagnose multicentric primary lung cancers of different histological type. However, it is often difficult to differentiate between multiple primary lung cancers and intrapulmonary metastases having the same histological type. In particular, in cases of multiple tumors classified as squamous cell carcinoma (such as cases C–F), differentiation based on pathological features alone is extremely difficult. Even when the morphological and immunohistological features are non-homogeneous among different parts of the tumors (e.g., cases A and B), the driver mutation is ubiquitously retained within the tumors of the same clone [16,17]. Therefore, distinction of clonality on the basis of mutation analysis is more specific and definitive than histological examination.

Detterbeck et al. reviewed the clinical and pathological criteria to distinguish second primary tumors from metastatic tumors [21]. They reported that it is impracticable to define criteria that conclusively establish the identical nature of tumors; merely finding observable similarities between tumors is insufficient. Using the method described, comprehensive mutation analysis is initially performed to identify the driver mutations in each cancer, which are subsequently compared to define their clonal origin. These criteria are definitive and reliable. Moreover, the decision criteria are generally clear and intuitive. In fact, this method yielded clear genetic diagnosis in all patients. In other words, no equivocal or ambiguous diagnosis was obtained in any of the cases. In our previous study, we had demonstrated that this method allows bronchoscopic biopsy samples and other small samples to be used for discrimination between primary and metastatic tumors [1]. Thus, our method may enable both flexible and rational decision-making based on accurate diagnosis. For example, a preoperative diagnosis of metastatic tumors may make it possible to avoid surgery, whereas a preoperative diagnosis of primary tumors would lead to surgical treatment. This novel approach may help resolve the dilemma of misdiagnosis in the clinical setting. Thus, we anticipate that it will come to be utilized as a standard diagnostic approach in daily clinical practice in the near future.

When selecting treatment methods for multiple lung cancers, it is necessary to consider the cancer type will markedly affect the prognosis. In cases D–F that have lymph node metastasis, a factor responsible for progression to an advanced stage was identified in the two tumors. Furthermore, the tumors exhibit different mutation profiles and PD-L1 staining properties. Therefore, the lesions targeted for treatment and the options selected for subsequent treatment (e.g., molecular-targeted drugs and immune checkpoint inhibitors) vary depending on the type of tumor that has metastasized to the lymph nodes. This suggests that accurate understanding of the pathology gained by performing a genetic diagnosis can exert a powerful effect on the clinical outcome. Although the use of immunotherapy has revolutionized the treatment of non-small-cell lung cancer, patterns of immunostaining with PD-L1, a biomarker for treatment response, may vary in tumor cells across individual primary tumors (e.g., (,) cases E and F) [22]. At present, molecularly targeted therapies are also rapidly evolving. The development of novel molecularly targeted therapies would enable the treatment to be specifically tailored to the features of mutations detected in individual cancers. Thus, in patients with multiple lung cancers, performing a mutation analysis helps select the medical treatment most likely to be effective.

5. Conclusions

In cases of multiple lung cancers, identifying the differences in the mutation profiles of multiple tumors will help determine their clonal origin and enable a distinction to be drawn between primary and metastatic tumors with great specificity, even in cases in which pathological distinction is impossible or equivocal. In addition, performing genetic diagnosis in addition to pathological diagnosis can help obtain a more accurate understanding of the pathology of multiple lung cancers and the lymphatic metastases. This approach may lead to the provision of treatment specifically tailored to the features of individual cases.

Author Contributions: T.G., Y.H., R.H. and T.N. wrote the manuscript. T.G., T.N., D.S., R.H., S.O. and Y.Y. performed the surgery. T.O., D.S. and R.H. carried out the pathological examination. Y.H., K.A., T.G., T.N., Y.Y., H.M., R.H., S.O. and M.O. participated in the genomic analyses. M.O. and Y.H. edited the final manuscript. All authors have read and agreed to the published version of the manuscript.

Acknowledgments: The authors greatly appreciate Hidetoshi Shigetomo, Yumi Kubota, Ritsuko Yokouchi, Yumiko Kakizaki, Toshiharu Tsutsui and Yoshihiro Miyashita for helpful scientific discussion.

References

1. Goto, T.; Hirotsu, Y.; Mochizuki, H.; Nakagomi, T.; Shikata, D.; Yokoyama, Y.; Oyama, T.; Amemiya, K.; Okimoto, K.; Omata, M. Mutational analysis of multiple lung cancers: Discrimination between primary and metastatic lung cancers by genomic profile. *Oncotarget* **2017**, *8*, 31133–31143. [CrossRef] [PubMed]
2. Gibbs, A.R.; Thunnissen, F.B. Histological typing of lung and pleural tumours: Third edition. *J. Clin. Pathol.* **2001**, *54*, 498–499. [CrossRef]
3. Chansky, K.; Detterbeck, F.C.; Nicholson, A.G.; Rusch, V.W.; Vallieres, E.; Groome, P.; Kennedy, C.; Krasnik, M.; Peake, M.; Shemanski, L.; et al. The IASLC Lung Cancer Staging Project: External Validation of the Revision of the TNM Stage Groupings in the Eighth Edition of the TNM Classification of Lung Cancer. *J. Thorac. Oncol.* **2017**, *12*, 1109–1121. [CrossRef]
4. Cancer Genome Atlas Research Network. Comprehensive molecular profiling of lung adenocarcinoma. *Nature* **2014**, *511*, 543–550. [CrossRef] [PubMed]
5. Cancer Genome Atlas Research Network. Comprehensive genomic characterization of squamous cell lung cancers. *Nature* **2012**, *489*, 519–525. [CrossRef] [PubMed]
6. Clinical Lung Cancer Genome Project (CLCGP); Network Genomic Medicine (NGM). A genomics-based classification of human lung tumors. *Sci. Transl. Med.* **2013**, *5*, 209ra153.
7. Rudin, C.M.; Durinck, S.; Stawiski, E.W.; Poirier, J.T.; Modrusan, Z.; Shames, D.S.; Bergbower, E.A.; Guan, Y.; Shin, J.; Guillory, J.; et al. Comprehensive genomic analysis identifies SOX2 as a frequently amplified gene in small-cell lung cancer. *Nat. Genet.* **2012**, *44*, 1111–1116. [CrossRef]
8. Peifer, M.; Fernandez-Cuesta, L.; Sos, M.L.; George, J.; Seidel, D.; Kasper, L.H.; Plenker, D.; Leenders, F.; Sun, R.; Zander, T.; et al. Integrative genome analyses identify key somatic driver mutations of small-cell lung cancer. *Nat. Genet.* **2012**, *44*, 1104–1110. [CrossRef]
9. Imielinski, M.; Berger, A.H.; Hammerman, P.S.; Hernandez, B.; Pugh, T.J.; Hodis, E.; Cho, J.; Suh, J.; Capelletti, M.; Sivachenko, A.; et al. Mapping the hallmarks of lung adenocarcinoma with massively parallel sequencing. *Cell* **2012**, *150*, 1107–1120. [CrossRef]
10. Govindan, R.; Ding, L.; Griffith, M.; Subramanian, J.; Dees, N.D.; Kanchi, K.L.; Maher, C.A.; Fulton, R.; Fulton, L.; Wallis, J.; et al. Genomic landscape of non-small cell lung cancer in smokers and never-smokers. *Cell* **2012**, *150*, 1121–1134. [CrossRef]
11. Forbes, S.A.; Beare, D.; Boutselakis, H.; Bamford, S.; Bindal, N.; Tate, J.; Cole, C.G.; Ward, S.; Dawson, E.; Ponting, L.; et al. COSMIC: Somatic cancer genetics at high-resolution. *Nucleic Acids Res.* **2017**, *45*, D777–D783. [CrossRef]
12. Goto, T.; Hirotsu, Y.; Oyama, T.; Amemiya, K.; Omata, M. Analysis of tumor-derived DNA in plasma and bone marrow fluid in lung cancer patients. *Med. Oncol.* **2016**, *33*, 29. [CrossRef] [PubMed]
13. Nakagomi, T.; Goto, T.; Hirotsu, Y.; Shikata, D.; Yokoyama, Y.; Higuchi, R.; Otake, S.; Amemiya, K.; Oyama, T.; Mochizuki, H.; et al. Genomic Characteristics of Invasive Mucinous Adenocarcinomas of the Lung and Potential Therapeutic Targets of B7-H3. *Cancers* **2018**, *10*, 487. [CrossRef]

14. Goto, T.; Hirotsu, Y.; Amemiya, K.; Mochizuki, H.; Omata, M. Understanding Intratumor Heterogeneity and Evolution in NSCLC and Potential New Therapeutic Approach. *Cancers* **2018**, *10*, 212. [CrossRef] [PubMed
15. Jamal-Hanjani, M.; Wilson, G.A.; McGranahan, N.; Birkbak, N.J.; Watkins, T.B.K.; Veeriah, S.; Shafi, S.; Johnson, D.H.; Mitter, R.; Rosenthal, R.; et al. Tracking the Evolution of Non-Small-Cell Lung Cancer. *N. Engl. J. Med.* **2017**, *376*, 2109–2121. [CrossRef]
16. Goto, T.; Hirotsu, Y.; Mochizuki, H.; Nakagomi, T.; Oyama, T.; Amemiya, K.; Omata, M. Stepwise addition of genetic changes correlated with histological change from "well-differentiated" to "sarcomatoid" phenotypes: A case report. *BMC Cancer* **2017**, *17*, 65. [CrossRef] [PubMed]
17. Yatabe, Y.; Matsuo, K.; Mitsudomi, T. Heterogeneous distribution of EGFR mutations is extremely rare in lung adenocarcinoma. *J. Clin. Oncol.* **2011**, *29*, 2972–2977. [CrossRef]
18. Swanton, C. Intratumor heterogeneity: Evolution through space and time. *Cancer Res.* **2012**, *72*, 4875–4882. [CrossRef]
19. Yap, T.A.; Gerlinger, M.; Futreal, P.A.; Pusztai, L.; Swanton, C. Intratumor heterogeneity: Seeing the wood for the trees. *Sci. Transl. Med.* **2012**, *4*, 127ps10. [CrossRef]
20. Gerlinger, M.; Rowan, A.J.; Horswell, S.; Larkin, J.; Endesfelder, D.; Gronroos, E.; Martinez, P.; Matthews, N.; Stewart, A.; Tarpey, P.; et al. Intratumor heterogeneity and branched evolution revealed by multiregion sequencing. *N. Engl. J. Med.* **2012**, *366*, 883–892. [CrossRef]
21. Detterbeck, F.C.; Nicholson, A.G.; Franklin, W.A.; Marom, E.M.; Travis, W.D.; Girard, N.; Arenberg, D.A.; Bolejack, V.; Donington, J.S.; Mazzone, P.J.; et al. The IASLC Lung Cancer Staging Project: Summary of Proposals for Revisions of the Classification of Lung Cancers with Multiple Pulmonary Sites of Involvement in the Forthcoming Eighth Edition of the TNM Classification. *J. Thorac. Oncol.* **2016**, *11*, 639–650. [CrossRef [PubMed]
22. Goto, T. Radiation as an In Situ Auto-Vaccination: Current Perspectives and Challenges. *Vaccines* **2019**, 100. [CrossRef] [PubMed]

9

HIP1R Expression and its Association with PD-1 Pathway Blockade Response in Refractory Advanced Non-Small Cell Lung Cancer: A Gene Set Enrichment Analysis

Young Wha Koh [1,*], Jae-Ho Han [1], Seokjin Haam [2] and Hyun Woo Lee [3]

1 Department of Pathology, Ajou University School of Medicine, Suwon 16499, Korea; hanpathol@naver.com
2 Department of Thoracic and Cardiovascular Surgery, Ajou University School of Medicine, Suwon 16499, Korea; haamsj@aumc.ac.kr
3 Department of Hematology-Oncology, Ajou University School of Medicine, Suwon 16499, Korea; leehw@ajou.ac.kr
* Correspondence: youngwha9556@gmail.com

Abstract: Huntingtin-interacting protein 1-related protein (HIP1R) plays an important role in the regulation of programmed death-ligand 1 (PD-L1). The aim of this study was to investigate the expression of HIP1R and confirm its predictive or prognostic roles in anti-PD-1 therapy in nonsmall cell lung cancer (NSCLC) patients. HIP1R and PD-L1 immunohistochemical expression was examined in 52 refractory advanced NSCLC patients treated with anti-PD-1 inhibitors. We performed gene set enrichment analysis (GSEA) to detect HIP1R-specific gene sets. Patients in the PD-1 inhibitor responder group had lower HIP1R expression by univariate logistic regression analysis (odds ratio (OR) = 0.235, $p = 0.015$) and multivariate logistic regression analysis (OR = 0.209, $p = 0.014$). Patients with high HIP1R expression had poorer progression-free survival (PFS) than patients with low HIP1R expression in univariate analysis ($p = 0.037$) and multivariate Cox analysis (hazard ratio = 2.098, $p = 0.019$). The web-based mRNA dataset also showed that high HIP1R expression correlated with inferior overall survival in lung adenocarcinoma ($p = 0.026$). GSEA revealed that HIP1R levels correlate with a set of genes that reflect PD-L1-related immune pathways. HIP1R expression may be a promising predictor for determination of patient responses to anti-PD-1 treatment.

Keywords: nonsmall cell lung cancer; HIP1R; PD-L1; biomarker

---

1. Introduction

Emergence of immune checkpoint inhibitors was a turning point in the treatment of advanced nonsmall cell lung cancer (NSCLC). Therapies targeting the programmed cell death protein 1 (PD-1) checkpoint, such as nivolumab and pembrolizumab, have yielded impressive responsive rates in advanced NSCLC patients otherwise refractory to multiples lines of therapy [1–3]. However, the overall response rate for PD-1 inhibitor therapy is approximately 15–20% in unselected patients with NSCLC, and between 15% and 45% in patients with PD-L1-expressing NSCLC [4]. We need a biomarker that can more accurately predict the response to PD-1 inhibitors.

Expression of programmed death ligand-1 (PD-L1), the PD-1 ligand, is currently the most widely used biomarker for PD-1 inhibition. To identify patients who preferentially respond to PD-1 blockade, we need to better understand how the PD-1 pathway is regulated. Recently, several mechanisms have been reported to underlie PD-1 pathway regulation. CKLF-like MARVEL transmembrane-domain-containing 6 (CMTM6) regulates the PD-1 pathway by maintaining the expression of PD-L1, and CMTM6 is a predictor of the response to PD-1 inhibitors [5,6]. F-box only protein 38 (FBXO38) mediates PD-1 ubiquitination of T cells, and knockout of FBXO38 in such cells induces tumor progression in a mouse model due to increased PD-1 expression by tumor-infiltrating T cells [7]. AXL expression displays a positive correlation with PD-L1 expression in lung adenocarcinoma with epidermal growth factor receptor (EGFR) mutation, and abolition of AXL kinase activity inhibits *PD-L1* mRNA expression in a lung adenocarcinoma cell line with EGFR mutation [8].

Recent research has uncovered new strategies to remove specific unwanted proteins by using cellular protein degradation mechanisms, including lysosome-targeting molecules [9], proteolysis-targeting chimeras (PROTACs) [10], and tag-based degradation systems (dTAG) [11]. Wang et al. reported that Huntingtin-interacting protein 1-related protein (HIP1R) promotes lysosomal degradation of PD-L1, inhibits HIP1R-induced PD-L1 accumulation, and alters T cell–mediated cytotoxicity in a human colorectal cancer cell line [12]. A chimeric peptide including a lysosomal sorting signal and the HIP1R PD-L1-binding sequence significantly inhibits PD-L1 protein expression [12]. Although immune checkpoint inhibition is the most popular treatment for lung cancer, relationships involving HIP1R and immune checkpoint inhibitors in lung cancer have not been studied.

The present study was conducted to determine whether HIP1R protein expression affects the response of NSCLC patients to anti-PD-1 inhibitors and their prognosis. The relationship between HIP1R and PD-L1 was also evaluated, employing immunohistochemical and web-based mRNA expression data. In addition, we performed gene set enrichment analysis (GSEA) on RNA-sequencing data from The Cancer Genome Atlas (TCGA) to confirm the molecular pathways associated with HIP1R expression.

2. Materials and Methods

2.1. Patients

We retrospectively selected 52 advanced NSCLC patients who were administered PD-1 inhibitor from 2016 to 2019, and they previously received one or two lines of chemotherapy. This study was approved by the Institutional Review Board of Ajou University School of Medicine. Informed consent was waived due to the retrospective nature of the study (AJIRB-BMR-KSP-19-050 and 2019-03-26).

Patients treated with PD-1 inhibitor were assigned to either a responder group (complete response, partial response, or stable disease) or a nonresponder group (disease progression), according to the response evaluation criteria for solid tumors (RECIST) version 1.1 [13].

2.2. Immunohistochemical Staining and HIP1R Expression Scoring

One board-certified pathologist (YWK) reviewed hematoxylin and eosin (H&E)-stained tissue samples to determine a definitive pathologic diagnosis according to the 2015 World Health Organization Classification of Lung Tumors [14]. All patients were pathologically staged according to the eighth edition of the TNM classification.

HIP1R immunohistochemical (IHC) staining was performed with a Benchmark XT automatic IHC staining device (Ventana Medical Systems, Tucson, AZ, USA). The samples were incubated with an anti-HIP1R antibody (dilution 1:1000, 16814-1-AP, polyclonal, Proteintech, Rosemont, IL, USA). We used a human placenta tissue as positive control according to the manufacturer's recommendations (Figure S1). We also evaluated the intensity of HIP1R staining on a four-point intensity scale: 0 (no staining), 1 (light yellow = faint staining), 2 (yellow-brown = moderate staining)' and 3 (brown = strong staining) (Figure 1). We also evaluated the percentages (0–100%) of cytoplasmic versus membranous localization of HIP1R. We used H-scores to interpret HIP1R staining [15], where H-score = [1 × (% cells 1+) + 2 × (% cells 2+) + 3 × (% cells 3+)]. H-scores (0–300) were obtained by multiplying the percentage of cells by the intensity score.

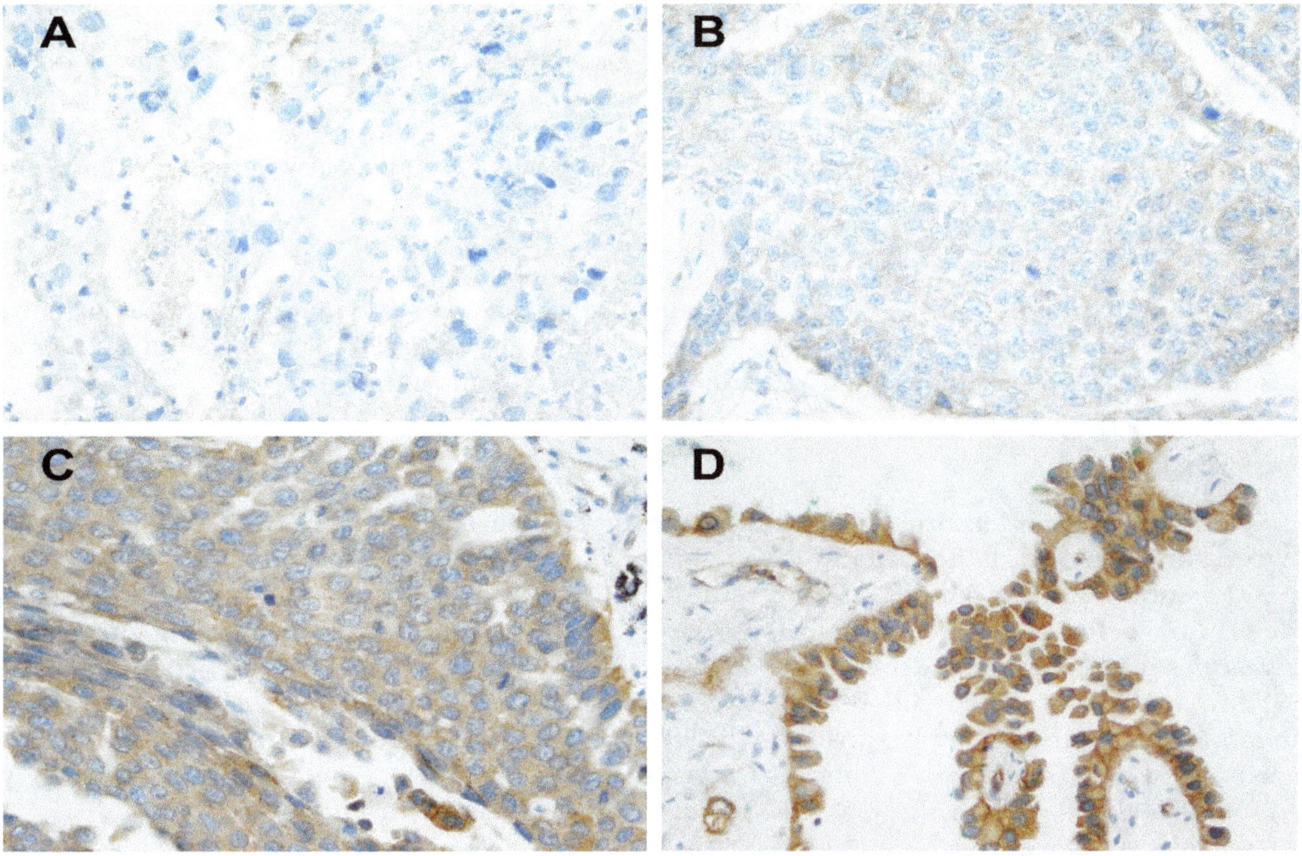

Figure 1. Huntingtin-interacting protein 1-related protein (HIP1R) expression in nonsmall cell carcinoma. (**A**) No staining of HIP1R, x400. (**B**) Faint HIP1R staining, X400. (**C**) Moderate HIP1R staining, X400. (**D**) Strong HIP1R staining, X400.

2.3. Immunohistochemical Staining and PD-L1 Expression Scoring

Two PD-L1 antibodies (clone name SP263 or 22C3) were used to detect PD-L1 expression. Sp263 was a companion diagnostic assay for OPDIVO® (nivolumab), and 22c3 was a companion diagnostic assay for KEYTRUDA® (pembrolizumab). We performed SP263 and/or 22C3 assays prior to PD-1 inhibitor treatment for all NSCLC patients. Thirteen (25%) of the 52 specimens were tested for both SP263 and 22C3, 27 (51.9%) for only SP263, and 12 (23.1%) for only 22C3. Two PD-L1 tests used prediluted antibody (ready to use) according to the protocol. The SP263 assay was performed using a VENTANA BenchMark ULTRA instrument (Roche, Basel, Switzerland), and the 22C3 assay was conducted using the Dako Link-48 platform (Dako, Carpinteria, California, US), as recommended by the manufacturers [16]. PD-L1 intensity was also evaluated on a four-point intensity scale (0, none; 1, faint; 2, moderate; and 3, strong), and the percentage of membranous expression of PD-L1 was determined (Figures S2 and S3). When both the 22C3 and SP263 tests were conducted, mean values were used. High PD-L1 expression was defined as $\geq$ 50% of definitive tumor cells exhibiting PD-L1 staining, because 50% was the cut-off used for NSCLC [17].

2.4. Web-Based mRNA Profiling, GSEA, and Kaplan Meier Analysis

The mRNA sequencing data of 517 lung adenocarcinoma patients and 501 lung squamous cell carcinoma patients were downloaded from The Cancer Genome Atlas (TCGA) cBioportal (http://cbioportal.org) [18]. We conducted correlation analysis involving PD-L1 and HIP1R mRNA sequencing data.

GSEA is a method of analyzing associations between gene expression and biological information. We conducted GSEA using GSEA version 4.0.3 from the Broad Institute at MIT and Harvard (http:

//www.broadinstitute.org/gsea/index.jsp) [19]. TCGA mRNA sequencing data derived from lung adenocarcinoma and lung squamous cell carcinoma patients was used. Depending on the median value, it is divided into low and high HIP1R. Hallmark gene sets representing well-defined biological states or processes were used for GSEA. 1000 permutations were used for estimating nominal p values. If the p value was less than 0.05 and the False Discovery Rate (FDR) was less than 0.25, the findings were considered statistically significant.

We conducted survival analyses using an online Kaplan Meier plotter tool [20]. The online Kaplan Meier plotter tool provides mRNA expression data of cancer patients and allows for survival analysis. Survival analyses were performed in 719 patients with lung adenocarcinoma and 524 lung squamous cell carcinoma cases according to their HIP1R mRNA expression.

2.5. Statistical Analyses

Spearman's rank order correlation coefficient analysis was used to measure monotonic relationships between continuous variables. Mann Whitney U-tests were used to compare differences between two independent groups. Univariate and multivariate logistic regression analyses were performed to determine factors that predicted a response to PD-1 inhibitors. Receiver operating curve (ROC) analysis was used to determine the cut-off values for HIP1R expression. The progression-free survival (PFS) or overall survival (OS) difference between the cohorts was determined using the log-rank test. Univariate and multivariate prognostic analyses were performed for PFS using a Cox proportional hazards regression model. SPSS Statistics for Windows (Version 25.0, IBM, Armonk, NY, USA) was used for all analyses, and p values <0.05 were considered to be statistically significant.

3. Results

3.1. Patient Demographics

Detailed patient and tumor characteristics are summarized in Table 1. Forty-six tissues were collected from lung lesions, and six were obtained from metastatic sites. Twenty-seven (51.9%) patients had been treated with nivolumab, and 25 (48.1%) patients received pembrolizumab. All patients were refractory to conventional treatments such as chemotherapy, radiotherapy, or target therapy. Therefore, they received PD-1 inhibitor as a second line or later setting. Twenty-seven (51.9%) patients were classified as responders, and 25 (48.1%) were classified as nonresponders. Four patients were treated with epidermal growth factor receptor (EGFR) inhibitors before PD-1 inhibitor administration. Patients with anaplastic lymphoma kinase (ALK) fusion were not identified in the present study.

3.2. Relationships Between HIP1R and PD-L1 Analyzed by IHC and mRNA Expression

We performed correlation analysis of HIP1R and PD-L1 expression using IHC techniques. There was no statistically significant correlation between HIP1R and PD-L1 expression ($p = 0.905$, Figure 2A).

Correlation analyses of HIP1R and PD-L1 expression were performed using mRNA data. From the TCGA dataset, HIP1R mRNA expression levels were negatively correlated with PD-L1 mRNA levels in adenocarcinoma and squamous cell carcinoma. (Spearman's rho = −0.233, $p < 0.001$, Figure 2B; Spearman's rho = −0.224, $p < 0.001$, Figure 2C).

Table 1. Demographic and clinical characteristics of patients.

Variable	Number (%)
Age, Median (Range) (Years)	64 (38–85)
Male Sex	43 (82.7%)
Smoking Sistory	31 (73.8%)
Histologic Subtype	
Adenocarcinoma	22 (42.3%)
Squamous Cell Carcinoma	19 (36.5%)
Pleomorphic Carcinoma	4 (7.7%)
NSCLC, NOS	7 (13.5%)
Clinical Stage at Diagnosis	
III	13 (25%)
IV	39 (75%)
Genetic Alteration Status	
EGFR-Mutated	4 (9.1%)
ALK-Rearranged	0 (0%)
Wild Type	44 (92.3%)
Type of PD-1 Blockade	
Nivolumab	27 (51.9%)
Pembrolizumab	25 (48.1%)
PD-L1 Expression	
Low (<50%)	17 (32.7%)
High (≥50%)	35 (67.3%)
Response to PD-1 Blockade	
Responder	27 (51.9%)
Nonresponder	25 (48.1%)

Smoking history was collected for 42 patients. EGFR test was performed in 44 patients. ALK test was performed in 47 patients. Abbreviations: epidermal growth factor receptor; EGFR, nonsmall-cell lung cancer—not otherwise specified; NSCLC, NOS, programmed cell death protein 1, PD-1; programmed death-ligand 1, PD-L1.

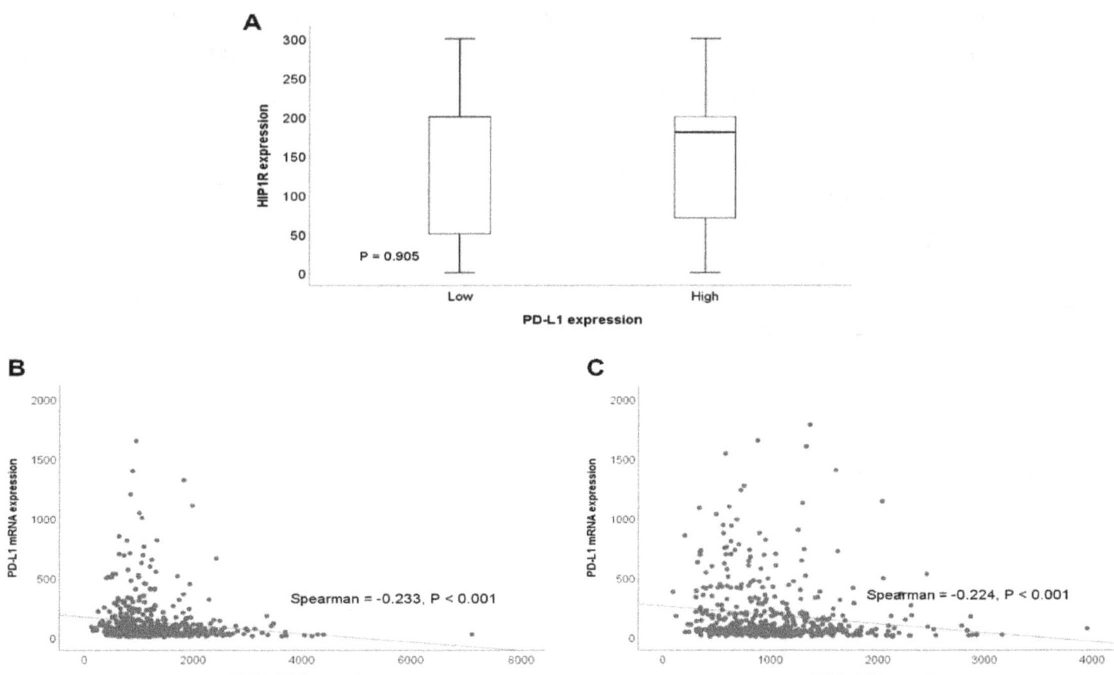

Figure 2. Correlation analyses involving Huntingtin-interacting protein 1-related protein (HIP1R) and programmed death-ligand 1 (PD-L1) expression. (**A**) Correlation between HIP1R and PD-L1 detected immunohistochemically. (**B**) Correlation between HIP1R and PD-L1 mRNA expression in lung adenocarcinoma. (**C**) Correlation between HIP1R and PD-L1 mRNA expression in lung squamous cell carcinoma.

3.3. Associations Involving HIP1R, PD-L1, Clinicopathologic Parameters, and Response to PD-1 Inhibitors

ROC analysis was performed to determine the cut-off value for HIP1R expression. Cut-off was determined as the value corresponding to the maximum joint sensitivity and specificity of the ROC curve. The area under the curve (AUC) was 0.659 for the expression of HIP1R, and the cut-off value was 180 (66% sensitivity and 68% specificity, Figure 3).

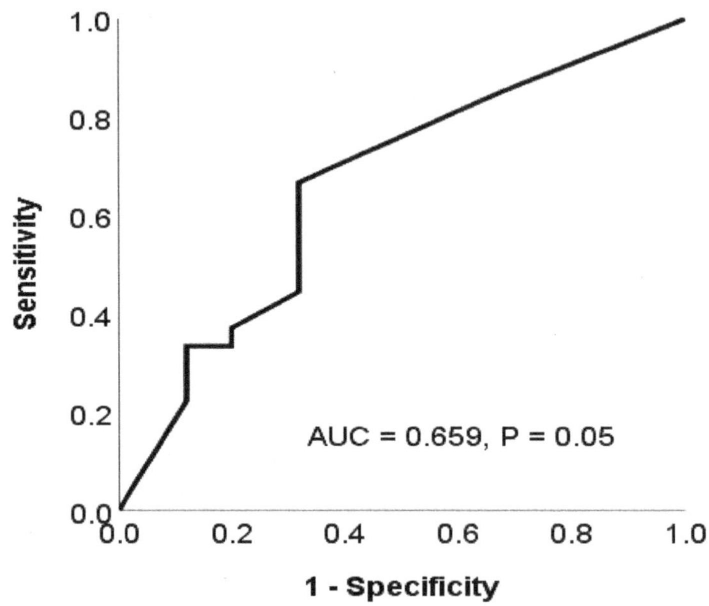

Figure 3. Receiver operating characteristic (ROC) and area under the curve (AUC) analysis of HIP1R expression.

We explored the predictive capacity of HIP1R, PD-L1, and clinicopathologic factors in terms of responses to PD-1 inhibition. By univariate analysis, the expression of HIP1R was found to be a predictor of the response to anti-PD-1 therapy (OR) = 0.235, $p = 0.015$; Table 2). PD-L1 expression was also found to be a predictor of the response to anti-PD-1 therapy (OR = 4.062, $p = 0.028$; Table 2). By multivariate analysis, the expression of HIP1R was an independent predictor of anti-PD-1 therapy response (OR = 0.209, $p = 0.014$, Table 2).

Table 2. Univariate and multivariate logistic regression analysis for predicting clinical response to PD-1 blockade.

	Univariate Analysis			Multivariate Analysis		
Covariate	OR	95% CI	*p*-Value †	OR	95% CI	*p*-Value †
Age (≥65 Years vs. <65 Years)	1.591	0.532–4.757	0.406			
Sex (Male vs. Female)	2.526	0.558–11.44	0.229			
Smoking History (+ vs. −)	3.238	0.720–14.56	0.126			
Presence of EGFR Mutation (+ vs. −)	0.222	0.021–2.330	0.210			
Type of PD-1 Blockade (Nivolumab vs. Pembrolizumab)	1.875	0.622–5.649	0.264			
PD-L1 (>50% vs. ≤50%)	4.062	1.166–14.15	0.028	4.664	1.198–18.15	0.026
HIP1R (>180 vs. ≤180)	0.235	0.074–0.751	0.015	0.209	0.060–0.731	0.014

† logistic regression analysis. Abbreviations: confidence interval; CI, epidermal growth factor receptor; EGFR, Huntingtin Interacting Protein 1 Related; HIP1R, odd ratio; OR, programmed cell death protein 1, PD-1; programmed death-ligand 1, PD-L1.

3.4. GSEA According to HIP1R mRNA Expression

We performed GSEA to identify gene sets associated with HIP1R mRNA expression in the TCGA mRNA data of lung adenocarcinoma and lung squamous cell carcinoma cases. In lung adenocarcinoma, we identified the top 20 most prominent pathways that were upregulated in the low HIP1R mRNA expression group (Table S1). Four of the 20 were immune-related gene sets and were statistically significant (HALLMARK_ALLOGRAFT_REJECTION, HALLMARK_INFLAMMATORY_RESPONSE, HALLMARK_IL6_JAK_STAT3_SIGNALING, and HALLMARK_IL2_STAT5_SIGNALING) (Figure 4). HALLMARK_INTERFERON_GAMMA_RESPONSE is also upregulated in the low HIP1R mRNA expression group, although the statistical significance was marginal ($p = 0.063$). Core enrichment gene lists for HALLMARK_ALLOGRAFT_REJECTION, HALLMARK_INFLAMMATORY_RESPONSE, HALLMARK_IL6_JAK_STAT3_SIGNALING and HALLMARK_IL2_STAT5_SIGNALING are summarized in Tables S2–S5. In lung squamous cell carcinoma, there were no statistically significant immune-related gene sets associated with HIP1R mRNA expression (Table S6).

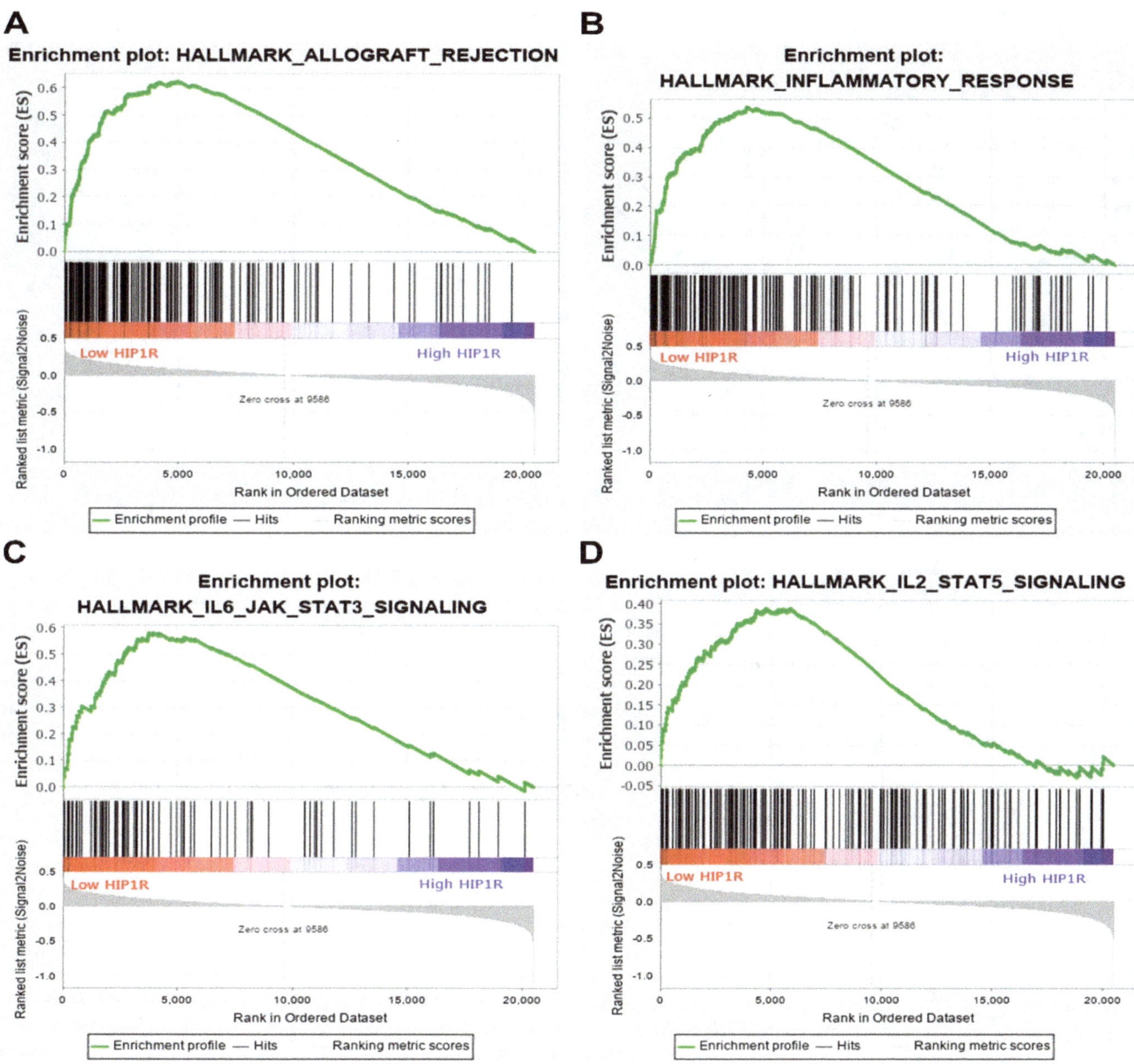

Figure 4. Gene set enrichment analysis (GSEA) according to HIP1R mRNA expression. (**A**) HALL MARK_ALLOGRAFT_REJECTION pathway; (**B**) HALLMARK_INFLAMMATORY_RESPONSE pathway; (**C**) HALLMARK_IL6_JAK_STAT3_SIGNALING pathway; (**D**) HALLMARK _IL2_STAT5_SIGNALING pathway.

3.5. Prognostic Significance of HIP1R and PD-L1

Patients with high HIP1R expression had inferior PFS to patients with low HIP1R expression ($p = 0.037$, Figure 5A). Patients with high HIP1R expression also showed an inferior OS than patients with low HIP1R expression, however the statistical significance was not reached ($p = 0.11$, Figure 5B). Patients with high PD-L1 expression had superior PFS or OS than patients with low PD-L1 expression ($p = 0.028$, Figure 5C and $p = 0.031$, Figure 5D, respectively). Furthermore, patients with high HIP1R expression and low PD-L1 expression had lower PFS or OS than patients with other expression patterns ($p < 0.001$, Figure 5E and $p = 0.001$, Figure 5F, respectively). In multivariate analysis, high HIP1R expression was an independent prognostic factor for PFS (HR = 2.098, $p = 0.019$, Table 3).

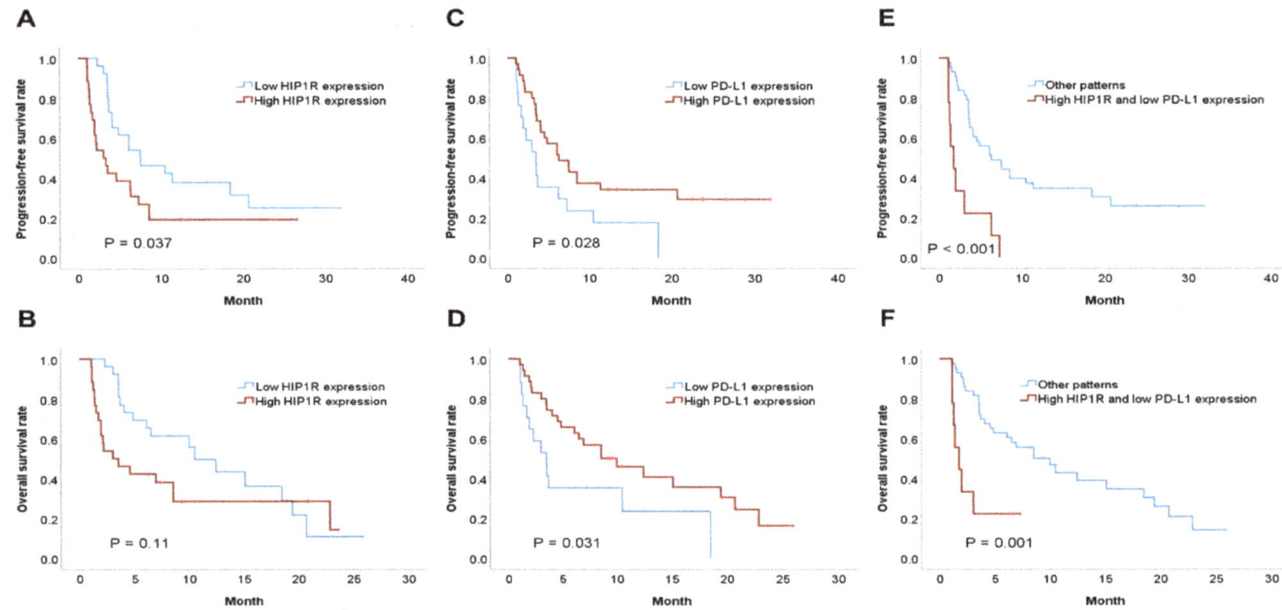

Figure 5. Comparison of survival rates according to HIP1R and PD-L1 expression. (**A**) Progression-free survival (PFS) and expression of HIP1R. (**B**) Overall survival (OS) and expression of HIP1R (**C**) PFS and PD-L1. (**D**) OS and PD-L1. (**E**) PFS, HIP1R, and PD-L1. (**F**) OS, HIP1R, and PD-L1.

Table 3. Univariate and multivariate analyses of progression-free survival.

	Univariate Analysis			Multivariate Analysis		
Covariate	HR	95% CI	*p*-Value †	HR	95% CI	*p*-Value †
Age (≥65 Years vs. <65 Years)	1.120	0.597–2.101	0.724			
Sex (Male vs. Female)	0.553	0.251–1.218	0.141			
Smoking History (+ vs. −)	1.121	0.517–2.429	0.773			
Presence of EGFR Mutation (+ vs. −)	1.603	0.482–5.329	0.441			
Type of PD-1 Blockade (Nivolumab vs. Pembrolizumab)	1.482	0.785–2.800	0.225			
PD-L1 (>50% vs. ≤50%)	0.489	0.254–0.942	0.032	0.432	0.222–0.844	0.014
HIP1R (>180 vs. ≤180)	1.935	1.027–3.648	0.041	2.098	1.136–4.133	0.019

† Cox proportional hazards regression model. Abbreviations: CI, confidence interval; EGFR, epidermal growth factor receptor; HIP1R, Huntingtin Interacting Protein 1 Related; HR, hazard ratio; PD-1, programmed cell death protein 1; PD-L1, programmed death-ligand 1.

We used a Kaplan Meier plotter tool and performed survival analysis according to HIP1R mRNA expression in lung adenocarcinoma and lung squamous cell carcinoma patients. The group with high HIP1R mRNA expression exhibited poorer OS in patients with adenocarcinoma ($p = 0.026$, Figure S4A). However, in lung squamous cell carcinoma, HIP1R mRNA expression was not correlated with OS ($p = 0.63$, Figure S4B)

4. Discussion

This study had several novel discoveries. First, we found that the expression of HIP1R was an independent predictive factor for anti-PD-1 treatment response by NSCLC patients. Second, the expression of HIP1R was an independent prognostic factor of PFS in patients treated with anti-PD-1 inhibitors. Third, GSEA revealed that *HIP1R* mRNA expression was tightly correlated with immune-related gene sets in lung adenocarcinoma. These GSEA results suggested that *HIP1R* mRNA expression plays an important role in regulating the expression of PD-L1.

GSEA revealed that low *HIP1R* mRNA expression was closely associated with allograft rejection, inflammatory responses, IL6-JAK-STAT3, IL2-STAT5, and interferon gamma response pathways in lung adenocarcinoma. PD-L1 expression is correlated with marked expression of adaptive immune responses (CD8+ T-cells) [21]. In our study, CD8 was also included in the core enrichment gene list of HALLMARK_ALLOGRAFT_REJECTION. Previous studies have also reported that the IL6-JAK-STAT3 pathway induces PD-L1 upregulation. IL-6 is positively correlated with PD-L1 expression in human hepatocellular carcinoma (HCC) cells, and IL-6 induces PD-L1 stability through glycosylation in a HCC cell line [22]. Glioblastoma-derived IL6 is required for up-regulation of myeloid PD-L1 in glioblastoma through a STAT3-dependent mechanism [23]. Combined blockade of IL6 and PD-L1 signaling achieves synergistic antitumor immune responses in colon carcinoma and murine melanoma models [24]. PD-L1 expression is also regulated by interferon gamma signaling in a melanoma cell line [25]. GSEA suggested that HIP1R expression plays an important role in adaptive immune responses associated with PD-L1.

In the present study, no correlation was identified between HIP1R and PD-L1 protein expression, However, HIP1R mRNA expression was negatively correlated with the mRNA expression level of PD-L1 in adenocarcinoma and squamous cell carcinoma. There are several possible explanations for this discrepancy. Post-transcriptional and post-translational modifications affect the level of protein expression [26]. Proteins can have significantly different half-lives in vivo [27]. There were no cases of surgery in our study, therefore the only sample we received was a biopsy. We cannot conduct additional experiments for mRNA testing of HIP1R and PD-L1, because very little tumor tissue remains in paraffin tissue.

Patients with high HIP1R mRNA expression exhibited poor clinical outcomes in web-based mRNA data of adenocarcinoma cases; however, HIP1R mRNA expression was not correlated with OS in squamous cell carcinoma. From our IHC data, HIP1R expression was correlated with poor clinical outcomes. However, we did perform subgroup analysis according to histologic type because of our small sample size. HIP1R levels also correlate with a set of genes that reflect PD-L1-related immune pathways in GSEA analysis of adenocarcinoma cases; however, there were no statistically significant immune-related gene sets associated with HIP1R mRNA expression in squamous cell carcinoma. Currently, lung adenocarcinoma and squamous cell carcinoma are known to involve different biologic mechanisms and prognoses. Therefore, the role of HIP1R in adaptive immune responses and its effect on clinical outcomes may vary depending on the histological type.

Despite some surprising discoveries, our study has certain limitations. First, our cohort was small. We performed multivariate logistic regression and prognostic analyses on only 52 samples. However, the web-based mRNA dataset also revealed results similar to ours. These results encourage further investigations involving larger populations. Second, we used an IHC method to detect HIP1R protein expression. There is no information regarding standardization, reliability, and reproducibility of IHC staining. We used the same antibody that Wang et al. used [12]. However, Wang et al. used HIP1R antibody (16814-1-AP) in Western Blott (WB) and immunofluorescence alone. Only recently has HIP1R attracted attention in cancer research, so few studies have been done on HIP1R. Therefore, there are no antibodies that are commonly used in immunohistochemistry. In the catalog of HIP1R antibody (16814-1-AP), it can be used in IHC, immunoprecipitation (IP), WB, and ELISA. According to the manufacturer's guidelines, this antibody was validated by western blot in HeLa cells and human liver tissue. We used a human placenta tissue as positive control as recommended. An automatic IHC staining device (Benchmark XT) may improve the reproducibility of IHC staining. The H-scoring method is widely used for immunochemical staining, and is known to have relatively high reproducibility among pathologists [28,29]. Third, we examined the protein expression of HIP1R and PD-L1 in refractory advanced NSCLC; however, the mRNA profiles of HIP1R and PD-L1 were not evaluated. Because protein expression of HIP1R did not correlate with PD-L1 expression, the relationship between HIP1R and PD-L1 mRNA expression profile is very important. To verify the results of GSEA, we should evaluate the mRNA expression profiles of HIP1R. However, the sample we have is a small biopsy, and we have already performed several immunohistochemical stainings for diagnosis and ALK and EGFR mutation tests. Therefore, currently, very little tumor tissue remains in paraffin tissue and we cannot conduct additional experiments for mRNA testing. To confirm our experiments, future research should measure the mRNA expression level of HIP1R on many samples and investigate the relationship with the PD-1 blocker and PD-L1 expression.

In conclusion, we examined the expression of HIP1R in 52 refractory NSCLC samples from patients treated with PD-1 inhibitors. HIP1R expression was an independent biomarker predicting patient response to PD-1 inhibitors. High HIP1R expression was an independent predictor of poor PFS. In addition, HIP1R mRNA expression was significantly correlated with immune-related gene sets in lung adenocarcinoma. These immune-related gene sets are known to play important roles in PD-L1 regulation. Based on our findings, HIP1R expression may be a promising predictor for the therapeutic determination of responses to anti-PD-1 treatment.

Supplementary Materials:
Table S1. Gene sets within the top 20-ranked list related to low HIP1R in adenocarcinoma patients; Table S2. Core enrichment gene list of HALLMARK_ALLOGRAFT_REJECTION; Table S3. Core enrichment gene list of HALLMARK _INFLAMMATORY_RESPONSE; Table S4. Core enrichment gene list of HALLMARK_IL6_JAK_STAT3_SIGNALING; Table S5. Core enrichment gene list of HALLMARK_IL2_STAT5_SIGNALING; Table S6. Gene sets within the top 20-ranked list related to low HIP1R in squamous cell carcinoma patients; Figure S1. HIP1R expression in positive control. Positive HIP1R expression in placental tissue, X400; Figure S2. PD-L1 sp263 expression in nonsmall cell carcinoma. (A) No staining of PD-L1 sp263, x400. (B) Faint PD-L1 sp263 staining, x400. (C) Moderate PD-L1 sp263 staining, x400. (D) Strong PD-L1 sp263 staining, x400; Figure S3. PD-L1 22c3 expression in nonsmall cell carcinoma. (A) No staining of PD-L1 22c3, x400. (B) Faint PD-L1 22c3 staining, x400. (C) Moderate PD-L1 22c3 staining, x400. (D) Strong PD-L1 22c3 staining, x400; Figure S4. Comparison of survival rates, according to HIP1R mRNA expression in patients with nonsmall cell carcinoma. (A) Overall survival (OS) and HIP1R in lung adenocarcinoma. (B) OS and HIP1R in lung squamous cell carcinoma.

Author Contributions: Conceptualization, Y.W.K.; formal analysis, Y.W.K.; funding acquisition, Y.W.K.; investigation, Y.W.K., J.-H.H., S.H., and H.W.L.; methodology, Y.W.K., J.-H.H., S.H., and H.W.L.; resources, Y.W.K.; supervision, Y.W.K.; visualization, Y.W.K.; writing—original draft, Y.W.K., J.-H.H., S.H., and H.W.L.; writing—review and editing, Y.W.K., J.-H.H, S.H., and H.W.L. All authors have read and agreed to the published version of the manuscript.

References

1. Garon, E.B.; Rizvi, N.A.; Hui, R.; Leighl, N.; Balmanoukian, A.S.; Eder, J.P.; Patnaik, A.; Aggarwal, C.; Gubens, M.; Horn, L.; et al. Pembrolizumab for the treatment of nonsmall-cell lung cancer. *New Engl. J. Med.* **2015**, *372*, 2018–2028. [CrossRef] [PubMed]
2. Gettinger, S.; Rizvi, N.A.; Chow, L.Q.; Borghaei, H.; Brahmer, J.; Ready, N.; Gerber, D.E.; Shepherd, F.A.; Antonia, S.; Goldman, J.W.; et al. Nivolumab Monotherapy for First-Line Treatment of Advanced NonSmall-Cell Lung Cancer. *J. Clin. Oncol. Off. J. Am. Soc. Clin. Oncol.* **2016**, *34*, 2980–2987. [CrossRef] [PubMed]
3. Herbst, R.S.; Baas, P.; Kim, D.W.; Felip, E.; Perez-Gracia, J.L.; Han, J.Y.; Molina, J.; Kim, J.H.; Arvis, C.D.; Ahn, M.J.; et al. Pembrolizumab versus docetaxel for previously treated, PD-L1-positive, advanced nonsmall-cell lung cancer (KEYNOTE-010): A randomised controlled trial. *Lancet* **2016**, *387*, 1540–1550. [CrossRef]
4. Shukuya, T.; Carbone, D.P. Predictive Markers for the Efficacy of Anti-PD-1/PD-L1 Antibodies in Lung Cancer. *J. Thorac. Oncol. Off. Publ. Int. Assoc. Study Lung Cancer* **2016**, *11*, 976–988. [CrossRef] [PubMed]

5. Mezzadra, R.; Sun, C.; Jae, L.T.; Gomez-Eerland, R.; de Vries, E.; Wu, W.; Logtenberg, M.E.W.; Slagter, M.; Rozeman, E.A.; Hofland, I.; et al. Identification of CMTM6 and CMTM4 as PD-L1 protein regulators. *Nature* **2017**, *549*, 106–110. [CrossRef]
6. Koh, Y.W.; Han, J.H.; Haam, S.; Jung, J.; Lee, H.W. Increased CMTM6 can predict the clinical response to PD-1 inhibitors in nonsmall cell lung cancer patients. *Oncoimmunology* **2019**, *8*, e1629261. [CrossRef]
7. Meng, X.; Liu, X.; Guo, X.; Jiang, S.; Chen, T.; Hu, Z.; Liu, H.; Bai, Y.; Xue, M.; Hu, R.; et al. FBXO38 mediates PD-1 ubiquitination and regulates anti-tumour immunity of T cells. *Nature* **2018**, *564*, 130–135. [CrossRef]
8. Tsukita, Y.; Fujino, N.; Miyauchi, E.; Saito, R.; Fujishima, F.; Itakura, K.; Kyogoku, Y.; Okutomo, K.; Yamada, M.; Okazaki, T.; et al. Axl kinase drives immune checkpoint and chemokine signalling pathways in lung adenocarcinomas. *Mol. Cancer* **2019**, *18*, 24. [CrossRef]
9. Bauer, P.O.; Goswami, A.; Wong, H.K.; Okuno, M.; Kurosawa, M.; Yamada, M.; Miyazaki, H.; Matsumoto, G.; Kino, Y.; Nagai, Y.; et al. Harnessing chaperone-mediated autophagy for the selective degradation of mutant huntingtin protein. *Nat. Biotechnol.* **2010**, *28*, 256–263. [CrossRef]
10. Sakamoto, K.M.; Kim, K.B.; Kumagai, A.; Mercurio, F.; Crews, C.M.; Deshaies, R.J. Protacs: Chimeric molecules that target proteins to the Skp1-Cullin-F box complex for ubiquitination and degradation. *Proc. Natl. Acad. Sci. USA* **2001**, *98*, 8554–8559. [CrossRef]
11. Nabet, B.; Roberts, J.M.; Buckley, D.L.; Paulk, J.; Dastjerdi, S.; Yang, A.; Leggett, A.L.; Erb, M.A.; Lawlor, M.A.; Souza, A.; et al. The dTAG system for immediate and target-specific protein degradation. *Nat. Chem. Biol.* **2018**, *14*, 431–441. [CrossRef] [PubMed]
12. Wang, H.; Yao, H.; Li, C.; Shi, H.; Lan, J.; Li, Z.; Zhang, Y.; Liang, L.; Fang, J.Y.; Xu, J. HIP1R targets PD-L1 to lysosomal degradation to alter T cell-mediated cytotoxicity. *Nat. Chem. Biol.* **2019**, *15*, 42–50. [CrossRef] [PubMed]
13. Eisenhauer, E.A.; Therasse, P.; Bogaerts, J.; Schwartz, L.H.; Sargent, D.; Ford, R.; Dancey, J.; Arbuck, S.; Gwyther, S.; Mooney, M.; et al. New response evaluation criteria in solid tumours: Revised RECIST guideline (version 1.1). *Eur. J. Cancer* **2009**, *45*, 228–247. [CrossRef]
14. Travis, W.D.; Brambilla, E.; Nicholson, A.G.; Yatabe, Y.; Austin, J.H.; Beasley, M.B.; Chirieac, L.R.; Dacic, S.; Duhig, E.; Flieder, D.B.; et al. The 2015 World Health Organization Classification of Lung Tumors: Impact of Genetic, Clinical and Radiologic Advances Since the 2004 Classification. *J. Thorac. Oncol. Official Publ. Int. Assoc. Study Lung Cancer* **2015**, *10*, 1243–1260. [CrossRef] [PubMed]
15. McCarty, K.S., Jr.; Szabo, E.; Flowers, J.L.; Cox, E.B.; Leight, G.S.; Miller, L.; Konrath, J.; Soper, J.T.; Budwit, D.A.; Creasman, W.T.; et al. Use of a monoclonal anti-estrogen receptor antibody in the immunohistochemical evaluation of human tumors. *Cancer Res.* **1986**, *46*, 4244s–4248s.
16. Munari, E.; Rossi, G.; Zamboni, G.; Lunardi, G.; Marconi, M.; Sommaggio, M.; Netto, G.J.; Hoque, M.O.; Brunelli, M.; Martignoni, G.; et al. PD-L1 Assays 22C3 and SP263 are Not Interchangeable in NonSmall Cell Lung Cancer When Considering Clinically Relevant Cutoffs: An Interclone Evaluation by Differently Trained Pathologists. *Am. J. Surg. Pathol.* **2018**, *42*, 1384–1389. [CrossRef]
17. Büttner, R.; Gosney, J.R.; Skov, B.G.; Adam, J.; Motoi, N.; Bloom, K.J.; Dietel, M.; Longshore, J.W.; López-Ríos, F.; Penault-Llorca, F.; et al. Programmed Death-Ligand 1 Immunohistochemistry Testing: A Review of Analytical Assays and Clinical Implementation in NonSmall-Cell Lung Cancer. *J. Clin. Oncol. Off. J. Am. Soc. Clin. Oncol.* **2017**, *35*, 3867–3876. [CrossRef]
18. Cerami, E.; Gao, J.; Dogrusoz, U.; Gross, B.E.; Sumer, S.O.; Aksoy, B.A.; Jacobsen, A.; Byrne, C.J.; Heuer, M.L.; Larsson, E.; et al. The cBio cancer genomics portal: An open platform for exploring multidimensional cancer genomics data. *Cancer Discov.* **2012**, *2*, 401–404. [CrossRef]
19. Subramanian, A.; Tamayo, P.; Mootha, V.K.; Mukherjee, S.; Ebert, B.L.; Gillette, M.A.; Paulovich, A.; Pomeroy, S.L.; Golub, T.R.; Lander, E.S.; et al. Gene set enrichment analysis: A knowledge-based approach for interpreting genome-wide expression profiles. *Proc. Natl. Acad. Sci. USA* **2005**, *102*, 15545–15550. [CrossRef]
20. Gyorffy, B.; Surowiak, P.; Budczies, J.; Lanczky, A. Online survival analysis software to assess the prognostic value of biomarkers using transcriptomic data in nonsmall-cell lung cancer. *PLoS ONE* **2013**, *8*, e82241. [CrossRef]
21. Huang, C.Y.; Wang, Y.; Luo, G.Y.; Han, F.; Li, Y.Q.; Zhou, Z.G.; Xu, G.L. Relationship between PD-L1 Expression and CD8+ T-cell Immune Responses in Hepatocellular Carcinoma. *J. Immunother.* **2017**, *40*, 323–333. [CrossRef] [PubMed]

22. Chan, L.C.; Li, C.W.; Xia, W.; Hsu, J.M.; Lee, H.H.; Cha, J.H.; Wang, H.L.; Yang, W.H.; Yen, E.Y.; Chang, W.C.; et al. IL-6/JAK1 pathway drives PD-L1 Y112 phosphorylation to promote cancer immune evasion. *J. Clin. Investig.* **2019**, *129*, 3324–3338. [CrossRef] [PubMed]
23. Lamano, J.B.; Lamano, J.B.; Li, Y.D.; DiDomenico, J.D.; Choy, W.; Veliceasa, D.; Oyon, D.E.; Fakurnejad, S.; Ampie, L.; Kesavabhotla, K.; et al. Glioblastoma-Derived IL6 Induces Immunosuppressive Peripheral Myeloid Cell PD-L1 and Promotes Tumor Growth. *Clin. Cancer Res. Off. J. Am. Assoc. Cancer Res.* **2019**, *25*, 3643–3657. [CrossRef] [PubMed]
24. Tsukamoto, H.; Fujieda, K.; Miyashita, A.; Fukushima, S.; Ikeda, T.; Kubo, Y.; Senju, S.; Ihn, H.; Nishimura, Y.; Oshiumi, H. Combined Blockade of IL6 and PD-1/PD-L1 Signaling Abrogates Mutual Regulation of Their Immunosuppressive Effects in the Tumor Microenvironment. *Cancer Res.* **2018**, *78*, 5011–5022. [CrossRef]
25. Garcia-Diaz, A.; Shin, D.S.; Moreno, B.H.; Saco, J.; Escuin-Ordinas, H.; Rodriguez, G.A.; Zaretsky, J.M.; Sun, L.; Hugo, W.; Wang, X.; et al. Interferon Receptor Signaling Pathways Regulating PD-L1 and PD-L2 Expression. *Cell Rep.* **2017**, *19*, 1189–1201. [CrossRef]
26. Greenbaum, D.; Colangelo, C.; Williams, K.; Gerstein, M. Comparing protein abundance and mRNA expression levels on a genomic scale. *Genome Biol.* **2003**, *4*, 117. [CrossRef]
27. Nie, L.; Wu, G.; Zhang, W. Correlation of mRNA expression and protein abundance affected by multiple sequence features related to translational efficiency in Desulfovibrio vulgaris: A quantitative analysis. *Genetics* **2006**, *174*, 2229–2243. [CrossRef]
28. Aviles-Salas, A.; Muniz-Hernandez, S.; Maldonado-Martinez, H.A.; Chanona-Vilchis, J.G.; Ramirez-Tirado, L.A.; HernaNdez-Pedro, N.; Dorantes-Heredia, R.; Rui, Z.M.J.M.; Motola-Kuba, D.; Arrieta, O. Reproducibility of the EGFR immunohistochemistry scores for tumor samples from patients with advanced nonsmall cell lung cancer. *Oncol. Lett.* **2017**, *13*, 912–920. [CrossRef]
29. Detre, S.; Jotti, G.S.; Dowsett, M. A "quickscore" method for immunohistochemical semiquantitation: Validation for oestrogen receptor in breast carcinomas. *J. Clin. Pathol.* **1995**, *48*, 876–878. [CrossRef]

10

Endocrinopathies Associated with Immune Checkpoint Inhibitor Cancer Treatment

Naoko Okura [1], Mai Asano [2], Junji Uchino [1,*], Yoshie Morimoto [1], Masahiro Iwasaku [1], Yoshiko Kaneko [1], Tadaaki Yamada [1], Michiaki Fukui [2] and Koichi Takayama [1]

1 Department of Pulmonary Medicine, Graduate School of Medical Science, Kyoto Prefectural University of Medicine, Kyoto 602-8566, Japan; ku-n07@koto.kpu-m.ac.jp (N.O.); yoshie-m@koto.kpu-m.ac.jp (Y.M.); miwasaku@koto.kpu-m.ac.jp (M.I.); kaneko-y@koto.kpu-m.ac.jp (Y.K.); tayamada@koto.kpu-m.ac.jp (T.Y.); takayama@koto.kpu-m.ac.jp (K.T.)

2 Department of Endocrinology and Metabolism, Graduate School of Medical Science, Kyoto Prefectural University of Medicine, Kyoto 602-8566, Japan; maias@koto.kpu-m.ac.jp (M.A.); michiaki@koto.kpu-m.ac.jp (M.F.)

* Correspondence: uchino@koto.kpu-m.ac.jp

Abstract: Treatment with immune checkpoint inhibitors has shown efficacy against a variety of cancer types. The effects of nivolumab and pembrolizumab on lung cancer have been reported, and further therapeutic advances are ongoing. The side effects of immune checkpoint inhibitors are very different from those of conventional cytocidal anticancer drugs and molecular targeted drugs, and they involve various organs such as the digestive and respiratory organs, thyroid and pituitary glands, and skin. The generic term for such adverse events is immune-related adverse events (irAEs). They are relatively infrequent, and, if mild, treatment with immune checkpoint inhibitors can be continued with careful control. However, early detection and appropriate treatment are critical, as moderate-to-severe irAEs are associated with markedly reduced organ function and quality of life, with fatal consequences in some cases. Of these, endocrinopathies caused by immune checkpoint inhibitors are sometimes difficult to distinguish from nonspecific symptoms in patients with advanced cancer and may have serious outcomes when the diagnosis is delayed. Therefore, it is necessary to anticipate and appropriately address the onset of endocrinopathies during treatment with immune checkpoint inhibitors. Here, we present a review of endocrine disorders caused by immune checkpoint inhibitor treatment.

Keywords: immune checkpoint inhibitors; immune-related adverse events; endocrine disorders; tumor-bearing patients

1. Introduction

In 2011, the Food and Drug Administration (FDA) approved the immune checkpoint inhibitor (ICI) ipilimumab, an anti-cytotoxic T-lymphocyte antigen-4 (anti-CTLA-4) antibody, for the treatment of malignant melanoma. Since then, anti-programmed cell death 1 (anti-PD-1) antibodies, such as nivolumab and pembrolizumab, and anti-programmed death ligand 1 (PD-L1) antibodies, such as atezolizumab and durvalumab, have been developed and approved for lung cancer treatment [1]. The effectiveness of cancer immunotherapy using these drugs can also be observed in cases receiving combined treatment with cytotoxic anticancer drugs and radiotherapy, and further expansion of the indications is expected in future.

CTLA-4 is a protein expressed on the surfaces of activated T-cells, and it inhibits T-cell activation after binding to antigen-presenting cells [2,3]. Anti-CTLA-4 antibodies bind to CTLA-4 and block the inhibitory receptors of activated T-cells, thus exerting antitumor effects. They also bind to the surface

CTLA-4 in regulatory T-cells (Tregs), thus reducing the immunosuppressive function of Tregs and enhancing tumor immune responses [4]. Furthermore, they are thought to reduce Tregs in tumor tissue via antibody-dependent cellular cytotoxicity (ADCC) and induce tumor cell death [5–7].

PD-1 is expressed on the surfaces of activated T-cells, and its binding with one of its ligands, PD-L1, inhibits T-cell activation [8]. Anti-PD-1 and anti-PD-L1 antibodies block the inhibitory system's signal to T-cells by obstructing such bindings, thus exerting antitumor effects. Therefore, while ICIs exhibit antitumor effects via a novel mechanism, immune adjustments do not work correctly in all cases, and side effects resembling autoimmune and inflammatory diseases have been reported. These types of adverse events, termed immune-related adverse events (irAEs), are characteristic side effects of ICI treatment, being distinct from the side effects of conventional anticancer drug treatment [9]. IrAEs involve almost the entire body, including the skin, gastrointestinal tract, and liver. In particular, endocrinopathy is a relatively frequent irAE [10,11].

Hypopituitarism, adrenocortical dysfunction, thyroid dysfunction, and type 1 diabetes mellitus are common endocrine disorders caused by ICI treatment [12]. Moreover, a small association between hypoparathyroidism and ICI treatment has been reported [13–16]. Pituitary dysfunction is frequent in patients receiving anti-CTLA-4 antibodies, while thyroid dysfunction is prevalent in patients receiving anti-PD-1/anti-PD-L1 antibodies [9,12]. Adrenal insufficiency is infrequent in patients treated with either drug [9,12]. Many symptoms of adrenal insufficiency, such as anorexia and malaise, are nonspecific and often observed in tumor-bearing patients. However, adrenal insufficiency can progress to fatal disease states such as adrenal crisis, and early detection and treatment according to the cause are necessary. Finally, although the frequency of type I diabetes mellitus associated with ICI treatment is small, clinicians should be aware that some cases can develop fulminant disease and should take the necessary actions in the early stages. It is important to be aware that symptoms such as fatigue caused by endocrinopathy may be misidentified as caused by the underlying cancer, and that endocrinopathy may occur with this drug when using immune checkpoint inhibitors. Table 1 shows the major ICIs indications and irAEs.

Table 1. Indication and major endocrinopathies of immune checkpoint inhibitors (ICIs).

Target	Drug	Indication	Major Endocrinopathies
Anti CTLA-4 antibody	Ipilimumab	Malignant melanoma	Hypopituitarism
		Renal cell cancer	
Anti-PD-1 antibody	Nivolumab	Malignant melanoma	Hypothyroidism Hyperthyroidism
		Non-small cell lung cancer	
		Renal cell cancer	
		Hodgkin lymphoma	
		Head and neck cancer	
		Gastric cancer	
		Malignant mesothelioma	
		Colorectal cancer with high-frequency microsatellite instability (MSI-High)	
		Esophageal cancer	
	Pembrolizumab	Non-small cell lung cancer	Hypothyroidism Hyperthyroidism
		Hodgkin lymphoma	
		Urothelial cancer	
		Solid cancers with high-frequency microsatellite instability (MSI-High)	
		Renal cell cancer	
		Head and neck cancer	
Anti PD-L1 antibody	Atezolizumab	Non-small cell lung cancer	Hypothyroidism
		Small cell lung cancer	
		Breast cancer	
	Durvalumab	Non-small cell lung cancer	Hypothyroidism Hyperthyroidism
	Avelumab	Merkel cell carcinoma renal cell cancer	Hypothyroidism

PD-1, programmed cell death 1; PD-L1, programmed death ligand 1; CTLA-4, cytotoxic T-lymphocyte antigen-4.

Here we present a review of endocrine disorders caused by ICI treatment.

2. Hypopituitarism

Hypopituitarism as an irAE is more common in patients receiving anti-CTLA-4 antibodies than in those receiving anti-PD-1/anti-PD-L1 antibodies, with the reported incidences being approximately 10% and ≤1% [17–22]. In addition, it has been reported that the incidence of hypophituitarism is higher with the concomitant use of anti-CTLA-4, and anti-PD-1/PD-L1 antibodies are more common than the use of a single agent [12]. Hypopituitarism caused by ICI treatment is classified into hypophysitis and isolated adrenocorticotropic (ACTH) deficiency. Pituitary gland enlargement is seen in hypophysitis, which causes hyposecretion of several anterior pituitary hormones, including thyroid-stimulating hormone (TSH), gonadotropins, and ACTH. On the other hand, the pituitary gland does not enlarge in ACTH deficiency, wherein the secretory capacity of only ACTH is reduced. There are very few reports of posterior pituitary dysfunction [17,23]. Although both patterns of dysfunction can occur in patients receiving anti-CTLA-4 antibodies, the use of anti-PD-1/anti-PD-L1 antibodies has been associated with ACTH deficiency in most cases [17,20,24]. Hypopituitarism often develops 4–10 weeks after treatment initiation due to anti-CTLA-4 antibodies [12]. An association between the incidence and the dose has also been noted, with one report showing a two-fold higher incidence in patients receiving high-dose ipilimumab (10 mg/kg) than in those receiving low-dose ipilimumab (3 mg/kg) [19]. Moreover, the higher dose (10 mg/kg) resulted in more adverse events than did the lower dose (3 mg/kg). However, significantly longer survival associated with the higher dose has been documented in some reports, and an association between irAE development and treatment efficacy has been pointed out [18,24]. Hypopituitarism also occurs within months to 1 year after treatment initiation due to anti-PD-1/anti-PD-L1 antibodies, and it may even develop after discontinuation of the drug [25–27]. It should be noted that ACTH hyposecretion always develops in all cases of hypopituitarism due to ICI treatment. The symptoms of ICI-induced hypopituitarism include anorexia and malaise due to secondary adrenal insufficiency, weight loss, gastrointestinal symptoms (nausea, vomiting, and diarrhea), hypotension, and hypoglycemia. In addition, headache, visual field impairment, and visual impairment occur in cases of hypophysitis with high-grade enlargement of the pituitary gland. In blood examination, abnormal findings such as hyponatremia and eosinophilia are recognized.

If hypopituitarism is suspected, it is necessary to measure the hormones secreted by the anterior pituitary gland and target organs. With regard to hypophysitis, diffuse enlargement and swelling of the pituitary gland and pituitary stalk with enhancement on contrast-enhanced magnetic resonance imaging are observed in more than half of the cases [17]. Subsequently, the enlarged pituitary gland gradually shrinks in the acute phase, and pituitary function is partially or completely lost [28,29]. During long-term observations, (median follow-up, 33 months) in one study, many of the thyroid and gonadal dysfunctions were found to be reversible, whereas ACTH hyposecretion was irreversible in most cases [29]. The pathogenesis of hypopituitarism due to ICI treatment remains unclear. In autopsied cases of pituitary dysfunction caused by tremelimumab, anti-CTLA-4 antibody, necrotic changes, and lymphocytic infiltrates with fibrosis were observed in the anterior pituitary gland. In addition, complement component 4 fragment (C4d) deposition associated with complement activation was observed; this suggested the involvement of both type IV and type II allergic reactions [17].

3. Adrenal Insufficiency

Adrenal insufficiency caused by ICI treatment includes primary and secondary adrenal insufficiency caused by hypopituitarism. Most cases are considered to have secondary adrenal insufficiency, and primary adrenal insufficiency is thought to be less frequent, with a reported incidence of 1.4% (95% confidence interval (CI): 0.9–2.2) for ipilimumab, 2.0% (95% CI: 0.9–4.3) for nivolumab, and 5.2% (95% CI: 2.9–9.2) to 7.6% (95% CI: 1.2–36.8) for nivolumab or pembrolizumab combined with ipilimumab [12]. The time of onset is estimated as one to several months after the start of treatment [22,30]. The symptoms of adrenal insufficiency are nonspecific and include fatigue, anorexia, abdominal pain, nausea, weight loss, hypotension, and hypoglycemia. The appearance of hyponatremia, eosinophilia, and neutropenia suggests the development of adrenal insufficiency. A low morning serum cortisol level despite an elevated plasma ACTH level suggests primary adrenal insufficiency, whereas a low plasma ACTH level suggests secondary adrenal insufficiency. Serum cortisol levels of ≥18 μg/dL are considered to indicate the absence of adrenal dysfunction, while adrenal dysfunction is represented by serum cortisol levels of <4 μg/dL. When the serum cortisol level is ≥4 μg/dL and <18 μg/dL, a rapid ACTH tolerance test or an insulin-hypoglycemia test can confirm the diagnosis [31]. Bilateral adrenal enlargement on abdominal computed tomography (CT) and fluorodeoxyglucose (FDG) uptake in the bilateral adrenal glands on positron emission tomography (PET) have been reported; however, similar findings may be observed in cases of adrenal metastasis, which warrant careful judgment [32]. With regard to the pathogenesis of primary adrenal insufficiency caused by ICI treatment, adrenal autoantibodies have been detected in one case of pembrolizumab-induced adrenal insufficiency, although several points remain to be clarified [31].

4. Thyroid Dysfunction

Among endocrinopathies occurring as irAEs, thyroid dysfunction is the most frequent. Although thyroid dysfunction is mainly caused by thyrotoxicosis, while hypothyroidism is caused by destructive thyroiditis, the occurrence of Basedow's disease after the administration of anti CTLA-4 antibodies has also been reported [33,34]. The reported incidence of thyroid dysfunction with the use of anti-PD-1 antibodies is 5–10%. The incidence of thyroid dysfunction is higher with the use of anti-PD-L1 antibodies (0–5%) and anti-CTLA-4 antibodies (0–5%) [19–21]. In a previous systematic review and meta-analysis, increased use of combination treatment was observed, with hypothyroidism occurring in 16.4% cases treated with nivolumab combined with ipilimumab [12]. Moreover, the incidence of hypothyroidism was significantly higher with ICI treatment than with chemotherapy and placebo treatment [12]. In other studies, thyroid dysfunction was more frequent in cases treated with anti-thyroglobulin (Tg) antibody (anti-TgAb) and anti-thyroid peroxidase antibody (anti-TPOAb) than in cases treated without these antibodies before nivolumab treatment initiation; this finding may be beneficial for predicting the onset of thyroid dysfunction [35,36]. Destructive thyroiditis occurs within a few weeks after ICI treatment initiation in many cases, and it may present with thyrotoxicosis [37–39]. Subsequently, patients may exhibit a transition to hypothyroidism within 3–6 weeks [37–40]. In a previous study, 12 of 99 patients who received pembrolizumab developed thyrotoxicosis, and transition to hypothyroidism occurred in nine of the 12 patients [39]. Another study found thyrotoxicosis in six of 10 patients who developed indolent thyroiditis after pembrolizumab treatment initiation; all six patients exhibited a transition to hypothyroidism after four weeks [38].

Symptoms of thyrotoxicosis include palpitations, sweating, fever, diarrhea, tremors, weight loss, and general fatigue. Neck pain is generally not observed. Blood tests show a decreased serum TSH level, elevated serum free T3 (FT3) and free T4 (FT4) levels, and negativity for thyroid receptor antibody (TRAb). Quite often, anti-TgAb and anti-TPOAb are positive [30,36]. In addition, there are many cases in which the increased serum Tg level is recognized by destruction of the thyroid gland, and it is said that the Tg level normalizes upon transitioning to hypothyroidism [40]. Thyroid echography frequently shows decreased blood flow and an internal heterogeneous low signal intensity. FDG-PET also shows increased uptake, while thyroid scintigraphy shows decreased iodine uptake [38].

Hypothyroidism may develop after thyrotoxicosis or simultaneously with the onset of thyroiditis. If the latter occurs, positivity for anti-TgAb and anti-TPOAb is seen in several cases [37]. Major symptoms include general fatigue, loss of appetite, constipation, bradycardia, and weight gain. Blood tests show elevated serum TSH and decreased serum FT4 and FT3 levels. In mild cases, a slightly high TSH level may result in a state of occult hypothyroidism. Thyroid echography may show decreased blood flow, parenchymal hypointensity, and atrophy. Hypothyroidism secondary to hypopituitarism must be ruled out in patients showing hypothyroidism. Hypopituitarism can be suspected when serum FT4 levels are low and TSH levels are low to normal. Differentiation should be cautious because low serum FT3 levels also occur in the end stages of malignancy and in low T3 syndrome complicating severe infections. In low T3 syndrome, the serum FT3 level is low and the serum FT4 level is normal or slightly decreased, while the serum TSH level is normal.

The mechanism by which ICIs cause thyroid dysfunction has not been clarified, but it has been suggested that the expression of PD-L1 and programmed death ligand 2 in the thyroid tissue plays a role [41].

5. Type 1 Diabetes Mellitus

Type 1 diabetes induced by ICI treatment results from the destruction of β-cells by ICIs and is reportedly more frequent with the use of anti-PD1/anti-PD-L1 antibodies. However, the reported incidences are 2.0% and 0.4% with nivolumab and pembrolizumab; thus, it seems to be a less common irAE [12]. The incidence of type I diabetes after ipilimumab treatment is even lower [20,42]. However, fulminant type I diabetes mellitus can worsen rapidly and prove fatal, and it is necessary to consider the possibility of this complication when administering ICIs. The time from anti-PD-1 therapy initiation to the onset of type 1 diabetes has been reported to be 13–504 days [43]. Symptoms include dry mouth, polydipsia, and polyuria due to hyperglycemia in mild-to-moderate cases. Severe disease is associated with ketosis, ketoacidosis, general fatigue, and disturbed consciousness, with further progression resulting in coma.

Fulminant type I diabetes mellitus exhibits a hyperacute onset over several days, and endogenous insulin is depleted at the time of diagnosis [44]. On the other hand, type I diabetes mellitus develops relatively slowly over the course of several weeks.

Because β-cell dysfunction is generally irreversible, it is important to make a diagnosis and initiate treatment before the development of ketoacidosis. Diabetes mellitus should be suspected when symptoms of hyperglycemia appear and fasting blood sugar and random blood sugar levels exceed 126 and 200 mg/mL, respectively. In such cases, definite diagnosis and diagnosis of the disease type should be performed.

Blood glucose levels may be elevated to approximately 200–300 mg/dL, although elevation to approximately 1000 mg/dL is also possible. The HbA1c level is also elevated, notwithstanding it is lower relative to the blood glucose level. The C peptide level gradually decreases in serum and urine, and anti-glutamic acid decarboxylase antibodies are generally absent.

6. Treatment

6.1. Hypopituitarism

Table 2 presents management strategies for hypopituitarism according to the Common Terminology Criteria for Adverse Events (CTCAE) grade. Treatment generally involves hormone replacement therapy. ACTH deficiency is treated with hydrocortisone (10 to 20 mg/day). High doses of glucocorticoids have been reported to improve pituitary enlargement [24,45]. On the other hand, it has been reported that high doses of glucocorticoids do not contribute to restoration of the secretory capacity of ACTH and are associated with relatively high mortality [24,45]. High-dose glucocorticoids are recommended only if the condition is associated with headache and pituitary enlargement with visual field damage. When both TSH and ACTH secretion disorders are present, hydrocortisone replacement therapy must be preceded by hormone replacement therapy. The use of ICIs in patients with treatment-induced hypopituitarism should be discontinued until treatment stabilizes their general condition.

Table 2. Management of hypopituitarism induced by immune checkpoint inhibitors.

CTCAE Grade	Management	Treatment of Adverse Event
Grade 1	• Hormone supplementation as needed	• Consider consultation with an endocrinologist • If adrenal insufficiency is suspected, start hydrocortisone 10–20 mg BID • Start testosterone or estrogen replacement therapy if needed
Grade 2	• Stop ICI treatment until symptoms stabilize by hormone supplementation • After amelioration of symptoms, resume administration of ICI	• Consult an endocrinologist • Consider pituitary imaging • Perform hormone replacement therapy as performed for Grade 1 events • Perform frequent thyroid function and other hormonal tests until baseline levels are achieved
Grade 3	• Same as above	• Consult an endocrinologist • Consider pituitary imaging • Perform a pituitary function test on hospitalization • If adrenal insufficiency is present, start hydrocortisone 15–30 mg BID • Perform hormone replacement therapy as performed for Grade 1 events • Perform frequent thyroid function and other hormonal tests until baseline levels are achieved
Grade 4	• Stop ICI treatment • Resume administration after recovery from crisis and stabilization of symptoms	• Perform full-body management during hospitalization • Consult an endocrinologist • Immediately start administration of hydrocortisone 100–200 mg BID • Physiological saline infusion under cardiac function monitoring • Consider pituitary imaging • Perform frequent thyroid function and other hormonal tests until baseline levels are achieved

CTCAE, Common Terminology Criteria for Adverse Events; ICI, immune checkpoint inhibitor; BID, bis in die

6.2. *Adrenal Insufficiency*

Table 3 presents management strategies for adrenal insufficiency according to the CTCAE grade. The condition should be managed according to its severity. Hydrocortisone (10–20 mg/day) replacement therapy should be initiated for patients with only laboratory abnormalities or mild symptoms that permit activities of daily living [46]. In case of adrenal crisis, systemic management and early administration of hydrocortisone are necessary. In all cases, consultation with an endocrinologist is recommended for medical care. If primary adrenal insufficiency due to ICI treatment occurs, the drugs should be discontinued and administered after stabilization of the patient's general condition by treatment.

Table 3. Management of adrenal insufficiency induced by immune checkpoint inhibitors.

CTCAE Grade	Management	Treatment of Adverse Event
Grade 1	• Hormone supplementation as needed • After amelioration of symptoms, resume administration of ICI	• Consult an endocrinologist • If adrenal insufficiency is suspected, start hydrocortisone 10–20 mg BID
Grade 2	• Stop ICI treatment until symptoms stabilize by hormone supplementation • After amelioration of symptoms, resume administration of ICI	• Consult an endocrinologist • Perform hormone replacement therapy as performed for Grade 1 events • Perform frequent hormonal tests until baseline levels are achieved
Grade 3	• Same as above	• Consult an endocrinologist • Perform an adrenal function test on hospitalization • If adrenal insufficiency is present, start hydrocortisone 15–30 mg BID
Grade 4	• Stop ICI treatment • Resume administration after recovery from crisis and stabilization of symptoms	• Perform full-body management during hospitalization • Consult an endocrinologist • Immediately start administration of hydrocortisone 100–200 mg BID • Physiological saline infusion under cardiac function monitoring • Perform an adrenal function test after the general condition has stabilized

CTCAE, Common Terminology Criteria for Adverse Events; ICI, immune checkpoint inhibitor.

6.3. *Thyroid Dysfunction*

Tables 4 and 5 show the management strategies for hyperthyroidism and hypothyroidism, respectively, according to the CTCAE grade. For thyrotoxicosis caused by destructive thyroiditis, antithyroid drugs are not necessary because the duration of symptoms is usually short. When symptoms such as tremors and motivation are recognized, symptomatic treatment with a β-blocker is required. Antithyroid drugs are reserved for patients with Basedow's disease.

Table 4. Management of hyperthyroidism induced by immune checkpoint inhibitors.

CTCAE Grade	Management	Treatment of Adverse Event
Grade 1	• Continue ICI treatment	• Continue to monitor TSH and FT4 levels until hyperthyroidism disappears
Grade 2	• Stop ICI treatment until the symptoms ameliorate or test values become normal • After amelioration of symptoms, resume administration of ICI	• Consult an endocrinologist • Perform a thyroid function test every 2–3 weeks • If the thyroid poisoning does not resolve after 6–8 weeks, Graves' disease is differentiated
Grade 3 or 4	• Same as above	• Consult an endocrinologist • Start administration of β-blocker • Conduct clinical tests every 1–3 weeks • In case of thyroid crisis, treat the patient in the intensive care unit

CTCAE, Common Terminology Criteria for Adverse Events; ICI, immune checkpoint inhibitor; TSH, thyroid-stimulating hormone; FT4, free T4.

Table 5. Management of hypothyroidism induced by immune checkpoint inhibitors.

CTCAE Grade	Management	Treatment of Adverse Event
Grade 1	• Continue ICI treatment	• Continue to monitor TSH, FT3, and FT4 levels every 2–3 weeks
Grade 2	• Stop ICI treatment until the symptoms ameliorate or test values become normal • After amelioration of symptoms, resume administration of ICI	• Consult an endocrinologist • Start thyroid hormone replacement therapy if symptoms are present or the TSH level is high • If thyroid function is stable, perform a thyroid function test every 6 weeks
Grade 3 or 4	• Same as above	• Consult an endocrinologist • Start administration of β-blocker • In case of myxedema coma, treat the patient in the intensive care unit • Following stabilization of symptoms, treat as per the protocol for Grade 2 events

CTCAE, Common Terminology Criteria for Adverse Events; ICI, immune checkpoint inhibitor; TSH, thyroid-stimulating hormone; FT4, free T4; FT3, free T3.

In case of hypothyroidism, if the TSH level is <10 mIU/L and no symptoms are observed, ICI administration is continued and serum TSH, FT4, and FT3 levels are monitored. If the TSH level is ≥10 mIU/L and moderate symptoms are present, thyroid hormone replacement therapy is planned [37]. In case of concomitant adrenal insufficiency, careful monitoring is required, and thyroid hormone replacement should be preceded by the administration of hydrocortisone if the adrenal insufficiency worsens.

ICI treatment can be resumed when treatment with or without thyroid hormone replacement therapy results in amelioration of symptoms.

6.4. Type 1 Diabetes Mellitus

Insulin therapy is the mainstay of treatment for type 1 diabetes mellitus due to ICI treatment, and immediate treatment must be initiated. If ketosis or ketoacidosis is present, immediate-acting insulin should be continuously administered, along with intravenous saline infusion and electrolyte management. After the ketosis or ketoacidosis has improved, the patient can be switched to insulin therapy. Once insulin treatment reduces the blood glucose levels, ICI treatment can be resumed.

7. Adrenal Insufficiency in Tumor-Bearing Patients

As noted above, primary/secondary adrenal insufficiency is a less common but potentially fatal irAE, and it often includes adrenal crisis, in patients receiving ICIs. On the other hand, symptoms are often nonspecific, such as anorexia and malaise, which are also common symptoms in cancer patients. Adrenal insufficiency is also a common condition in cancer patients, and efforts must be made to detect it at an early stage.

Causes of adrenal insufficiency other than ICI treatment in cancer patients include steroid withdrawal syndrome, adrenal metastases from primary disease, and autoimmune adrenalitis.

Long-term corticosteroid treatment may be used for various purposes in cancer patients, including palliation of symptoms such as fatigue, resolution of cerebral edema, and treatment of drug-induced or radioactive organ damage. In addition, they are often administered during anticancer drug therapy. Long-term corticosteroid use causes hypothalamic–pituitary–adrenal suppression and adrenal atrophy. Steroid withdrawal syndrome may occur when steroids are suddenly reduced or discontinued, and many patients present with clinical features of acute adrenal insufficiency. It is necessary to pay attention to sudden dose reduction and discontinuation in patients who have been receiving long-term steroid treatment, and steroid withdrawal syndrome should be suspected when symptoms indicating adrenal insufficiency are observed. In case of steroid withdrawal syndrome, the symptoms rapidly disappear when the steroid dose is increased in most cases.

Moreover, when physical stresses such as diarrhea, trauma, and dehydration occur in patients receiving long-term corticosteroid treatment, relative steroid deficiency may develop and result in adrenal insufficiency symptoms. The causative disease should be treated, and the dose of the steroid drug should be increased. Failure to take appropriate measures may result in adrenal crisis and potentially fatal conditions. On the other hand, in cancer patients, metastatic adrenal tumors may cause adrenal insufficiency. A previous study involving autopsy of malignant tumors found adrenal metastasis in approximately 3% cases [47]. Further, chronic primary adrenocortical insufficiency due to metastatic adrenal tumors is rare and has been reported to occur in approximately 1% patients [47]. Even in cases of metastatic adrenal tumors, cortisol secretion is preserved until approximately 90% of the bilateral adrenal glands are destroyed, and the typical symptoms may not appear in many cases, which complicates diagnosis [48].

8. Adrenal Crisis

Adrenal crisis can occur when infection and injury are complicated by adrenocortical insufficiency, and it progresses to a fatal disease state via absolute and relative steroid deficiency. Primary/secondary adrenal insufficiency due to ICI treatment may also lead to adrenal crisis, and early diagnosis and appropriate measures should be implemented at onset. The initial symptoms of adrenal crisis, like those of adrenal insufficiency, are nonspecific and include general malaise, anesthesia, loss of appetite, weight loss, nausea, abdominal pain, and fever. However, after >12 h, consciousness disturbance and hypotension can occur.

Blood tests often show hyponatremia, hyperkalemia, hypoglycemia, dehydration, and eosinophilia. When adrenal crisis is suspected on the basis of the medical history and test results, immediate measures should be taken while excluding other conditions such as sepsis. Initial treatment includes infusion of a large volume of saline, glucose solution, and hydrocortisone. Measurements of blood cortisol and ACTH are useful for diagnosis.

9. Conclusions

In summary, endocrine dysfunction is a frequent irAE associated with ICI treatment. Anti-CTLA-4 antibodies often cause hypopituitarism, while anti-PD-1/anti-PD-L1 antibodies cause thyroid dysfunction. Primary adrenal insufficiency and type I diabetes mellitus are less frequent with all ICIs. Hypopituitarism may also cause secondary adrenal insufficiency via ACTH hyposecretion. Symptoms of adrenal insufficiency are nonspecific and common also in cancer patients; therefore, diagnosis may be difficult. Moreover, symptoms of adrenal insufficiency in cancer patients often have a background other than irAE caused by ICI in tumor bearing patients. While adrenal insufficiency leads to adrenal crisis in severe cases, type 1 diabetes mellitus may progress to fulminant disease; thus, both conditions should be detected and treated at the early stages. As the indications of ICIs expand, the number of irAEs episodes also tends to increase as shown in Figure 1. In the future, early detection and proper management of endocrine dysfunction should be considered important for the treatment using ICI as mentioned above.

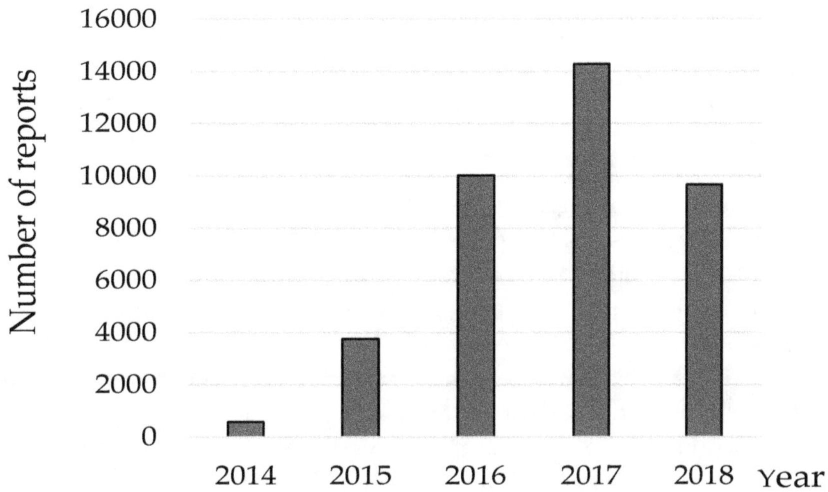

Figure 1. Adopted from Reference [49]. Food and Drug Administration (FDA)-reported numbers of immune-related Adverse Events (irAEs) with anti programmed cell death 1 (PD-1)/ programmed death ligand 1 (PD-L1) antibody monotherapy versus anti PD-1/PD-L1 antibody plus anti cytotoxic T-lymphocyte antigen-4 (CTLA-4) antibody combination treatment. (Number of reports up to June in 2018).

Author Contributions: Writing—original draft preparation, N.O., M.A., and J.U.; writing—review and editing, J.U., Y.M., M.I., Y.K., and T.Y.; supervision, M.F. and K.T. All authors have read and agreed to the published version of the manuscript.

References

1. Ribas, A.; Wolchok, J.D. Cancer immunotherapy using checkpoint blockade. *Science* **2018**, *359*, 1350–1355. [CrossRef]
2. Salomon, B.; Bluestone, J.A.C. Omplexities of Cd28/B7: Ctla-4 C Ostimulatory P Athways In A Utoimmunity And T Ransplantation. *Annu. Rev. Immunol.* **2001**, *19*, 225–252. [CrossRef] [PubMed]
3. Teft, W.A.; Kirchhof, M.G.; Madrenas, J. A molecular perspective of ctla-4 function. *Annu. Rev. Immunol.* **2006**, *24*, 65–97. [CrossRef] [PubMed]
4. Quezada, S.A.; Simpson, T.R.; Peggs, K.S.; Merghoub, T.; Vider, J.; Fan, X.; Blasberg, R.; Yagita, H.; Muranski, P.; Antony, P.A.; et al. Tumor-reactive CD4+ T cells develop cytotoxic activity and eradicate large established melanoma after transfer into lymphopenic hosts. *J. Exp. Med.* **2010**, *207*, 637–650. [CrossRef] [PubMed]
5. Bulliard, Y.; Jolicoeur, R.; Windman, M.; Rue, S.M.; Ettenberg, S.; Knee, D.A.; Wilson, N.S.; Dranoff, G.; Brogdon, J.L. Activating fc γ receptors contribute to the antitumor activities of immunoregulatory receptor-targeting antibodies. *J. Exp. Med.* **2013**, *210*, 1685–1693. [CrossRef]
6. Selby, M.J.; Engelhardt, J.J.; Quigley, M.; Henning, K.A.; Chen, T.; Srinivasan, M.; Korman, A.J. Anti-CTLA-4 antibodies of IgG2a isotype enhance antitumor activity through reduction of intratumoral regulatory T cells. *Cancer Immunol. Res.* **2013**, *1*, 32–42. [CrossRef] [PubMed]
7. Simpson, T.R.; Li, F.; Montalvo-Ortiz, W.; Sepulveda, M.A.; Bergerhoff, K.; Arce, F.; Roddie, C.; Henry, J.Y.; Yagita, H.; Wolchok, J.D.; et al. Fc-dependent depletion of tumor-infiltrating regulatory t cells co-defines the efficacy of anti-CTLA-4 therapy against melanoma. *J. Exp. Med.* **2013**, *210*, 1695–1710. [CrossRef]
8. Freeman, G.J.; Long, A.J.; Iwai, Y.; Bourque, K.; Chernova, T.; Nishimura, H.; Fitz, L.J.; Malenkovich, N.; Okazaki, T.; Byrne, M.C.; et al. Engagement of the PD-1 immunoinhibitory receptor by a novel B7 family member leads to negative regulation of lymphocyte activation. *J. Exp. Med.* **2000**, *192*, 1027–1034. [CrossRef]

9. Chang, L.S.; Barroso-Sousa, R.; Tolaney, S.M.; Hodi, F.S.; Kaiser, U.B.; Min, L. Endocrine toxicity of cancer immunotherapy targeting immune checkpoints. *Endocr. Rev.* **2018**, *40*, 17–65. [CrossRef]
10. Davies, M.; Duffield, E.A. Safety of checkpoint inhibitors for cancer treatment: Strategies for patient monitoring and management of immune-mediated adverse events. *ImmunoTargets Ther.* **2017**, *6*, 51–71. [CrossRef]
11. Postow, M.A. Managing Immune Checkpoint-Blocking Antibody Side Effects. *Am. Soc. Clin. Oncol. Educ. B* **2015**, *76*–83. [CrossRef] [PubMed]
12. De Filette, J.; Andreescu, C.E.; Cools, F.; Bravenboer, B.; Velkeniers, B. A Systematic Review and Meta-Analysis of Endocrine-Related Adverse Events Associated with Immune Checkpoint Inhibitors. *Horm. Metab. Res.* **2019**, *51*, 145–156. [CrossRef] [PubMed]
13. Win, M.A.; Thein, K.Z.; Qdaisat, A.; Yeung, S.C.J. Acute symptomatic hypocalcemia from immune checkpoint therapy-induced hypoparathyroidism. *Am. J. Emerg. Med.* **2017**, *35*, 1039.e5–1039.e7. [CrossRef]
14. Umeguchi, H.; Takenoshita, H.; Inoue, H.; Kurihara, Y.; Sakaguchi, C.; Yano, S.; Hasuzawa, N.; Sakamoto, S.; Sakamoto, R.; Ashida, K. Autoimmune-Related Primary Hypoparathyroidism Possibly Induced by the Administration of Pembrolizumab: A Case Report. *J. Oncol. Pract.* **2018**, *14*, 449–451. [CrossRef] [PubMed]
15. Trinh, B.; Sanchez, G.O.; Herzig, P.; Läubli, H. Inflammation-induced hypoparathyroidism triggered by combination immune checkpoint blockade for melanoma. *J. Immunother. Cancer* **2019**, *7*. [CrossRef] [PubMed]
16. Piranavan, P.; Li, Y.; Brown, E.; Kemp, E.H.; Trivedi, N. Immune Checkpoint Inhibitor-Induced Hypoparathyroidism Associated with Calcium-Sensing Receptor-Activating Autoantibodies. *J. Clin. Endocrinol. Metab.* **2018**, *104*, 550–556. [CrossRef] [PubMed]
17. Caturegli, P.; Di Dalmazi, G.; Lombardi, M.; Grosso, F.; Larman, H.B.; Larman, T.; Taverna, G.; Cosottini, M.; Lupi, I. Hypophysitis Secondary to Cytotoxic T-Lymphocyte–Associated Protein 4 Blockade: Insights into Pathogenesis from an Autopsy Series. *Am. J. Pathol.* **2016**, *186*, 3225–3235. [CrossRef]
18. Bertrand, A.; Kostine, M.; Barnetche, T.; Truchetet, M.E.; Schaeverbeke, T. Immune related adverse events associated with anti-CTLA-4 antibodies: Systematic review and meta-analysis. *BMC Med.* **2015**, *13*. [CrossRef]
19. Byun, D.J.; Wolchok, J.D.; Rosenberg, L.M.; Girotra, M. Cancer immunotherapy-immune checkpoint blockade and associated endocrinopathies. *Nat. Rev. Endocrinol.* **2017**, *13*, 195–207. [CrossRef]
20. Barroso-Sousa, R.; Barry, W.T.; Garrido-Castro, A.C.; Hodi, F.S.; Min, L.; Krop, I.E.; Tolaney, S.M. Incidence of endocrine dysfunction following the use of different immune checkpoint inhibitor regimens a systematic review and meta-analysis. *JAMA Oncol.* **2018**, *4*, 173–182. [CrossRef]
21. González-Rodríguez, E.; Rodríguez-Abreu, D. Immune Checkpoint Inhibitors: Review and Management of Endocrine Adverse Events. *Oncologist* **2016**, *21*, 804–816. [CrossRef] [PubMed]
22. Cukier, P.; Santini, F.C.; Scaranti, M.; Hoff, A.O. Endocrine side effects of cancer immunotherapy. *Endocr. Relat. Cancer* **2017**, *24*, T331–T347. [CrossRef] [PubMed]
23. Zhao, C.; Tella, S.H.; Rivero, J.D.e.l.; Kommalapati, A.; Ebenuwa, I.; Gulley, J.; Strauss, J.; Brownell, I. Anti-PD-L1 treatment induced central diabetes insipidus. *J. Clin. Endocrinol. Metab.* **2018**, *103*, 365–369. [CrossRef] [PubMed]
24. Faje, A.; Reynolds, K.; Zubiri, L.; Lawrence, D.; Cohen, J.V.; Sullivan, R.J.; Nachtigall, L.; Tritos, N. Hypophysitis secondary to nivolumab and pembrolizumab is a clinical entity distinct from ipilimumab-associated hypophysitis. *Eur. J. Endocrinol.* **2019**, *181*, 211–219. [CrossRef]
25. Kanie, K.; Iguchi, G.; Bando, H.; Fujita, Y.; Odake, Y.; Yoshida, K.; Matsumoto, R.; Fukuoka, H.; Ogawa, W.; Takahashi, Y. Two Cases of Atezolizumab-Induced Hypophysitis. *J. Endocr. Soc.* **2018**, *2*, 91–95. [CrossRef]
26. Cho, K.Y.; Miyoshi, H.; Nakamura, A.; Kurita, T.; Atsumi, T. Hyponatremia can be a powerful predictor of the development of isolated ACTH deficiency associated with nivolumab treatment. *Endocr. J.* **2017**, *64*, 235–236. [CrossRef]
27. Okano, Y.; Satoh, T.; Horiguchi, K.; Toyoda, M.; Osaki, A.; Matsumoto, S.; Tomaru, T.; Nakajima, Y.; Ishii, S.; Ozawa, A.; et al. Nivolumab-induced hypophysitis in a patient with advanced malignant melanoma. *Endocr. J.* **2016**, *63*, 905–912. [CrossRef]
28. Albarel, F.; Gaudy, C.; Castinetti, F.; Carré, T.; Morange, I.; Conte-Devolx, B.; Grob, J.J.; Brue, T. Long-term follow-up of ipilimumab-induced hypophysitis, a common adverse event of the anti-CTLA-4 antibody in melanoma. *Eur. J. Endocrinol.* **2015**, *172*, 195–204. [CrossRef]

29. Ryder, M.; Callahan, M.; Postow, M.A.; Wolchok, J.; Fagin, J.A. Endocrine-related adverse events following ipilimumab in patients with advanced melanoma: A comprehensive retrospective review from a single institution. *Endocr. Relat. Cancer* **2014**, *21*, 371–381. [CrossRef]
30. Trainer, H.; Hulse, P.; Higham, C.E.; Trainer, P.; Lorigan, P. Hyponatraemia secondary to nivolumab-induced primary adrenal failure. *Endocrinol. Diabetes Metab. Case Rep.* **2016**, *2016*. [CrossRef]
31. Paepegaey, A.-C.; Lheure, C.; Ratour, C.; Lethielleux, G.; Clerc, J.; Bertherat, J.; Kramkimel, N.; Groussin, L. Polyendocrinopathy Resulting From Pembrolizumab in a Patient With a Malignant Melanoma. *J. Endocr. Soc.* **2017**, *1*, 646–649. [CrossRef]
32. Min, L.; Ibrahim, N. Ipilimumab-induced autoimmune adrenalitis. *Lancet Diabetes Endocrinol.* **2013**, *1*, e15. [CrossRef]
33. Inaba, H.; Ariyasu, H.; Okuhira, H.; Yamamoto, Y.; Akamatsu, H.; Katsuda, M.; Jinnin, M.; Hara, I.; Akamizu, T. Endocrine dysfunctions during treatment of immune-checkpoint inhibitors. *Trends Immunother.* **2018**, *2*. [CrossRef]
34. Gan, E.H.; Mitchell, A.L.; Plummer, R.; Pearce, S.; Perros, P. Tremelimumab-Induced Graves Hyperthyroidism. *Eur. Thyroid J.* **2017**, *6*, 167–170. [CrossRef] [PubMed]
35. Kimbara, S.; Fujiwara, Y.; Iwama, S.; Ohashi, K.; Kuchiba, A.; Arima, H.; Yamazaki, N.; Kitano, S.; Yamamoto, N.; Ohe, Y. Association of antithyroglobulin antibodies with the development of thyroid dysfunction induced by nivolumab. *Cancer Sci.* **2018**, *109*, 3583–3590. [CrossRef]
36. Kobayashi, T.; Iwama, S.; Yasuda, Y.; Okada, N.; Tsunekawa, T.; Onoue, T.; Takagi, H.; Hagiwara, D.; Ito, Y.; Morishita, Y.; et al. Patients With Antithyroid Antibodies Are Prone To Develop Destructive Thyroiditis by Nivolumab: A Prospective Study. *J. Endocr. Soc.* **2018**, *2*, 241–251. [CrossRef]
37. Alhusseini, M.; Samantray, J. Hypothyroidism in Cancer Patients on Immune Checkpoint Inhibitors with anti-PD1 Agents: Insights on Underlying Mechanisms. *Exp. Clin. Endocrinol. Diabetes* **2017**, *125*, 267–269. [CrossRef]
38. Orlov, S.; Salari, F.; Kashat, L.; Walfish, P.G. Induction of painless thyroiditis in patients receiving programmed death 1 receptor immunotherapy for metastatic malignancies. *J. Clin. Endocrinol. Metab.* **2015**, *100*, 1738–1741. [CrossRef]
39. De Filette, J.; Jansen, Y.; Schreuer, M.; Everaert, H.; Velkeniers, B.; Neyns, B.; Bravenboer, B. Incidence of thyroid-related adverse events in melanoma patients treated with pembrolizumab. *J. Clin. Endocrinol. Metab.* **2016**, *101*, 4431–4439. [CrossRef]
40. Delivanis, D.A.; Gustafson, M.P.; Bornschlegl, S.; Merten, M.M.; Kottschade, L.; Withers, S.; Dietz, A.B.; Ryder, M. Pembrolizumab-induced thyroiditis: Comprehensive clinical review and insights into underlying involved mechanisms. *J. Clin. Endocrinol. Metab.* **2017**, *102*, 2770–2780. [CrossRef]
41. Yamauchi, I.; Sakane, Y.; Fukuda, Y.; Fujii, T.; Taura, D.; Hirata, M.; Hirota, K.; Ueda, Y.; Kanai, Y.; Yamashita, Y.; et al. Clinical Features of Nivolumab-Induced Thyroiditis: A Case Series Study. *Thyroid* **2017**, *27*, 894–901. [CrossRef] [PubMed]
42. Shiba, M.; Inaba, H.; Ariyasu, H.; Kawai, S.; Inagaki, Y.; Matsuno, S.; Iwakura, H.; Yamamoto, Y.; Nishi, M.; Akamizu, T. Fulminant type 1 diabetes mellitus accompanied by positive conversion of anti-insulin antibody after the administration of anti-CTLA-4 antibody following the discontinuation of anti-PD-1 antibody. *Intern. Med.* **2018**, *57*, 2029–2034. [CrossRef]
43. Baden, M.Y.; Imagawa, A.; Abiru, N.; Awata, T.; Ikegami, H.; Uchigata, Y.; Oikawa, Y.; Osawa, H.; Kajio, H.; Kawasaki, E.; et al. Characteristics and clinical course of type 1 diabetes mellitus related to anti-programmed cell death-1 therapy. *Diabetol. Int.* **2019**, *10*, 58–66. [CrossRef] [PubMed]
44. Imagawa, A.; Hanafusa, T.; Awata, T.; Ikegami, H.; Uchigata, Y.; Osawa, H.; Kawasaki, E.; Kawabata, Y.; Kobayashi, T.; Shimada, A.; et al. Report of the Committee of the Japan Diabetes Society on the Research of Fulminant and Acute-onset Type 1 Diabetes Mellitus: New diagnostic criteria of fulminant type 1 diabetes mellitus (2012). *J. Diabetes Investig.* **2012**, *3*, 536–539. [CrossRef] [PubMed]
45. Min, L.; Hodi, F.S.; Giobbie-Hurder, A.; Ott, P.A.; Luke, J.J.; Donahue, H.; Davis, M.; Carroll, R.S.; Kaiser, U.B. Systemic high-dose corticosteroid treatment does not improve the outcome of ipilimumab-related hypophysitis: A retrospective cohort study. *Clin. Cancer Res.* **2015**, *21*, 749–755. [CrossRef] [PubMed]
46. Yanase, T.; Tajima, T.; Katabami, T.; Iwasaki, Y.; Tanahashi, Y.; Sugawara, A.; Hasegawa, T.; Mune, T.; Oki, Y.; Nakagawa, Y.; et al. Diagnosis and treatment of adrenal insufficiency including adrenal crisis: A Japan endocrine society clinical practice guideline. *Endocr. J.* **2016**, *63*, 765–784. [CrossRef] [PubMed]

47. Lam, K.-Y.; Lo, C.-Y. Metastatic tumours of the adrenal glands: A 30-year experience in a teaching hospital. *Clin. Endocrinol. (Oxf).* **2002**, *56*, 95–101. [CrossRef]
48. Barker, N.W. The pathologic anatomy in twenty-eight cases of Addison's disease. *Arch. Pathol.* **1929**, *8*, 432–450.
49. Raschi, E.; Mazzarella, A.; Antonazzo, I.C.; Bendinelli, N.; Forcesi, E.; Tuccori, M.; Moretti, U.; Poluzzi, E.; De Ponti, F. Toxicities with Immune Checkpoint Inhibitors: Emerging Priorities From Disproportionality Analysis of the FDA Adverse Event Reporting System. *Target Oncol.* **2019**, *14*, 205–221. [CrossRef]

11

Prognostic Value of Tumor Size in Resected Stage IIIA-N2 Non-Small-Cell Lung Cancer

Chih-Yu Chen [1,2], Bing-Ru Wu [1,2], Chia-Hung Chen [1,2], Wen-Chien Cheng [1,2], Wei-Chun Chen [1,3,4], Wei-Chih Liao [1,2,4,*], Chih-Yi Chen [5], Te-Chun Hsia [1,3,4] and Chih-Yen Tu [1,2]

1 Division of Pulmonary and Critical Care Medicine, Department of Internal Medicine, China Medical University Hospital, Taichung 40447, Taiwan; cychen0808@gmail.com (C.-Y.C.); d18351@mail.cmuh.org.tw (B.-R.W.); d7996@mail.cmuh.org.tw (C.-H.C.); d14321@mail.cmuh.org.tw (W.-C.C.); d8040@mail.cmuh.org.tw (W.-C.C.); d1914@mail.cmuh.org.tw (T.-C.H.); d7855@mail.cmuh.org.tw (C.-Y.T.)
2 School of Medicine, China Medical University, Taichung 40402, Taiwan
3 Department of Respiratory Therapy, China Medical University, Taichung 40402, Taiwan
4 Hyperbaric oxygen therapy center, China Medical University Hospital, Taichung 40447, Taiwan
5 Department of Surgery, Chung Shan Medical University Hospital, Taichung 40201, Taiwan; cshy1566@csh.org.tw
* Correspondence: weichih.liao@gmail.com

Abstract: The eighth edition of the American Joint Committee on Cancer (AJCC) staging system for lung cancer was introduced in 2017 and included major revisions, especially of stage III. For the subgroup stage IIIA-N2 non-small-cell lung cancer (NSCLC), surgical resection remains controversial due to heterogeneous disease entity. The aim of this study was to evaluate the clinicopathologic features and prognostic factors of patients with completely resected stage IIIA-N2 NSCLC. We retrospectively evaluated 77 consecutive patients with pathologic stage IIIA-N2 NSCLC (AJCC eighth edition) who underwent surgical resection with curative intent in China Medical University Hospital between 2006 and 2014. Survival analysis was conducted, using the Kaplan–Meier method. Prognostic factors predicting overall survival (OS) and disease-free survival (DFS) were analyzed, using log-rank tests and multivariate Cox proportional hazards models. Of the 77 patients with pathologic stage IIIA-N2 NSCLC examined, 35 (45.5%) were diagnosed before surgery and 42 (54.5%) were diagnosed unexpectedly during surgery. The mean age of patients was 59 years, and the mean length of follow-up was 38.1 months. The overall one-, three-, and five-year OS rates were 91.9%, 61.3%, and 33.5%, respectively. Multivariate analysis showed that tumor size <3 cm (hazards ratio (HR): 0.373, $p = 0.003$) and video-assisted thoracoscopic surgery (VATS) approach (HR: 0.383, $p = 0.014$) were significant predictors for improved OS. For patients with surgically treated, pathologic stage IIIA-N2 NSCLC, tumor size <3 cm and the VATS approach seemed to be associated with better prognosis.

Keywords: non-small-cell lung cancer; stage IIIA-N2; surgery

1. Introduction

Lung cancer is the most commonly diagnosed cancer and the leading cause of cancer death in the world. In 2018, an estimated 2.1 million new cases (1,368,524 in men and 725,352 in women) of lung and bronchial cancer were diagnosed, and 1.8 million individuals (1,184,947 in men and 576,060 in women) were expected to die of the tumor [1]. Despite recent advances in molecularly targeted therapy and immunotherapy, the long-term survival of patients with lung cancer remains poor, and the five-year-survival rate is below 20% [2,3]. While more than 80% of tumors were unresectable, surgical resection is the major treatment modality for curative intent, with the five-year survival rate being about 60% [4].

The most important prognostic factor for lung cancer is the stage at presentation, which also guides the clinical management of these patients. Based on a global database of lung-cancer cases assembled by the International Association for the Study of Lung Cancer (IASLC) [5], the eighth edition of the American Joint Committee on Cancer (AJCC) staging system for lung cancer was published in 2017 [6], and it was implemented in clinical practice worldwide in 2018 [7]. In addition to the reclassification of extra-thoracic disease into M1b and M1c, the most significant change distinguishing the eighth edition from the seventh edition is the modification of T classification, which may result in different stage allocations. In the eighth edition, stages T1–T4 are redefined according to tumor size (T1a $\leq$ 1 cm; 1 cm < T1b < 2 cm; 2 cm < T1c < 3 cm; 3 cm < T2a < 4 cm; 4 cm < T2b < 5 cm; 5 cm < T3 < 7 cm; T4 > 7 cm). For patients with former stage IIIA-N2 disease, the reclassification of tumor size more than 5 cm shifting from T2b to T3 (> 5 cm but < 7 cm) and from T3 to T4 (> 7 cm) results in a change of stage from IIIA to IIIB.

Due to heterogeneous disease entity, the role of surgical resection for patients with former stage IIIA-N2 non-small-cell lung cancer (NSCLC) remains controversial. According to the guidelines [7,8], multidisciplinary team assessment prior to treatment is warranted to evaluate the resectability, depending on single N2 lymph node station involvement and/or small lymph node size (<3 cm). The treatment options include resection, followed by adjuvant chemotherapy; induction therapy, followed by surgery; definitive concurrent chemoradiation; and consolidation therapy with Durvalumab. However, despite the complexity in treatment planning and major changes in T description and stage allocation of the eighth edition, the guidelines do not address the consequent changes to treatment algorithms for patients with clinical stage IIIA-N2 NSCLC. Furthermore, the role of surgical resection with curative intent in such patients has not been well evaluated. Hence, the aim of this study was to evaluate the clinical features and surgical–pathological factors that affect the prognosis of patients with resected stage IIIA-N2 NSCLC.

2. Materials and Methods

This study was approved by the Institutional Review Board of China Medical University Hospital (CMUH109-REC1-037, date of approval: 11 March 2020), and informed consent was waived because of the retrospective nature of the study.

2.1. Inclusion Criteria

From 1 January 2006 to 31 December 2014, 748 patients with lung cancer underwent surgical resection with mediastinal lymph node dissection or sampling at China Medical University Hospital. The tumor-node-metastasis (TNM) staging system was reclassified according to the eighth edition of the AJCC staging system. A total of 77 (10.3%) patients with stage IIIA-N2 NSCLC who underwent surgical resection with curative intent were enrolled in the study. Smoking status was classified as ever (including current and former smoker) or never smoker. Family history of cancer was defined as any first-degree relative diagnosed with any form of cancer. The preoperative staging workup included complete blood count, serum biochemistry, carcinoembryonic antigen (CEA), chest radiography, chest computed tomography (CT) scan, bronchoscopy, and nuclear medicine exam. Patients with positive surgical tumor margin and incomplete medical record were excluded. There were weekly multidisciplinary lung cancer meetings where thoracic radiologists, radiation oncologist, surgeons, and pulmonologists from the China Medical University Hospital jointly reviewed and discussed the management plan of patients with lung cancer.

2.2. Surgical Technique

Only patients having the Eastern Cooperative Oncology Group (ECOG) performance of 0 or 1 were considered as surgical candidates, and all surgery was performed with curative intent. All patients underwent surgery either with preoperatively clinical N2 disease or unexpectedly during surgery. Tumor location was analyzed as dichotomous variables (lower versus upper or middle lobes; peripheral (outer one-third of lung field) versus central (inner two-thirds of lung fields)). Induction therapy was defined as preoperative chemotherapy and/or radiotherapy. Adjuvant therapy was defined as treatment with either chemotherapy, radiotherapy, or a combination of both after surgical resection. The type of surgery included standard (pneumonectomy, bilobectomy, or lobectomy) and limited resection (wedge resection or segmentectomy). Mediastinal lymph node dissection or sampling with a minimum of three different stations was performed according to the surgeon's experience, and all resected lymph nodes were labeled separately. All pulmonary resections were performed either through open thoracotomy or video-assisted thoracoscopic surgery (VATS).

2.3. *Histopathological Evaluation*

All surgical specimens were evaluated for pathologic staging. Histological typing was performed according to the World Health Organization classification. The recorded variables included tumor size, differentiation grade, visceral pleural involvement, lymphovascular permeation, perineural invasion, multiple N2 station, and N2 ratio. Multiple N2 station was defined as lymph node metastasis involving more than one N2 station. N2 ratio was calculated by dividing the total number of metastatic by the total number of N2 lymph nodes examined.

2.4. *Statistical Analysis*

All statistical analyses were performed by using MedCalc Statistical Software version 19.0.7 (MedCalc Software bvba, Ostend, Belgium; https://www.medcalc.org; 2019). Normally and non-normally distributed continuous data were expressed as mean (standard deviation (SD)) and median (interquartile range (IQR)), respectively. Categorical variables were reported as number (%). Overall survival (OS) was defined as the time from the date of pathological diagnosis until the date of death or last follow-up. Disease-free survival (DFS) was defined as the time from the date of pathological diagnosis until the date of recurrence, death, or last follow-up. Survival curves were estimated by using the Kaplan–Meier method. The prognostic factor analyses were performed by log-rank tests and Cox proportional-hazards regression model. Statistical analysis was considered to be significant when the p-value was < 0.05.

3. Results

3.1. *Demographic and Clinicopathologic Characteristics*

Of the 77 patients with pathologic stage IIIA-N2 NSCLC, 35 were male, and 42 were female, with a mean age of 59 years (SD, 12.2 years; range, 34 to 82 years). Thirty-five (45.5%) patients were diagnosed as N2 disease before surgery, and 42 (54.5%) were diagnosed unexpectedly during surgery. Forty-one (53.2%) patients underwent VATS, and 36 (46.8%) underwent open thoracotomy. The most common histology was adenocarcinoma (62, 80.5%), followed by squamous cell carcinoma (9, 11.7%). The mean size of tumor was 2.9 cm (SD, 1.0 cm). Forty-five (58.4%) patients had tumors of 3 cm or less in diameter, and 32 (41.6%) patients had tumors greater than 3 cm. With respect to lymph node involvement, multiple N2 station was seen in 21 (27.3%) patients and median N2 ratio was 33.3% (IQR, 13.8–50%). Sixty-five (84.4%) patients received adjuvant chemotherapy, of which 23 patients received postoperative radiotherapy. Demographic and clinicopathologic characteristics of the patients are shown in Table 1.

Table 1. Demographic and clinicopathologic characteristics of 77 patients with resected stage IIIA-N2 non-small-cell lung cancer.

Parameter	Value
Age, Mean (SD), y	59 (12.2)
Male, No. (%)	35 (45.5)
Ever smoker, No. (%)	29 (37.7)
Family History of Cancer, No. (%)	14 (18.2)
Comorbidities, No. (%)	
Hypertension	24 (31.2)
Cardiovascular Disease	8 (10.4)
Chronic Obstructive Pulmonary DiseaseLiver Disease	6 (7.8) 6 (7.8)
Chronic Kidney Disease	4 (5.2)
Diabetes Mellitus	10 (13.0)
Performance status, No. (%)	
ECOG 0	39 (50.6)
ECOG 1	38 (49.4)
Clinical N2, No. (%)	35 (45.5)
Surgical Procedure, No. (%)	
Limited Resection	8 (10.4)
Standard Resection	69 (89.6)
Surgical Approach, No. (%)	
VATS	41 (53.2)
Open Thoracotomy	36 (46.8)
Tumor size, mean (SD), cm	2.9 (1.0)
Tumor Size, No. (%)	
≤3 cm	45 (58.4)
3–5 cm	32 (41.6)
Histology, No. (%)	
Adenocarcinoma	62 (80.5)
Squamous Cell Carcinoma	9 (11.7)
Others	6 (7.8)
Differentiation, No. (%)	
Well–moderate	48 (62.3)
Poor	27 (35.1)
Unknown	2 (2.6)
CEA, Median (IQR), ng/mL	4.0 (2.3–13.1)
Visceral Pleural Involvement, No. (%)	35 (45.5)
Lymphovascular Permeation, No. (%)	66 (85.7)
Perineural Invasion, No. (%)	12 (15.6)
Number of Examined Lymph Nodes, Median (IQR)	14 (9–20)
Number of Positive Lymph Nodes, Median (IQR)	3 (1–6)
N2 Ratio, Median (IQR), %	33.3 (13.8–50.0)
Tumor Location, No. (%)	
Central Location	44 (57.1)
Lower Lobe Location	31 (40.3)
Multiple N2 Station, No. (%)	21 (27.3)
Induction therapy, No. (%)	10 (13.0)
Adjuvant Therapy, No. (%)	65 (84.4)
Postoperative Radiotherapy, No. (%)	23 (29.9)

SD, standard deviation; IQR, interquartile range; ECOG, Eastern Cooperative Oncology Group; VATS, video-assisted thoracoscopic surgery; CEA, carcinoembryonic antigen; y, years.

3.2. Overall Survival

Figure 1 depicts that the one-, three-, and five-year OS rates were 91.9%, 61.3%, and 33.5%, respectively. The mean length of follow-up was 38.1 months.

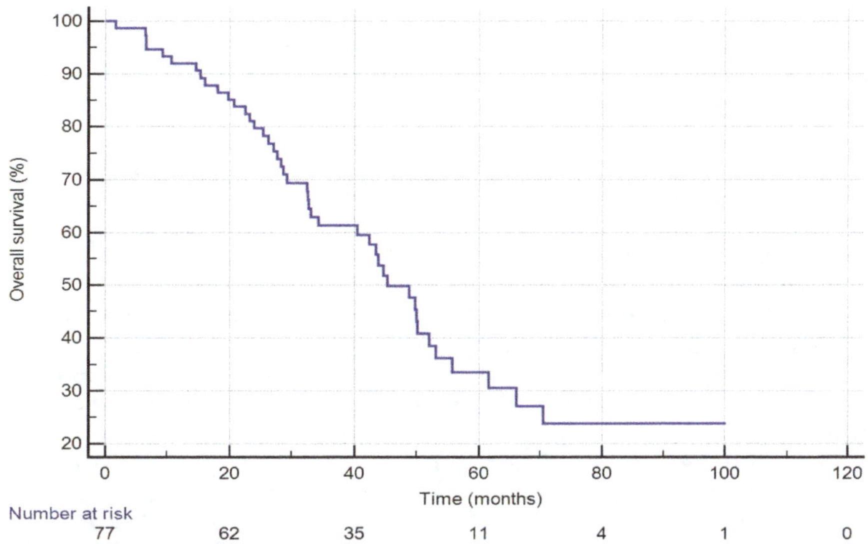

Figure 1. Overall-survival curves of 77 patients with completely resected stage IIIA-N2 non-small-cell lung cancer.

In univariate analysis, the median OS was significantly influenced by tumor size. The median OS was 52.0 months (95% CI: 45.3–66.1) in patients with tumors of 3 cm or less, worsening to 32.6 months (95% CI: 23.2–43.6) in patients with tumors greater than 3 cm (log-rank $p = 0.002$) and corresponding to a five-year OS rate of 43.3% and 21.7%, respectively (Figure 2). Moreover, patients with VATS approach had significantly better OS compared with those who received open thoracotomy (five-year OS: 63.5% vs. 18.3%; log-rank $p = 0.009$). On the other hand, OS rates were significantly worse in patients with elder age (versus those with age under 65 years, five-year OS: 24.2% vs. 39.0%; log-rank $p = 0.031$) and those with ECOG 1 (versus those with ECOG 0, 5-year OS: 19.3% vs. 49.4%; log-rank $p = 0.016$).

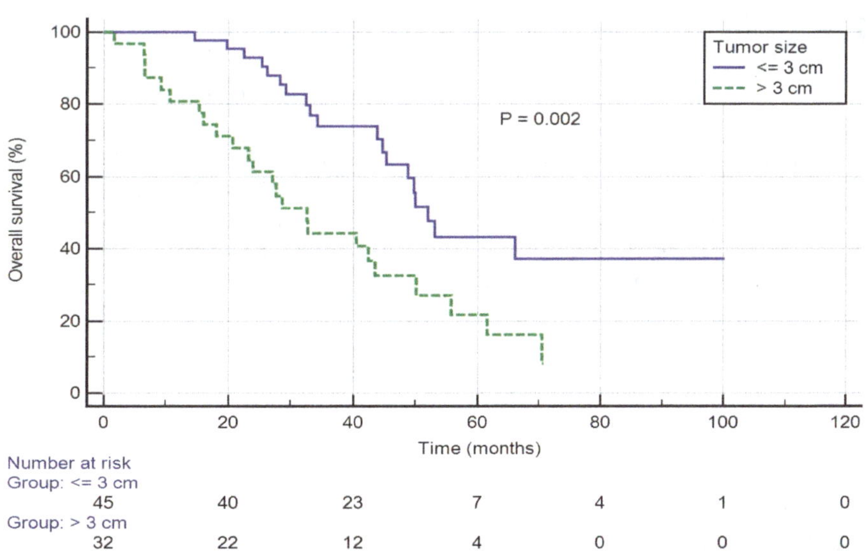

Figure 2. Overall survival curves of patients stratified by tumor size.

Multivariate analysis showed that tumor size <3 cm (HR: 0.373, 95% CI: 0.194–0.714, $p = 0.003$) and VATS approach (HR: 0.383, 95% CI: 0.178–0.824, $p = 0.014$) were significant predictors for OS. Univariate and multivariate data are shown in Tables 2 and 3.

Table 2. Univariate analysis of factors associated with overall survival.

Parameter	Hazard Ratio (95% CI)	*p*-Value
Age (≥65 y versus <65)	1.939 (1.050–3.582)	0.034
Gender (Male versus Female)	1.084 (0.582–2.020)	0.799
Ever Smoker (Yes versus No)	0.987 (0.526–1.851)	0.967
Family History of Cancer (Yes versus No)	0.681 (0.302–1.532)	0.352
Hypertension (Yes versus No)	0.630 (0.310–1.279)	0.201
Cardiovascular Disease (Yes versus No)	0.523 (0.161–1.692)	0.279
Chronic Obstructive Pulmonary Disease (Yes versus No)	2.094 (0.741–5.916)	0.163
Liver Disease (Yes versus No)	1.662 (0.698–3.960)	0.251
Chronic Kidney Disease (Yes versus No)	0.395 (0.054–2.877)	0.359
Diabetes Mellitus (Yes versus No)	1.040 (0.438–2.469)	0.930
Performance Status (ECOG 1 versus ECOG 0)	2.093 (1.133–3.867)	0.018
Clinical N2 (Yes versus Unsuspected)	0.963 (0.525–1.767)	0.903
Limited Resection (Yes versus Anatomical)	1.453 (0.612–3.449)	0.397
VATS (Yes versus Open Thoracotomy)	0.429 (0.223–0.824)	0.011
Tumor Size (≤3 versus 3–5)	0.390 (0.213–0.715)	0.002
Histology (Adenocarcinoma versus Others)	1.442 (0.689–3.018)	0.332
Differentiation (Poor versus Others)	0.618 (0.311–1.226)	0.168
CEA (≥3 versus <3)	1.593 (0.729–3.482)	0.243
Visceral Pleural Involvement (Yes versus No)	1.359 (0.743–2.486)	0.319
Lymphovascular Permeation (Yes versus No)	1.314 (0.513–3.352)	0.567
Perineural Invasion (Yes versus No)	0.483 (0.173–1.354)	0.166
N2 Ratio (≥40% versus <40%)	1.167 (0.632–2.154)	0.622
Central Location (Yes versus Peripheral)	1.061 (0.576–1.955)	0.848
Lower Lobe Location (Yes versus Upper or Middle)	1.408 (0.757–2.619)	0.280
Multiple N2 Station (Yes versus No)	1.056 (0.550–2.028)	0.870
Induction Therapy (Yes versus No)	0.793 (0.281–2.236)	0.660
Adjuvant Therapy (Yes versus No)	1.147 (0.483–2.725)	0.756
Postoperative Radiotherapy (Yes versus No)	0.551 (0.263–1.151)	0.113

Variables with *p*-values of less than 0.2 were tested in multivariate analysis. CI, confidence interval; ECOG, Eastern Cooperative Oncology Group; VATS, video-assisted thoracoscopic surgery; CEA, carcinoembryonic antigen.

Table 3. Multivariate analysis of factors associated with overall survival.

Parameter	Hazard Ratio (95% CI)	*p*-Value
Age (≥65 y versus <65)	1.576 (0.799–3.111)	0.190
Performance Status (ECOG 1 versus ECOG 0)	1.669 (0.878–3.173)	0.118
VATS (Yes versus Open Thoracotomy)	0.383 (0.178–0.824)	0.014
Tumor Size (≤3 versus 3–5)	0.373 (0.194–0.714)	0.003
Differentiation (Poor versus Others)	0.732 (0.358–1.499)	0.394
Perineural Invasion (Yes versus No)	0.681 (0.229–2.023)	0.489
Postoperative Radiotherapy (Yes versus No)	1.173 (0.501–2.745)	0.713

CI, confidence interval; ECOG, Eastern Cooperative Oncology Group; VATS, video-assisted thoracoscopic surgery.

3.3. Disease-Free Survival

The one-, three-, and five-year DFS rates were 53.4%, 24.5%, and 12.5%, respectively.

In univariate analysis, the median DFS was significantly influenced by tumor size. The median DFS was 18.4 months (95% CI: 11.9–33.6) in patients with tumors of 3 cm or less, worsening to 11.0 months (95% CI: 7.1–15.6) in patients with tumors greater than 3 cm (log-rank $p = 0.016$) and corresponding to a three-year DFS rate of 33.4% and 12.5%, respectively (Supplementary Materials Figure S1). There was a non-significant trend between poor prognosis and both clinical N2 disease (versus unsuspected N2 disease, three-year DFS: 16.2% vs. 31.1%; log-rank $p = 0.077$) and elevated CEA level (versus CEA level less than 3 ng/mL, three-year DFS: 18.2% vs. 33.3%; log-rank $p = 0.053$).

Multivariate analysis showed that tumor size <3 cm (HR: 0.451, 95% CI: 0.235–0.865, $p = 0.017$) and clinical N2 versus unsuspected N2 disease (HR: 2.525, 95% CI: 1.340–4.757, $p = 0.004$) were significant predictors for DFS. Both univariate and multivariate data are shown in Supplementary Materials Tables S1 and S2.

4. Discussion

The AJCC TNM staging system is the global standard for lung cancer staging [8]. Compared with the seventh edition, the eighth edition has been validated in several cohorts [9,10], demonstrating better survival stratification and prognosis prediction. With regard to the major changes in the T classification, former stage IIIA-N2 disease is further separated into stage IIIA and IIIB, based on tumor size, which is suggestive of distinct prognosis between the two subgroups. Sui et al. [9] retrospectively analyzed a Chinese cohort including 3599 patients with pathological stage IA to IIIA between 2005 and 2012. Of 772 former stage IIIA patients, stage migration to IIIB was found in 180 (23.3%) patients, and associated with lower five-year survival rate (26.1% vs. 41.7%, $p < 0.001$). Therefore, we focused on updated stage IIIA-N2 NSCLC, which represents a heterogenic group of patients and complex treatment modalities, including surgical resection.

The role of surgical resection for patients with stage IIIA-N2 NSCLC remains controversial, with different management preferences between Europe and America [11]. In Europe, surgeons tend to perform upfront resection, without induction therapy, for single-station, non-bulky N2 disease. The European Society for Medical Oncology (ESMO) guideline recommends that surgical resection, followed by adjuvant chemotherapy, is a reasonable treatment option for single-station N2 disease [8]. By contrast, in America, the standard treatment has been induction chemotherapy or chemoradiation, followed by surgical resection. A Cardiothoracic Surgery Network survey [12] demonstrated that more than 80% of thoracic surgeon preferred induction therapy for stage IIIA-N2 NSCLC, whereas only 12% preferred surgical resection followed by adjuvant therapy. For macroscopic single station N2 disease, 62% would consider surgical resection only if N2 clearance was achieved, whereas 18% considered this inoperable and offer definitive concurrent chemoradiation. Regarding the preference of induction therapy followed by surgical resection in America, considerations include better tolerance to full-dose chemotherapy preoperatively, better control of the systemic micro-metastases, assessment of treatment response before decision of surgery, and possible parenchymal sparing surgery [13]. Therefore, the approach of induction therapy is supported by the National Comprehensive Cancer Center Network (NCCN) guideline [7]. However, despite the high agreement and guideline recommendation, substantial variation in clinical practice existed in The Society of Thoracic Surgeons General Thoracic Surgery Database [14]. Of 3319 clinical stage III-N2 patients, 54% received direct surgical resection and 46% received induction therapy, with five-year survival rates of 36% and 35%, respectively. Considering the controversial role of surgical resection for patients with updated stage IIIA-N2 NSCLC, our study was aimed to investigate prognostic factors to guide therapeutic decisions.

For former stage IIIA-N2 NSCLC, previous studies have well demonstrated prognostic factors, including number of positive lymph nodes [15], microscopic N2 [16], single-station N2 [17–20], VATS approach [21], lobectomy approach [22], postoperative radiotherapy [23,24], and pathological response after induction therapy [25,26]. However, there is still some concern about changes of T classification and stage migration in the eighth edition. In the study, we presented a single-center retrospective study of 77 surgically resected IIIA-N2 NSCLC patients, staged according to the eighth edition of the AJCC staging system. Our first finding is that tumor size <3 cm was associated with better prognosis (HR: 0.373, $p = 0.003$). The possible reason is that tumor size was correlated with occult systemic micro-metastases. Yang et al. [27] reported that the proportions of cases with N0M0 status with tumor size <2 cm and >7 cm were 70.79% and 33.33%, respectively. Cho et al. [28] analyzed the data of 1821 patients with clinical N0-1 NSCLC, in which they found that tumor size >3 cm was a common predictor for unsuspected N2 and multiple-station N2 disease. Based on our finding and major changes of T classification, further large-scale studies are warranted to confirm the role of tumor size in patient selection and treatment strategy. Our second finding is that VATS approach was associated with better prognosis (HR: 0.383, $p = 0.014$). Previous studies showed similar results [21,26]. Despite the possible selection bias of our study, the consistency of these findings suggests that the VATS approach can be employed safely, without compromised prognosis.

Our 33.5% five-year OS rate is slightly lower than that of the IASLC database [5], in which the five-year OS rates for clinical and pathological stage IIIA disease are 36% and 41%, respectively. The relatively poorer prognosis in our patients highlights the importance of patient selection and the multimodality treatment approach. First, in patients with stage IIIA-N2 NSCLC undergoing surgical resection, the prognostic value of degree of lymph node involvement has been well documented. The ESMO guideline [8] highlights that single-station N2 disease is the most important features while evaluating resectability. Several studies [17–20] have also demonstrated that multiple-station N2 involvement indicates a poorer prognosis, regardless of whether the induction therapy is given: five-year OS rate is usually below 25%. Given the poorer prognosis and higher risk of systemic micro-metastases, upfront surgical resection should be avoided in patients with multiple-station N2 disease. However, in our study, 21 (27.3%) patients with multiple-station N2 disease received surgical resection, whereas only 10 (13%) patients received induction therapy. Second, regardless of whether to offer surgical resection, the implementation of multimodality treatment is of most importance [7,8]. There is pooled evidence in a network meta-analysis [29] where patients with stage IIIA-N2 NSCLC treated with single modality treatment of either surgery or radiotherapy alone seemed to have the worst outcomes. Nevertheless, in our study, 12 (15.6%) patients received surgical resection, only without adjuvant therapy. The lack of multimodality treatment would also explain the poorer outcome of the study.

Our study has some limitations. First, given the nature of retrospective analysis, patients in our study were highly selected by multidisciplinary team screening and not representative of all patients with stage IIIA-N2 NSCLC. In addition, it is not possible to answer the question whether upfront surgical resection is superior to other multimodality approaches. Second, the number of cases in our study was small. The uneven distribution of clinicopathologic characteristics (e.g., single- or multiple-station N2) and treatment approaches (e.g., induction therapy) complicated the interpretation, and the statistical power could be limited.

5. Conclusions

In conclusion, we retrospectively reviewed the clinical and pathological characteristics of patients with completely resected stage IIIA-N2 NSCLC, according to the eighth edition of the AJCC staging system. Tumor size <3 cm was the only independent factor for better OS and DFS. In addition, the VATS approach was also a good prognostic factor regarding OS rate. These findings may be helpful to identify patients with stage IIIA-N2 NSCLC eligible to surgical resection.

Author Contributions: Conceptualization, Chih-Yu Chen; Data curation, Wen-Chien Cheng and Wei-Chun Chen; Formal analysis, B.-R.W. and C.-H.C.; Methodology, C-H.C.; Software, Chih-Yu Chen; Supervision, T.-C.H. and C.-Y.T.; Validation, Chih-Yi Chen; Visualization, C-H.C.; Writing—original draft, Chih-Yu Chen; Writing—review & editing, W.-C.L. All authors have read and agreed to the published version of the manuscript.

Acknowledgments: The authors would like to thank the editor and reviewers for the editorial assistance and their valuable comments. This study is supported in part by the Taiwan Ministry of Health and Welfare Clinical Trial Center (MOHW109-TDU-B-212-114004).

References

1. Bray, F.; Ferlay, J.; Soerjomataram, I.; Siegel, R.L.; Torre, L.A.; Jemal, A. Global cancer statistics 2018: GLOBOCAN estimates of incidence and mortality worldwide for 36 cancers in 185 countries. *CA Cancer J. Clin.* **2018**, *68*, 394–424. [CrossRef] [PubMed]
2. Wang, B.Y.; Huang, J.Y.; Cheng, C.Y.; Lin, C.H.; Ko, J.; Liaw, Y.P. Lung cancer and prognosis in taiwan: A population-based cancer registry. *J. Thorac. Oncol.* **2013**, *8*, 1128–1135. [CrossRef] [PubMed]

3. Howlader, N.; Noone, A.; Krapcho, M.; Miller, D.; Brest, A.; Yu, M.; Ruhl, J.; Tatalovich, Z.; Mariotto, A.; Lewis, D.J.N.C.I. *SEER Cancer Statistics Review, 1975–2016*; National Cancer Institute: Bethesda, MD, USA, 2019.
4. Goya, T.; Asamura, H.; Yoshimura, H.; Kato, H.; Shimokata, K.; Tsuchiya, R.; Sohara, Y.; Miya, T.; Miyaoka, E. Prognosis of 6644 resected non-small cell lung cancers in Japan: A Japanese lung cancer registry study. *Lung Cancer* **2005**, *50*, 227–234. [CrossRef] [PubMed]
5. Goldstraw, P.; Chansky, K.; Crowley, J.; Rami-Porta, R.; Asamura, H.; Eberhardt, W.E.; Nicholson, A.G.; Groome, P.; Mitchell, A.; Bolejack, V. The IASLC Lung Cancer Staging Project: Proposals for Revision of the TNM Stage Groupings in the Forthcoming (Eighth) Edition of the TNM Classification for Lung Cancer. *J. Thorac. Oncol.* **2016**, *11*, 39–51. [CrossRef]
6. Detterbeck, F.C.; Boffa, D.J.; Kim, A.W.; Tanoue, L.T. The Eighth Edition Lung Cancer Stage Classification. *Chest* **2017**, *151*, 193–203. [CrossRef]
7. Ettinger, D.S.; Aisner, D.L.; Wood, D.E.; Akerley, W.; Bauman, J.; Chang, J.Y.; Chirieac, L.R.; D'Amico, T.A.; Dilling, T.J.; Dobelbower, M.; et al. NCCN Guidelines Insights: Non-Small Cell Lung Cancer, Version 5.2018. *J. Natl. Compr. Canc. Netw.* **2018**, *16*, 807–821. [CrossRef]
8. Postmus, P.E.; Kerr, K.M.; Oudkerk, M.; Senan, S.; Waller, D.A.; Vansteenkiste, J.; Escriu, C.; Peters, S. Early and locally advanced non-small-cell lung cancer (NSCLC): ESMO Clinical Practice Guidelines for diagnosis, treatment and follow-up. *Ann. Oncol.* **2017**, *28*, 1–21. [CrossRef]
9. Sui, X.; Jiang, W.; Chen, H.; Yang, F.; Wang, J.; Wang, Q. Validation of the Stage Groupings in the Eighth Edition of the TNM Classification for Lung Cancer. *J. Thorac. Oncol.* **2017**, *12*, 1679–1686. [CrossRef]
10. Yang, L.; Wang, S.; Zhou, Y.; Lai, S.; Xiao, G.; Gazdar, A.; Xie, Y. Evaluation of the 7(th) and 8(th) editions of the AJCC/UICC TNM staging systems for lung cancer in a large North American cohort. *Oncotarget* **2017**, *8*, 66784–66795. [CrossRef]
11. Rocco, G.; Nason, K.; Brunelli, A.; Varela, G.; Waddell, T.; Jones, D.R. Management of stage IIIA (N2) non-small cell lung cancer: A transatlantic perspective. *J. Thorac. Cardiovasc. Surg.* **2016**, *151*, 1235–1238. [CrossRef]
12. Veeramachaneni, N.K.; Feins, R.H.; Stephenson, B.J.; Edwards, L.J.; Fernandez, F.G. Management of stage IIIA non-small cell lung cancer by thoracic surgeons in North America. *Ann. Thorac. Surg.* **2012**, *94*, 922–926, discussion 926–928. [CrossRef] [PubMed]
13. Mehran, R. The role of surgery in patients with clinical n2 disease. *Thorac. Surg. Clin.* **2013**, *23*, 327–335. [CrossRef] [PubMed]
14. Boffa, D.; Fernandez, F.G.; Kim, S.; Kosinski, A.; Onaitis, M.W.; Cowper, P.; Jacobs, J.P.; Wright, C.D.; Putnam, J.B.; Furnary, A.P. Surgically Managed Clinical Stage IIIA-Clinical N2 Lung Cancer in The Society of Thoracic Surgeons Database. *Ann. Thorac. Surg.* **2017**, *104*, 395–403. [CrossRef] [PubMed]
15. Yoo, C.; Yoon, S.; Lee, D.H.; Park, S.I.; Kim, D.K.; Kim, Y.H.; Kim, H.R.; Choi, S.H.; Kim, W.S.; Choi, C.M.; et al. Prognostic Significance of the Number of Metastatic pN2 Lymph Nodes in Stage IIIA-N2 Non-Small-Cell Lung Cancer After Curative Resection. *Clin. Lung Cancer* **2015**, *16*, 203–212. [CrossRef] [PubMed]
16. Garelli, E.; Renaud, S.; Falcoz, P.E.; Weingertner, N.; Olland, A.; Santelmo, N.; Massard, G. Microscopic N2 disease exhibits a better prognosis in resected non-small-cell lung cancer. *Eur. J. Cardiothorac. Surg.* **2016**, *50*, 322–328. [CrossRef]
17. Cerfolio, R.J.; Bryant, A.S. Survival of patients with unsuspected N2 (stage IIIA) nonsmall-cell lung cancer. *Ann. Thorac. Surg.* **2008**, *86*, 362–366, discussion 366–367. [CrossRef]
18. Decaluwe, H.; De Leyn, P.; Vansteenkiste, J.; Dooms, C.; Van Raemdonck, D.; Nafteux, P.; Coosemans, W.; Lerut, T. Surgical multimodality treatment for baseline resectable stage IIIA-N2 non-small cell lung cancer. Degree of mediastinal lymph node involvement and impact on survival. *Eur. J. Cardiothorac. Surg.* **2009**, *36*, 433–439. [CrossRef]
19. Yoshino, I.; Yoshida, S.; Miyaoka, E.; Asamura, H.; Nomori, H.; Fujii, Y.; Nakanishi, Y.; Eguchi, K.; Mori, M.; Sawabata, N.; et al. Surgical outcome of stage IIIA- cN2/pN2 non-small-cell lung cancer patients in Japanese lung cancer registry study in 2004. *J. Thorac. Oncol.* **2012**, *7*, 850–855. [CrossRef]
20. Tsitsias, T.; Boulemden, A.; Ang, K.; Nakas, A.; Waller, D.A. The N2 paradox: Similar outcomes of pre- and postoperatively identified single-zone N2a positive non-small-cell lung cancer. *Eur. J. Cardiothorac. Surg.* **2014**, *45*, 882–887. [CrossRef]

21. Wang, S.; Zhou, W.; Zhang, H.; Zhao, M.; Chen, X. Feasibility and long-term efficacy of video-assisted thoracic surgery for unexpected pathologic N2 disease in non-small cell lung cancer. *Ann. Thorac. Med.* **2013**, *8*, 170–175. [CrossRef]
22. Jimenez, M.F.; Varela, G.; Novoa, N.M.; Aranda, J.L. Results of surgery for non-small cell lung cancer with N2 involvement unsuspected before thoracotomy. *Arch. Bronconeumol.* **2008**, *44*, 65–69. [CrossRef]
23. Robinson, C.G.; Patel, A.P.; Bradley, J.D.; DeWees, T.; Waqar, S.N.; Morgensztern, D.; Baggstrom, M.Q.; Govindan, R.; Bell, J.M.; Guthrie, T.J.; et al. Postoperative radiotherapy for pathologic N2 non-small-cell lung cancer treated with adjuvant chemotherapy: A review of the National Cancer Data Base. *J. Clin. Oncol.* **2015**, *33*, 870–876. [CrossRef] [PubMed]
24. Yang, C.F.; Kumar, A.; Gulack, B.C.; Mulvihill, M.S.; Hartwig, M.G.; Wang, X.; D'Amico, T.A.; Berry, M.F. Long-term outcomes after lobectomy for non-small cell lung cancer when unsuspected pN2 disease is found: A National Cancer Data Base analysis. *J. Thorac. Cardiovasc. Surg.* **2016**, *151*, 1380–1388. [CrossRef]
25. Cerfolio, R.J.; Maniscalco, L.; Bryant, A.S. The treatment of patients with stage IIIA non-small cell lung cancer from N2 disease: Who returns to the surgical arena and who survives. *Ann. Thorac. Surg.* **2008**, *86*, 912–920, discussion 912–920. [CrossRef] [PubMed]
26. Yang, C.F.; Adil, S.M.; Anderson, K.L.; Meyerhoff, R.R.; Turley, R.S.; Hartwig, M.G.; Harpole, D.H., Jr.; Tong, B.C.; Onaitis, M.W.; D'Amico, T.A.; et al. Impact of patient selection and treatment strategies on outcomes after lobectomy for biopsy-proven stage IIIA pN2 non-small cell lung cancer. *Eur. J. Cardiothorac. Surg.* **2016**, *49*, 1607–1613. [CrossRef] [PubMed]
27. Yang, F.; Chen, H.; Xiang, J.; Zhang, Y.; Zhou, J.; Hu, H.; Zhang, J.; Luo, X. Relationship between tumor size and disease stage in non-small cell lung cancer. *BMC Cancer* **2010**, *10*, 474. [CrossRef]
28. Cho, H.J.; Kim, S.R.; Kim, H.R.; Han, J.O.; Kim, Y.H.; Kim, D.K.; Park, S.I. Modern outcome and risk analysis of surgically resected occult N2 non-small cell lung cancer. *Ann. Thorac. Surg.* **2014**, *97*, 1920–1925. [CrossRef]
29. Zhao, Y.; Wang, W.; Liang, H.; Yang, C.J.; D'Amico, T.; Ng, C.S.H.; Liu, C.C.; Petersen, R.H.; Rocco, G.; Brunelli, A.; et al. The Optimal Treatment for Stage IIIA-N2 Non-Small Cell Lung Cancer: A Network Meta-Analysis. *Ann. Thorac. Surg.* **2019**, *107*, 1866–1875. [CrossRef]

12

PD-(L)1 Inhibitors in Combination with Chemotherapy as First-Line Treatment for Non-Small-Cell Lung Cancer

Jorge García-González [1,*,†], Juan Ruiz-Bañobre [1,*,†], Francisco J. Afonso-Afonso [2], Margarita Amenedo-Gancedo [3], María del Carmen Areses-Manrique [4], Begoña Campos-Balea [5], Joaquín Casal-Rubio [6], Natalia Fernández-Núñez [5], José Luis Fírvida Pérez [4], Martín Lázaro-Quintela [6], Diego Pérez Parente [7], Leonardo Crama [7], Pedro Ruiz-Gracia [7], Lucía Santomé-Couto [8] and Luis León-Mateos [1,*]

1 Medical Oncology Department, University Clinical Hospital of Santiago de Compostela and Translational Medical Oncology Group (Oncomet), Health Research Institute of Santiago de Compostela (IDIS), CIBERONC, 15706 Santiago de Compostela, Spain

2 Medical Oncology Department, Complexo Hospitalario Universitario de Ferrol, 15405 A Coruña, Spain; francisco.javier.afonso.afonso@sergas.es

3 Medical Oncology Department, Centro Oncológico de Galicia, 15009 A Coruña, Spain; margarita.amenedo@cog.es

4 Medical Oncology Department, Complexo Hospitalario Universitario de Ourense, 32005 Ourense, Spain; karmeleareses@hotmail.com (M.d.C.A.-M.); jlfirvidap@gmail.com (J.L.F.P.)

5 Medical Oncology Department, Hospital Universitario Lucus Augusti, 27003 Lugo, Spain; bcamposbalea@hotmail.com (B.C.-B.); fernandeznunez.ntalia@gmail.com (N.F.-N.)

6 Medical Oncology Department, Complexo Hospitalario Universitario de Vigo, 36213 Vigo, Spain; joaquin.casal.rubio@sergas.es (J.C.-R.); martin.lazaro.quintela@sergas.es (M.L.-Q.)

7 Lung Cancer Medical Department, Roche Farma S.A., 28042 Madrid, Spain; diego.perez@roche.com (D.P.P.); leonardo.crama@roche.com (L.C.); pedro.ruiz.pr1@roche.com (P.R.-G.)

8 Medical Oncology Department, Hospital POVISA, 36211 Vigo, Spain; lsantome@povisa.es

* Correspondence: jorgejose.garcia.gonzalez@sergas.es (J.G.-G.); jurruba@gmail.com (J.R.-B.); luis.leon.mateos@sergas.es (L.L.-M.)

† Shared first authors.

Abstract: The combination of programmed cell death-1 (PD-1)/programmed death ligand-1 (PD-L1) inhibitors with chemotherapy has emerged as a promising therapeutic option for advanced non-small-cell lung cancer (NSCLC). The aim of this meta-analysis was to evaluate the efficacy of the combined strategy in this setting. For this purpose, we performed a literature search of randomized controlled trials comparing PD-(L)1 inhibitors plus platinum-based chemotherapy versus chemotherapy alone in stage IV NSCLC patients. Seven clinical trials with 4562 patients were included. In the intention-to-treat wildtype population, PD-(L)1 inhibitor plus chemotherapy was significantly associated with improved progression-free survival (PFS) (Hazard ratio (HR) = 0.61, 95% confidence interval (CI): 0.57–0.65, $p < 0.001$) and overall survival (OS) (HR = 0.76, 95% CI: 0.67–0.86; $p < 0.001$) compared to chemotherapy. A significantly higher overall response rate (ORR) was also observed with the combined strategy (Odds ratio (OR) = 2.12, 95% CI: 1.70–2.63, $p < 0.001$). Furthermore, in all the analyzed subgroups, addition of PD-(L)1 inhibitors to chemotherapy significantly improved efficacy endpoints. Specifically, stratification according to PD-L1 expression revealed a benefit across all patients, regardless of their PFS status. In conclusion, PD-(L)1 blockade added to standard platinum-based chemotherapy significantly improved PFS, OS, and ORR in the up-front treatment of advanced NSCLC.

Keywords: non-small-cell lung cancer; immunotherapy; PD-1 inhibitors; PD-L1 inhibitors; chemotherapy; meta-analysis

1. Introduction

Lung cancer remains the leading cause of cancer-related death worldwide among men and the second among women [1]. Non-small-cell lung cancer (NSCLC), which is the most common type, accounts for 80% to 85% of all lung cancer diagnoses [2]. It is frequently diagnosed in the advanced stage, with 5-year survival rates ranging from 0% to 5% with chemotherapy, the only systemic therapeutic strategy available for decades [3]. In this regard, blockade of the programmed cell death-1 (PD-1)/programmed death ligand-1 (PD-L1) axis in particular has opened up a new horizon in the lung cancer therapeutic landscape, increasing overall survival (OS) not only in patients with advanced NSCLC but also in patients with stage III NSCLC and extensive-stage small-cell lung cancer [4–6].

Since 2015, three different PD-(L)1 inhibitors have been approved by the European Medicines Agency (EMA) and/or the U.S. Food and Drug Administration (FDA) for the treatment of metastatic NSCLC (mNSCLC) [7]: two anti-PD-1 antibodies (nivolumab and pembrolizumab) and one anti-PD-L1 antibody (atezolizumab), indicated for patients regardless of their PD-L1 expression status (nivolumab and atezolizumab) or for PD-L1-positive patients only (pembrolizumab). All of them have demonstrated an improvement in OS compared to docetaxel in second-line therapy [8–10]. In the first-line setting, results from the KEYNOTE 024 trial demonstrated that, compared with platinum-based chemotherapy, OS, progression-free survival (PFS), and overall response rate (ORR) were significantly improved in patients with PD-L1 expression on at least 50% of tumor cells and without oncogenic driver mutations [11,12]. Interestingly, an additional study assessing pembrolizumab efficacy versus chemotherapy using a PD-L1 tumor proportion score (TPS) of 1% or greater (KEYNOTE-042 [13]) demonstrated improved OS for the full cohort, which, despite being higher for higher PD-L1 expression, supported a potential extended role of pembrolizumab monotherapy as a standard first-line treatment for PD-L1-expressing advanced/metastatic NSCLC [14]. In contrast, nivolumab did not demonstrate statistically significant survival benefits in previously untreated PD-L1-positive mNSCLC (CheckMate-026 [15]).

Nevertheless, many patients with advanced NSCLC do not benefit from PD-(L)1 inhibitors, either in the first line or in the second or successive lines of treatment. The search for reliable predictive biomarkers of response to these drugs is therefore essential to improve patient outcomes.

The potential synergistic effects of combining chemotherapy and immunotherapy to improve the antitumor activity of anti-PD-(L)1 monotherapy were initially suggested in preclinical studies [16] (Apetoh, 2015 #16) and were further demonstrated in several clinical trials [4–6,17–25]. However, although promising outcomes have been reported, several questions remain unanswered, such as the potential real benefit for all patients at the expense of increased toxicity or the possible molecular factors that could predict the benefit of this combined therapeutic strategy.

The objective of this study was to evaluate the efficacy of the combined strategy by conducting a pairwise meta-analysis (MA) of the available information on PD-(L)1 inhibitors in combination with chemotherapy in the first-line treatment of patients with advanced NSCLC.

2. Materials and Methods

2.1. Search Strategies and Study Selection

We conducted a systematic search in PubMed to identify all eligible trials from inception until 1 January 2020, with no start date limit applied. Literature search terms used were "non-small cell lung cancer" (or "NSCLC"), "chemotherapy", "pembrolizumab", "nivolumab", "atezolizumab", "durvalumab", and all terms related to clinical trial registration (ClinicalTrials.gov, EU Clinical Trials Register, ISRCTN, and ANZCTR). An additional search of abstracts presented at the American Society of Clinical Oncology (ASCO), European Society for Medical Oncology (ESMO), American Association for Cancer Research for Medical Oncology (AACR), and World Conference on Lung Cancer (WCLC) was also performed.

2.2. Selection Criteria

Only phase III trials conducted in patients with advanced/metastatic stage IV NSCLC not previously treated for their metastatic disease and receiving at least one PD-(L)1 inhibitor in combination with a chemotherapeutic agent were eligible for inclusion. Efficacy outcomes regarding combinations of immunotherapy plus chemotherapy expressed as PFS or OS had to be provided. Observational studies, editorials, reviews, and commentaries were excluded.

2.3. Statistical Analysis

The DerSimonian–Laird random effects models for main and subgroup analyses was implemented, assessing heterogeneity of effect-size estimates from the individual studies by Cochran's Q test and the I^2 statistic. Additionally, MA corresponding to analysis of binary data of proportions was also performed using a DerSimonian–Laird random effects model without transformation of the proportion. A high level of heterogeneity was considered if I^2 was greater than 50%. Due to the relatively low number of trials involved in this MA, values and significance of heterogeneity must be considered as guidance only [26]. Statistical significance was reached for *p*-values less than 0.05. Analyses were not controlled for multiplicity; no alpha was assigned to the different analyses. The nature of this study is therefore exploratory, mainly in the subgroup analysis. Hazard ratios (HRs) and 95% confidence intervals (CIs) for OS and PFS from the overall population and subgroups from each individual trial of advanced NSCLC were calculated. For dichotomous data, odds ratios (ORs) were estimated. The MA was performed using Open Meta Analyst v. 10 (Center for Evidence Synthesis in Health, Brown University). Recommendations of the Cochrane Collaboration and the Preferred Reporting Items for Systematic Reviews and Meta-Analyses (PRISMA) guidelines were followed for this MA [27].

For the ORR, different endpoints, including complete response (CR), partial response (PR), stable disease (SD), and progressive disease (PD), were alternately modeled. These sensitivity analyses along with those for OS and PFS did not quantitatively alter the results and conclusions of the main analyses.

3. Results

3.1. Studies Included in the Meta-Analysis

A total of 80 records from PubMed were screened. Three additional studies presented at the WCLC and/or ESMO were also included. Study selection and exclusion criteria are summarized in Figure 1. Finally, seven clinical trials carried out with 4562 patients met the inclusion criteria and were included in the MA [17,20–25,28,29]. In the specific case of CheckMate-227, part 1 [30] was excluded because immunotherapy-plus-chemotherapy efficacy evaluation was not part of the main objectives; only part 2 was considered for this MA [21].

3.2. Study Characteristics

The specific characteristics of the studies included in the MA are summarized in Table 1. The control arm in all studies was platinum-based chemotherapy with pemetrexed (three studies [17,20,21,28]) or with nab-paclitaxel/paclitaxel (five studies [21–25,29]). In one three-arm trial (IMpower150 [24]), bevacizumab was added in the control and experimental arm. This study included two experimental arms: carboplatin, paclitaxel, and atezolizumab (arm A) and carboplatin, paclitaxel, bevacizumab, and atezolizumab (arm B) versus carboplatin, paclitaxel, and bevacizumab (arm C). No comparisons between arms A and C were performed because the HR may not reflect the actual effect of add-on immunotherapy (atezolizumab plus chemotherapy vs. bevacizumab plus chemotherapy).

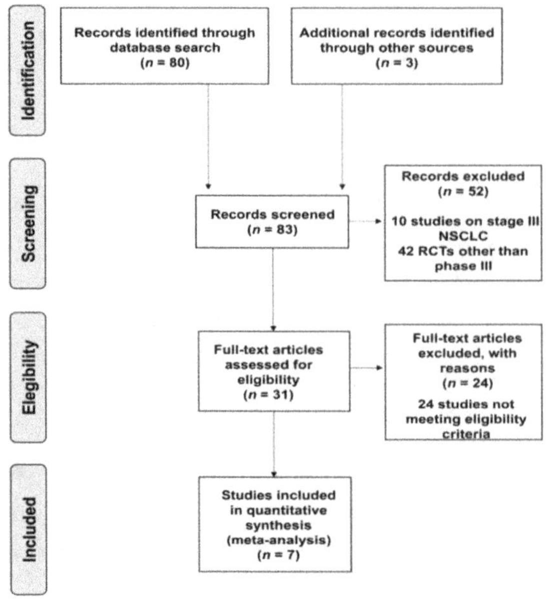

Figure 1. Flow chart of study selection (up to 1 January 2020). NSCLC, non-small-cell lung cancer; RCTs, randomized controlled trials.

Table 1. Characteristics and main outcomes of the studies included in the meta-analysis.

Study	Histology Expression	PD-L1 Expression	Primary Endpoint	Experimental Arm	Control Arm	Analysis Timing
IMpower130 [25]	Nonsquamous	All	PFS (ITT-WT *) OS (ITT-WT *)	Atezolizumab + (carboplatin + nab-paclitaxel) (*n* = 451)	Carboplatin + nab-paclitaxel (*n* = 228)	PFS: Final OS: Interim
IMpower150 [23,24]	Nonsquamous	All	PFS (ITT-WT *) OS (ITT-WT *)	Atezolizumab + (carboplatin + paclitaxel + bevacizumab) (*n* = 356)	Carboplatin + paclitaxel + bevacizumab (*n* = 336)	PFS: Final OS: Interim
KEYNOTE-189 [17,28]	Nonsquamous	All	PFS (ITT) OS (ITT)	Pembrolizumab + (carboplatin or cisplatin + pemetrexed) (*n* = 410)	Carboplatin or cisplatin + pemetrexed (*n* = 206)	PFS: Final OS: Interim
IMpower132 [20]	Nonsquamous	All	PFS (ITT) OS (ITT)	Atezolizumab + (carboplatin or cisplatin + pemetrexed) (*n* = 292)	Carboplatin or cisplatin + pemetrexed (*n* = 286)	PFS: Final OS: Interim
IMpower131 [29]	Squamous	All	PFS (ITT) OS (ITT)	Atezolizumab + (carboplatin + nab-paclitaxel) (*n* = 343)	Carboplatin + nab-paclitaxel (*n* = 340)	PFS: Final OS: Interim
KEYNOTE-407 [22]	Squamous	All	PFS (ITT) OS (ITT)	Pembrolizumab + (carboplatin + paclitaxel or nab-paclitaxel) (*n* = 278)	Carboplatin + paclitaxel or nab-paclitaxel (*n* = 281)	PFS: Final OS: Interim

* Patients with epidermal growth factor receptor (EGFR) or anaplastic lymphoma kinase (ALK) mutations excluded. PD-L1, programmed cell death-ligand 1; PFS, progression-free survival; OS, overall survival; ITT, intention-to-treat; WT, wildtype; +, plus (combination therapy).

Three studies tested anti-PD1 antibodies [17,21,22,28], and four studies tested anti-PD-L1 antibodies [20,23–25,29]. Patients with epidermal growth factor receptor (EGFR) or anaplastic lymphoma kinase (ALK) mutations were included in two clinical trials assessing atezolizumab [24,25]. Regarding the histology, four studies included patients with nonsquamous NSCLC [20,21,24,25], two included patients with squamous NSCLC [22,29], and one evaluated patients presenting both histological types [21] (note that the primary endpoint in CheckMate-227 part 2 was OS in nonsquamous mNSCLC patients only; however, both histological types were considered for this MA).

An all-comers design was used in all the studies, with NSCLC patients entering the trial regardless of their PD-L1 expression status. Stratification was performed based on this biomarker in all trials. Thus, subjects were classified as PD-L1-negative or PD-L1-positive, and within this group, investigators distinguished patients with high or low expression levels [20,25,29]. In the atezolizumab trials [20,23–25,29], levels were considered high (TC3 or IC3) when PD-L1 expression was recorded on at least 50% of tumor cells or at least 10% of tumor-infiltrating immune cells (TIICs) by immunohistochemistry; levels were considered low–intermediate, or TC1/2 or IC1/2, when expression was reported on at least 1% of tumor cells or TIICs and less than 50% of tumor cells or less than 10% of TIICs by immunohistochemistry; and PD-L1-negative status, or TC0 and IC0, was determined when expression was reported on less than 1% of tumor cells and TIICs. Similar criteria were followed in trials assessing pembrolizumab or nivolumab, but PD-L1 expression was only measured in tumor cells [17,21,22,28].

According to the eligibility criteria, none of the studies included patients who had received prior treatment for metastatic disease. However, in terms of therapy for nonmetastatic disease, although most of the studies included treatment-naïve patients, in those evaluating pembrolizumab (KEYNOTE-189 [17,28] and KEYNOTE-407 [22]) or atezolizumab [20,23–25,29], subjects had received previous therapies (Supplementary Table S1).

Coprimary endpoints for six clinical trials were PFS and OS [17,20,22–25,28,29]. The primary endpoint for CheckMate-227 part 2 was OS in nonsquamous NSCLC patients; PFS was assessed as a secondary endpoint [21]. Mature PFS data were reported in all the studies included in this MA [17,20–25,28,29], while final data for OS were available for only one of them [21]. Interim analyses were provided for the other six studies [17,20,22–25,28,29]. Both endpoints were evaluated in the intention-to-treat (ITT) population and specifically in the wildtype population (without EGFR or ALK mutations) in the IMpower130 [25] and IMpower150 studies [23,24] (see Supplementary Table S2 for the available information on patients with mutations in IMpower150). IMpower150 was the only study in which a subsequent subgroup analysis in patients with EGFR mutations or baseline liver metastasis was performed [23]. Additionally, one or both coprimary endpoints were analyzed according to different subgroups in all the studies included in the MA (PFS in six clinical trials [17,22–25,28,29] and OS in five studies [17,21,22,25,28,29]).

Patient population characteristics of all the studies included in the MA are shown in Supplementary Table S3.

3.3. *Efficacy Endpoints in the Overall Population*

Median PFS ranged from 4.8 to 6.8 months in the control arms and from 6.3 to 8.8 months in the treatment arms. Median OS ranged from 10.7 to 14.7 months in the control arms and from 14.2 to 22.0 months in the treatment arms. MA results demonstrated that the addition of a PD-(L)1 to chemotherapy was associated with improved PFS (PFS: $HR_{pooled} = 0.61$, 95% CI: 0.57–0.65, $p < 0.001$, Figure 2A) and OS (OS: $HR_{pooled} = 0.76$, 95% CI: 0.67–0.86; $p < 0.001$, Figure 2B) compared with chemotherapy alone. The objective response rate (ORR) was also significantly improved with the PD-(L)1 inhibitor–chemotherapy combination (odds ratio (OR_{pooled}) = 2.12, 95% CI: 1.70–2.63, $p < 0.001$, Supplementary Figure S1). The best ORR values were obtained in the IMpower150 (ORR = 56.4%) trial for nonsquamous NSCLC and KEYNOTE-407 for squamous NSCLC (57.9%). Notably, in terms of both OS and ORR, there was significant heterogeneity across the six trials ($I^2 = 52.07\%$, $p = 0.03$; $I^2 = 67.42\%$, $p = 0.005$).

3.4. *Subgroup Analysis*

Subgroup analyses according to sex (women vs. men), age (<65 years vs. ≥65 years), Eastern Cooperative Oncology Group performance status (ECOG-PS = 0 vs. ECOG-PS = 1), smoking status (never-smoker vs. current/former smoker), liver metastasis (yes vs. no), and PD-L1 expression (high vs. low vs. negative) were carried out. As shown in Figure 3, overall, the addition of PD-(L)1 blockade to chemotherapy significantly improved PFS in all the subgroups. Specifically, stratification according to PD-L1 expression revealed a benefit across all PD-L1 strata with a strong reduction in the risk of disease progression in those patients showing high expression levels ($HR_{pooled} = 0.412$, 95% CI: 0.34–0.5, $p < 0.001$). In terms of OS (Figure 3), although almost all subgroups benefited from the use of the PD-(L)1 inhibitor–chemotherapy combination, in certain cases, such as in never-smokers and PD-L1-low patients, results did not achieve statistical significance ($HR_{pooled} = 0.589$, 95% CI: 0.335–1.069, $p = 0.082$; $HR_{pooled} = 0.819$, 95% CI: 0.648–1.035, $p = 0.093$, respectively).

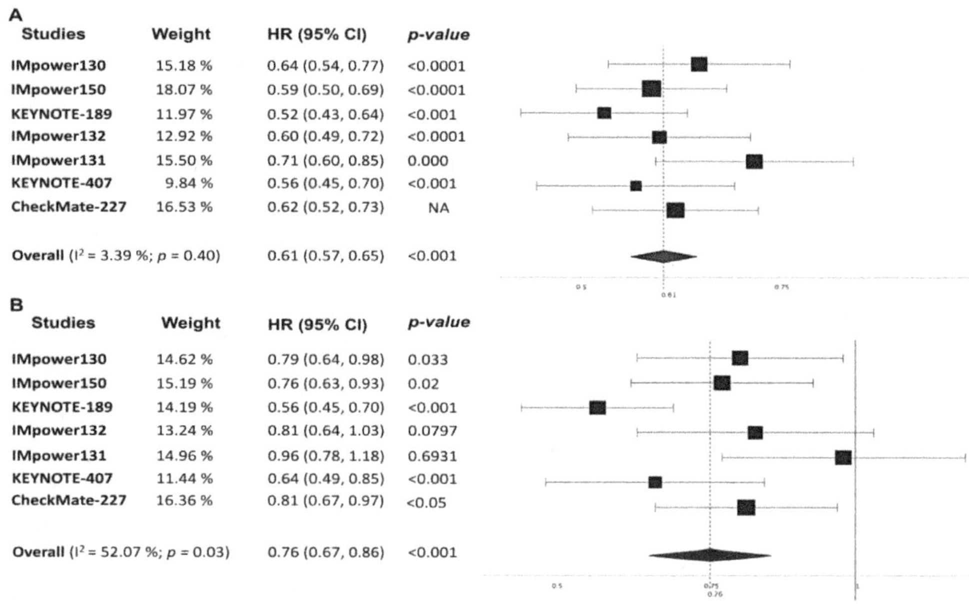

Figure 2. Forest plot of pooled hazard ratios for (**A**) progression-free survival (PFS) and (**B**) overall survival (OS) in patients who received programmed cell death-1 (PD-1)/programmed death ligand-1 (PD-L1) inhibitors plus chemotherapy vs. chemotherapy alone. HR, hazard ratio; CI, confidence interval.

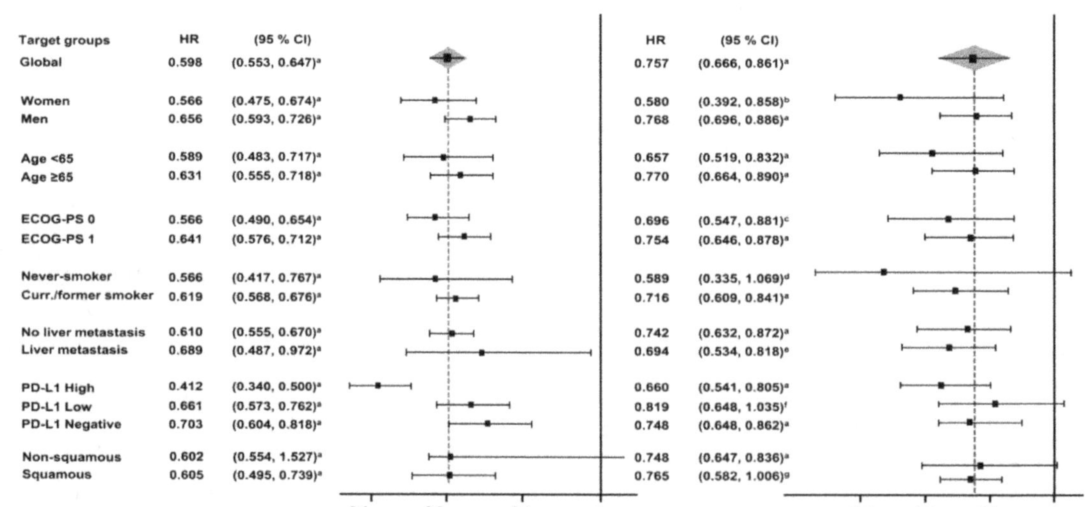

Figure 3. Forest plot of hazard ratios for progression-free survival (PFS) and overall survival (OS) in the subgroup analysis. PFS, progression-free survival; OS, overall survival. HR, hazard ratio; CI, confidence interval; Curr., current.; ^{a} $p < 0.001$; ^{b} $p = 0.006$; ^{c} $p = 0.003$; ^{d} $p = 0.082$; ^{e} $p = 0.007$; ^{f} $p = 0.093$; ^{g} $p = 0.055$.

Regarding patients with liver metastasis, a specific benefit with atezolizumab plus bevacizumab was observed both in terms of OS and PFS. Further details on the OS and PFS subgroup analyses are shown in Figures 4 and 5, respectively. Additional subgroup analyses based on the histology are available only for PFS and OS in Supplementary Figure S2.

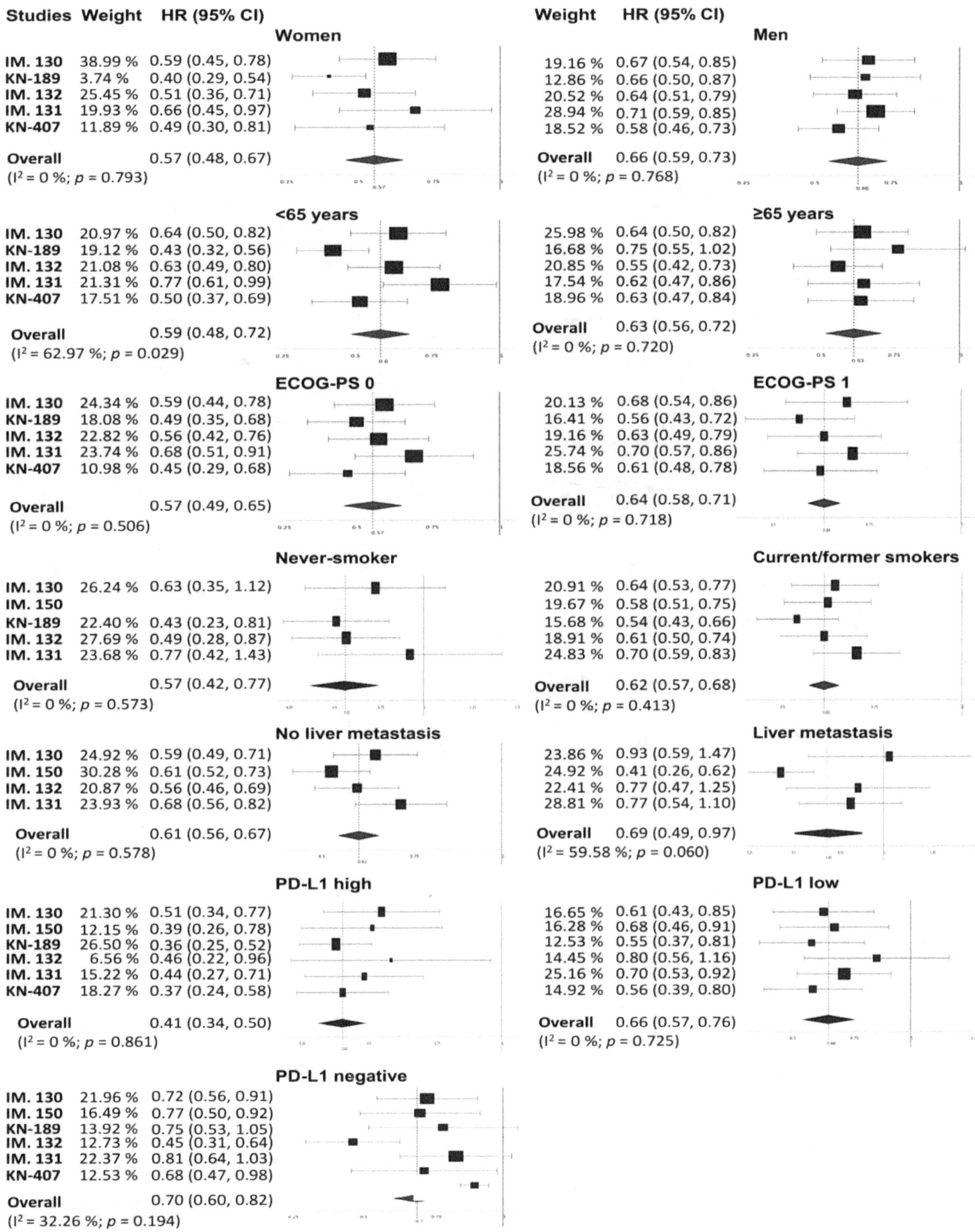

Figure 4. Forest plot of hazard ratios for progression-free survival (PFS) in the different patient subgroups. CI, confidence interval; ECOG-PS, Eastern Cooperative Oncology Group performance status; HR, hazard ratio; IM., IMpower; KN, KEYNOTE.

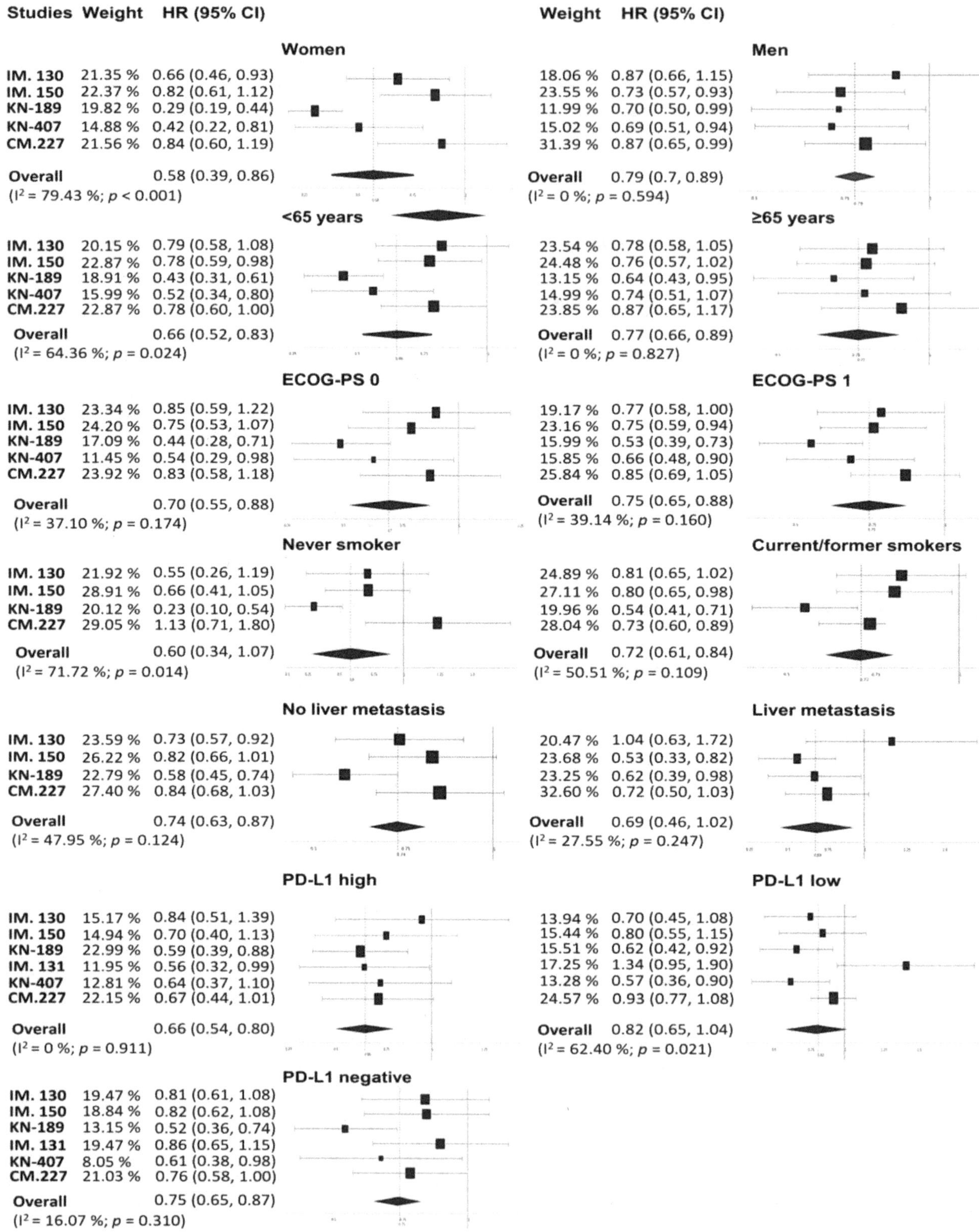

Figure 5. Forest plot of hazard ratios for overall survival (OS) in the different patient subgroups. CI, confidence interval; HR, hazard ratio; ECOG-PS, Eastern Cooperative Oncology Group performance status; IM., IMpower; KN, KEYNOTE; CM., CheckMate.

4. Discussion

The optimal treatment strategy for advanced NSCLC has been the focus of several randomized clinical trials. Promising immunotherapy results in the second or later lines of therapy resulted in the approval of atezolizumab, pembrolizumab, and nivolumab [31–35]. Several clinical trials subsequently evaluated PD-(L)1 inhibitor–chemotherapy strategies in front-line treatment, some of which are included in this MA.

Our results demonstrate an overall benefit—both in terms of PFS and OS—of the addition of PD-(L)1 blockade. Although statistical significance was reached for the pooled HR for OS, substantial heterogeneity (I^2 of 52.07%) across the seven trials was also identified. Furthermore, it is worth mentioning that the most recent data were considered for this MA in the vast majority of cases and that, to date, this is the first analysis to include results from CheckMate-227 part 2 [21]. Positive efficacy results have also been reported by Tun et al. [36], who included almost the same trials as those analyzed in this study (CheckMate-227 data were collected from part 1 [37]). Other meta-analyses have also reported improvements in the efficacy of the combined strategy. Differences in these may be explained by the trials included therein, such as the study by Chen et al., in which comparisons of immune checkpoint inhibitors against chemotherapy were also considered [38]; the study by Shen et al. [39] with broader inclusion criteria (e.g., studies that directly or indirectly investigated the ORR, the disease control response (DCR), or some safety endpoints); or the meta-analysis by Addeo et al. [40], in which studies using avelumab and durvalumab were also considered. Thus, our results support the evidence that a combination strategy of PD-(L)1 inhibitor plus chemotherapy may be beneficial compared to chemotherapy alone. Indeed, to date, the combination of pembrolizumab or atezolizumab with platinum-based chemotherapy, with or without bevacizumab, are EMA-approved options available for first-line treatment of advanced/metastatic NSCLC wildtype tumors.

With respect to subgroup analyses, overall benefits were reported across the different categories. Specifically, analysis in terms of PD-L1 marker yielded a statistically significant improvement in PFS regardless of the level of PD-L1 expression. In the case of OS, improvements were observed in patients with high PD-L1 expression and patients negative for this biomarker, but not in those with low levels, probably because of the moderate–high heterogeneity recorded in the pooled analysis ($I^2 = 67.01\%$; $p = 0.016$). It is also important to note that the studies included utilized different PD-L1 assay methods, possibly representing an additional confounding factor to be considered. Other subgroup analyses also resulted in important outcomes. Thus, this meta-analysis demonstrated that patients benefited from additional immunotherapy regardless of their age. It should be noted that the impact of advanced age on the effectiveness of immune checkpoint inhibitors has not been strongly established so far, highlighting the importance of these findings. Interestingly, combinations with pembrolizumab yielded the lowest HR values in terms of both PFS and OS in several subgroups, including women, patients <65 years, and patients with ECOG-PS = 0, pointing to a potential benefit in these individuals. With respect to liver metastasis, in the IMpower150 trial [23,24], improvements were reported both in terms of PFS and OS, suggesting a specific benefit with the atezolizumab and bevacizumab combination. Indeed, although other atezolizumab trials previously reported outcomes in patients with liver metastases, data from IMpower130 [41] and IMpower132 [42] showed no survival benefit with atezolizumab plus chemotherapy, supporting the benefits of adding the antiangiogenic agent in the combination [23]. Despite the fact that the updated KEYNOTE-189 analysis showed a clinical benefit of pembrolizumab-containing regimens over chemotherapy alone in patients with liver metastases (median OS 12.6 vs. 6.6, OS HR 0.62, 12-month OS rate 51% vs. 3%) [43], this baseline characteristic, in contrast with the IMpower trials, was not a stratification factor in the study.

Most clinical trials do not include advanced NSCLC patients with driver mutations. IMpower150 was the only study to include this type of patient, showing a positive trend in OS probably due to the addition of bevacizumab to the combination strategy, as previously discussed [43]. However, this therapeutic strategy for patients with EGFR/ALK mutations should be further confirmed in prospective, randomized studies.

This meta-analysis also has some limitations. First, as mentioned, the PD-L1 assay methods were not consistent across different studies. Thus, while PD-L1 immunohistochemistry was read on both tumor cells and tumor-infiltrating cells in the atezolizumab studies (IMpower) [20,24,25,29,43], PD-L1 expression was only measured on tumor cells in the trials assessing pembrolizumab (KEYNOTE) and nivolumab (CheckMate-227), [17,21,22,28]. Second, six of the included trials only provided interim analysis of the OS [17,20,22,24,25,28,29,43], which may misrepresent overall efficacy. Finally, the subgroup analysis was limited by the available information (PFS subgroup analyses were not assessed in CheckMate-227), and consequently caution must be exercised when interpreting the results. In this regard, certain limitations were also found with the available data of three of the studies, IMpower131, IMpower132, and CheckMate-227 part 2, whose results have only been published as congress abstracts and personal communications to date [20,21,29]. Despite these limitations, our results confirm those obtained in individual studies and are in line with the outcomes obtained in similar meta-analyses.

In conclusion, treatment with PD-(L)1 inhibitors resulted in significantly longer OS and PFS in stage IV NSCLC patients compared with chemotherapy alone. As a result, immunotherapy–chemotherapy combinations may be considered as a first-line strategy for these patients.

Supplementary Materials:
Figure S1: Forest plot of pooled odds ratios for overall response rate (ORR) in patients who received PD-(L)1 inhibitors plus chemotherapy vs. chemotherapy alone; Figure S2: Forest plot of pooled hazard ratios for (**A**) progression-free survival (PFS) and (**B**) overall survival in patients with nonsquamous or squamous NSCLC who received PD-(L)1 inhibitors plus chemotherapy vs. chemotherapy alone; Table S1: Treatments previously administered for nonmetastatic disease (data not available for atezolizumab studies); Table S2: Mutation status of IMpower150 [25,26] study patients; and Table S3: Characteristics of the patient population of the studies included in the meta-analysis.

Author Contributions: J.G.-G., J.R.-B., L.L.-M. and D.P.P. were responsible for data analyses and manuscript preparation and revision. F.J.A.-A., M.A.-G., M.d.C.A.-M., B.C.-B., J.C.-R., N.F.-N., J.L.F.P., M.L.-Q., D.P.P., L.C., P.R.-G., L.S.-C. contributed to manuscript preparation and approved the final version. All authors have read and agree to the published version of the manuscript.

Acknowledgments: The authors would like to thank Almudena Fuster-Matanzo from Medical Statistics Consulting S.L. (Valencia) for providing scientific support and medical writing services. J.R.-B. is supported by a Río Hortega fellowship from the Institute of Health Carlos III (CM19/00087).

Conflicts of Interest: J.G.-G. reports advisory and consultancy honoraria from Roche, Merck, Bristol-Myers Squibb, AstraZeneca, Lilly, Pfizer, and Boehringer; speaker honoraria from Roche; and travel/accommodation/expenses support from Roche, Merck, Bristol-Myers Squibb, and Boehringer. J.R.-B. reports advisory and consultancy honoraria from Boehringer; speaker honoraria from Roche; and travel/accommodation/expenses support from Bristol-Myers Squibb, Merck Sharp & Dohme, Ipsen, and PharmaMar. F.J.A.-A. reports advisory and consultancy honoraria from Roche, Merck, Bristol-Myers Squibb, AstraZeneca, Pfizer, Janssen, Ipsen, Boehringer, Takeda, and Sanofi; speaker honoraria from Lilly; and travel/accommodation/expenses support from Roche, Bristol-Myers Squibb, AstraZeneca, Pfizer, Ipsen, and Boehringer. M.A.-G. reports advisory honoraria from Clovis Oncology and Tesaro, as well as speaker honoraria from Astrazeneca, PharmaMar, and Roche. M.d.C.A.-M. reports advisory and consultancy honoraria from Roche, Merck, Bristol-Myers Squibb, and Boehringer. B.C.-B. reports advisory honoraria from Boehringer and Sanofi; speaker honoraria from Roche, Merck, Bristol-Myers Squibb, and AstraZeneca; and travel/accommodation/expenses support from Roche, Lilly, and Boehringer. N.F.-N. reports advisory and consultancy honoraria from Bristol-Myers Squibb, Bayer, and Boehringer; speaker honoraria from Roche, Bristol-Myers Squibb, AstraZeneca, Bayer, Janssen, Boehringer, and Sanofi; and travel/accommodation/expenses support from Roche, Bristol-Myers Squibb, Lilly, Pfizer, Bayer, and Sanofi. J.L.F.P. reports advisory, consultancy, and speaker honoraria from AstraZeneca, Bristol-Myers Squibb, Boehringer, Kyowa, Lilly, Merck, MSD, Novartis, Pfizer, Pierre Fabre, Takeda, and Roche. M.L.-Q. reports advisory and consultancy honoraria from Roche, Merck, Bristol-Myers Squibb, GSK, Ipsen, Boehringer, Takeda, Sanofi, and Tesaro; speaker honoraria from Roche, Merck, AstraZeneca, Lilly, Janssen, Ipsen, and Boehringer; and travel/accommodation/expenses support from Roche, Merck, Lilly, Pfizer, Ipsen, Boehringer, and Takeda. L.S.-C. reports advisory and consultancy honoraria from Bristol-Myers Squibb and Boehringer, speaker honoraria from Roche, and travel/accommodation/expenses support from Roche and Pfizer. L.L.M. reports advisory and consultancy honoraria from Roche/Genentech, AstraZeneca, Boehringer Ingelheim, Merck Sharp and Dohme, Takeda, Lilly, Bristol-Myers Squibb, and Ipsen. L.C., P.R.-G. and D.P.P. are full-time employees of Roche Farma S.A. at the time the study was conducted. The rest of the authors declare no conflicts of interest.

References

1. Torre, L.A.; Siegel, R.L.; Jemal, A. Lung Cancer Statistics. *Adv. Exp. Med. Biol.* **2016**, *893*, 1–19.
2. Planchard, D.; Popat, S.; Kerr, K.; Novello, S.; Smit, E.F.; Faivre-Finn, C.; Mok, T.S.; Reck, M.; Van Schil, P.E.; Hellmann, M.D.; et al. Metastatic non-small cell lung cancer: ESMO Clinical Practice Guidelines for diagnosis, treatment and follow-up. *Ann. Oncol.* **2018**, *29*, iv192–iv237. [CrossRef] [PubMed]
3. Goldstraw, P.; Chansky, K.; Crowley, J.; Rami-Porta, R.; Asamura, H.; Eberhardt, W.E.; Nicholson, A.G.; Groome, P.; Mitchell, A.; Bolejack, V. The IASLC Lung Cancer Staging Project: Proposals for Revision of the TNM Stage Groupings in the Forthcoming (Eighth) Edition of the TNM Classification for Lung Cancer. *J. Thorac. Oncol.* **2016**, *11*, 39–51. [CrossRef] [PubMed]
4. Antonia, S.J.; Villegas, A.; Daniel, D.; Vicente, D.; Murakami, S.; Hui, R.; Yokoi, T.; Chiappori, A.; Lee, K.H.; de Wit, M.; et al. Durvalumab after Chemoradiotherapy in Stage III Non-Small-Cell Lung Cancer. *N. Engl. J. Med.* **2017**, *377*, 1919–1929. [CrossRef] [PubMed]
5. Horn, L.; Mansfield, A.S.; Szczesna, A.; Havel, L.; Krzakowski, M.; Hochmair, M.J.; Huemer, F.; Losonczy, G.; Johnson, M.L.; Nishio, M.; et al. First-Line Atezolizumab plus Chemotherapy in Extensive-Stage Small-Cell Lung Cancer. *N. Engl. J. Med.* **2018**, *379*, 2220–2229. [CrossRef]
6. Paz-Ares, L.; Dvorkin, M.; Chen, Y.; Reinmuth, N.; Hotta, K.; Trukhin, D.; Statsenko, G.; Hochmair, M.J.; Ozguroglu, M.; Ji, J.H.; et al. Durvalumab plus platinum-etoposide versus platinum-etoposide in first-line treatment of extensive-stage small-cell lung cancer (CASPIAN): A randomised, controlled, open-label, phase 3 trial. *Lancet* **2019**, *394*, 1929–1939. [CrossRef]
7. Lu, M.; Su, Y. Immunotherapy in non-small cell lung cancer: The past, the present, and the future. *Thorac. Cancer* **2019**, *10*, 585–586. [CrossRef]
8. Fehrenbacher, L.; von Pawel, J.; Park, K.; Rittmeyer, A.; Gandara, D.R.; Ponce Aix, S.; Han, J.Y.; Gadgeel, S.M.; Hida, T.; Cortinovis, D.L.; et al. Updated Efficacy Analysis Including Secondary Population Results for OAK: A Randomized Phase III Study of Atezolizumab versus Docetaxel in Patients with Previously Treated Advanced Non-Small Cell Lung Cancer. *J. Thorac. Oncol.* **2018**, *13*, 1156–1170. [CrossRef]
9. Font, E.; Gettinger, S.N.; Burgio, M.; Antonia, S.J.; Holgado, E.; Spigel, D.R.; Arrieta, O.; Domine, M.; Aren, O.; Brahmer, J.; et al. 1301PD Three-year follow-up from CheckMate 017/057: Nivolumab versus docetaxel in patients with previously treated advanced non-small cell lung cancer (NSCLC). *Ann. Oncol.* **2017**. [CrossRef]
10. Herbst, R.; Baas, P.; Kim, D.-S.; Felip, E.; Perez-Gracia, J.L.; Han, J.-Y.; Molina, J.; Kim, J.-P.; Arvis, C.; Ahn, M.-J.; et al. Factors associated with better overall survival (OS) in patients with previously treated, PD-L1–expressing, advanced NSCLC: Multivariate analysis of KEYNOTE-010. *J. Clin. Oncol.* **2017**, *35*, 9090. [CrossRef]
11. Reck, M.; Rodriguez-Abreu, D.; Robinson, A.G.; Hui, R.; Csoszi, T.; Fulop, A.; Gottfried, M.; Peled, N.; Tafreshi, A.; Cuffe, S.; et al. Pembrolizumab versus Chemotherapy for PD-L1-Positive Non-Small-Cell Lung Cancer. *N. Engl. J. Med.* **2016**, *375*, 1823–1833. [CrossRef] [PubMed]
12. Reck, M.; Rodriguez-Abreu, D.; Robinson, A.G.; Hui, R.; Csoszi, T.; Fulop, A.; Gottfried, M.; Peled, N.; Tafreshi, A.; Cuffe, S.; et al. Updated Analysis of KEYNOTE-024: Pembrolizumab Versus Platinum-Based Chemotherapy for Advanced Non-Small-Cell Lung Cancer With PD-L1 Tumor Proportion Score of 50% or Greater. *J. Clin. Oncol.* **2019**, *37*, 537–546. [CrossRef] [PubMed]
13. Mok, T.S.K.; Wu, Y.L.; Kudaba, I.; Kowalski, D.M.; Cho, B.C.; Turna, H.Z.; Castro, G., Jr.; Srimuninnimit, V.; Laktionov, K.K.; Bondarenko, I.; et al. Pembrolizumab versus chemotherapy for previously untreated, PD-L1-expressing, locally advanced or metastatic non-small-cell lung cancer (KEYNOTE-042): A randomised, open-label, controlled, phase 3 trial. *Lancet* **2019**, *393*, 1819–1830. [CrossRef]
14. Lopes, G.; Wu, Y.-L.; Kudaba, I.; Kowalski, D.; Cho, B.C.; Castro, G.; Srimuninnimit, V.; Bondarenko, I.; Kubota, K.; Lubiniecki, G.M.; et al. Pembrolizumab (pembro) versus platinum-based chemotherapy (chemo) as first-line therapy for advanced/metastatic NSCLC with a PD-L1 tumor proportion score (TPS) ≥ 1%: Open-label, phase 3 KEYNOTE-042 study. *J. Clin. Oncol.* **2018**, *36*. [CrossRef]
15. Carbone, D.P.; Reck, M.; Paz-Ares, L.; Creelan, B.; Horn, L.; Steins, M.; Felip, E.; van den Heuvel, M.M.; Ciuleanu, T.E.; Badin, F.; et al. First-Line Nivolumab in Stage IV or Recurrent Non-Small-Cell Lung Cancer. *N. Engl. J. Med.* **2017**, *376*, 2415–2426. [CrossRef] [PubMed]
16. Apetoh, L.; Ladoire, S.; Coukos, G.; Ghiringhelli, F. Combining immunotherapy and anticancer agents: The right path to achieve cancer cure? *Ann. Oncol.* **2015**, *26*, 1813–1823. [CrossRef]

17. Gadgeel, S.M.; Garassino, M.C.; Esteban, E.; Speranza, G.; Felip, E.; Hochmair, M.J.; Powell, S.F.; Cheng, S.Y.; Bischoff, H.; Peled, N.; et al. KEYNOTE-189: Updated OS and progression after the next line of therapy (PFS2) with pembrolizumab (pembro) plus chemo with pemetrexed and platinum vs placebo plus chemo for metastatic nonsquamous NSCLC. *J. Clin. Oncol.* **2019**, *37*, 9013. [CrossRef]
18. Jotte, R.; Cappuzzo, F.; Vynnychenko, I.; Stroyakovskiy, D.; Rodriguez-Abreu, D.; Hussein, M.; Soo, R.; Conter, H.J.; Kozuki, T.; Huang, K.; et al. Atezolizumab in Combination With Carboplatin and Nab-Paclitaxel in Advanced Squamous Non-Small-Cell Lung Cancer (IMpower131): Results From a Randomized Phase III Trial. *J. Thorac. Oncol.* **2020**. [CrossRef]
19. Langer, C.J.; Gadgeel, S.M.; Borghaei, H.; Papadimitrakopoulou, V.A.; Patnaik, A.; Powell, S.F.; Gentzler, R.D.; Martins, R.G.; Stevenson, J.P.; Jalal, S.I.; et al. Carboplatin and pemetrexed with or without pembrolizumab for advanced, non-squamous non-small-cell lung cancer: A randomised, phase 2 cohort of the open-label KEYNOTE-021 study. *Lancet Oncol.* **2016**, *17*, 1497–1508. [CrossRef]
20. Papadimitrakopoulou, V.; Cobo, M.; Bordoni, R.; Dubray-Longeras, P.; Szalai, Z.; Ursol, G.; Novello, S.; Orlandi, F.; Ball, S.; Goldschmidt, J.; et al. OA05.07 IMpower132: PFS and Safety Results with 1L Atezolizumab + Carboplatin/Cisplatin + Pemetrexed in Stage IV Non-Squamous NSCLC. *J. Thorac. Oncol.* **2018**, *13*, S332–S333. [CrossRef]
21. Paz-Ares, L.; Ciuleanu, T.E.; Yu, X.; Salman, P.; Pluzanski, A.; Nagrial, A.; Havel, L.; Kowalyszyn, R.; Audigier-Valette, C.; Wu, Y.L.; et al. LBA3 Nivolumab (NIVO) + platinum-doublet chemotherapy (chemo) vs chemo as first-line (1L) treatment (tx) for advanced non-small cell lung cancer (aNSCLC): CheckMate 227 - part 2 final analysis. *Ann. Oncol.* **2019**, *30*, xi67–xi68. [CrossRef]
22. Paz-Ares, L.; Luft, A.; Vicente, D.; Tafreshi, A.; Gumus, M.; Mazieres, J.; Hermes, B.; Cay Senler, F.; Csoszi, T.; Fulop, A.; et al. Pembrolizumab plus Chemotherapy for Squamous Non-Small-Cell Lung Cancer. *N. Engl. J. Med.* **2018**, *379*, 2040–2051. [CrossRef]
23. Reck, M.; Mok, T.S.K.; Nishio, M.; Jotte, R.M.; Cappuzzo, F.; Orlandi, F.; Stroyakovskiy, D.; Nogami, N.; Rodriguez-Abreu, D.; Moro-Sibilot, D.; et al. Atezolizumab plus bevacizumab and chemotherapy in non-small-cell lung cancer (IMpower150): Key subgroup analyses of patients with EGFR mutations or baseline liver metastases in a randomised, open-label phase 3 trial. *Lancet Respir. Med.* **2019**, *7*, 387–401. [CrossRef]
24. Socinski, M.A.; Jotte, R.M.; Cappuzzo, F.; Orlandi, F.; Stroyakovskiy, D.; Nogami, N.; Rodriguez-Abreu, D.; Moro-Sibilot, D.; Thomas, C.A.; Barlesi, F.; et al. Atezolizumab for First-Line Treatment of Metastatic Nonsquamous NSCLC. *N. Engl. J. Med.* **2018**, *378*, 2288–2301. [CrossRef] [PubMed]
25. West, H.; McCleod, M.; Hussein, M.; Morabito, A.; Rittmeyer, A.; Conter, H.J.; Kopp, H.G.; Daniel, D.; McCune, S.; Mekhail, T.; et al. Atezolizumab in combination with carboplatin plus nab-paclitaxel chemotherapy compared with chemotherapy alone as first-line treatment for metastatic non-squamous non-small-cell lung cancer (IMpower130): A multicentre, randomised, open-label, phase 3 trial. *Lancet Oncol.* **2019**, *20*, 924–937. [CrossRef]
26. Cochrane Collaboration. *Cochrane Handbook for Systematic Reviews of Interventions*; John Wiley & Sons: Chichester, UK; Hoboken, NJ, USA, 2008.
27. Moher, D.; Liberati, A.; Tetzlaff, J.; Altman, D.G. Preferred reporting items for systematic reviews and meta-analyses: The PRISMA statement. *J. Clin. Epidemiol.* **2009**, *62*, 1006–1012. [CrossRef]
28. Gandhi, L.; Rodgríguez-Abreu, D.; Gadgeel, S.; Esteban, E.; Felip, E.; Angelis, F.D.; Domine, M.; Clingan, P.; Hochmair, M.J.; Powell, S.; et al. Abstract CT075: KEYNOTE-189: Randomized, double-blind, phase 3 study of pembrolizumab (pembro) or placebo plus pemetrexed (pem) and platinum as first-line therapy for metastatic NSCLC. *Cancer Res.* **2018**, *78*, CT075.
29. Jotte, R.M.; Cappuzzo, F.; Vynnychenko, I.; Stroyakovskiy, D.; Rodriguez Abreu, D.; Hussein, M.A.; Soo, R.A.; Conter, H.J.; Kozuki, T.; Silva, C.; et al. IMpower131: Primary PFS and safety analysis of a randomized phase III study of atezolizumab + carboplatin + paclitaxel or nab-paclitaxel vs carboplatin + nab-paclitaxel as 1L therapy in advanced squamous NSCLC. *J. Clin. Oncol.* **2018**, *36*, LBA9000. [CrossRef]
30. Hellmann, M.D.; Ciuleanu, T.E.; Pluzanski, A.; Lee, J.S.; Otterson, G.A.; Audigier-Valette, C.; Minenza, E.; Linardou, H.; Burgers, S.; Salman, P.; et al. Nivolumab plus Ipilimumab in Lung Cancer with a High Tumor Mutational Burden. *N. Engl. J. Med.* **2018**, *378*, 2093–2104. [CrossRef]

31. Conforti, F.; Pala, L.; Bagnardi, V.; De Pas, T.; Martinetti, M.; Viale, G.; Gelber, R.D.; Goldhirsch, A. Cancer immunotherapy efficacy and patients' sex: A systematic review and meta-analysis. *Lancet Oncol.* **2018**, *19*, 737–746. [CrossRef]
32. Tan, P.S.; Aguiar, P.; Haaland, B.; Lopes, G. Comparative effectiveness of immune-checkpoint inhibitors for previously treated advanced non-small cell lung cancer—A systematic review and network meta-analysis of 3024 participants. *Lung Cancer* **2018**, *115*, 84–88. [CrossRef]
33. You, W.; Liu, M.; Miao, J.D.; Liao, Y.Q.; Song, Y.B.; Cai, D.K.; Gao, Y.; Peng, H. A Network Meta-analysis Comparing the Efficacy and Safety of Anti-PD-1 with Anti-PD-L1 in Non-small Cell Lung Cancer. *J. Cancer* **2018**, *9*, 1200–1206. [CrossRef]
34. Zhou, G.-W.; Xiong, Y.; Chen, S.; Xia, F.; Li, Q.; Hu, J. Anti-PD-1/PD-L1 antibody therapy for pretreated advanced nonsmall-cell lung cancer: A meta-analysis of randomized clinical trials. *Medicine* **2016**, *95*, e4611. [CrossRef] [PubMed]
35. Zhao, Q.; Xie, R.; Lin, S.; You, X.; Weng, X. Anti-PD-1/PD-L1 Antibody Therapy for Pretreated Advanced or Metastatic Nonsmall Cell Lung Carcinomas and the Correlation between PD-L1 Expression and Treatment Effectiveness: An Update Meta-Analysis of Randomized Clinical Trials. *BioMed. Res. Int.* **2018**, *2018*, 3820956. [CrossRef] [PubMed]
36. Tun, A.M.; Thein, K.Z.; Thein, W.L.; Guevara, E. Checkpoint inhibitors plus chemotherapy for first-line treatment of advanced non-small cell lung cancer: A systematic review and meta-analysis of randomized controlled trials. *Future Sci. OA* **2019**, *5*, Fso421. [CrossRef]
37. Hellmann, M.D.; Paz-Ares, L.; Bernabe Caro, R.; Zurawski, B.; Kim, S.W.; Carcereny Costa, E.; Park, K.; Alexandru, A.; Lupinacci, L.; de la Mora Jimenez, E.; et al. Nivolumab plus Ipilimumab in Advanced Non-Small-Cell Lung Cancer. *N. Engl. J. Med.* **2019**, *381*, 2020–2031. [CrossRef]
38. Chen, Y.; Zhou, Y.; Tang, L.; Peng, X.; Jiang, H.; Wang, G.; Zhuang, W. Immune-Checkpoint Inhibitors as the First Line Treatment of Advanced Non-Small Cell Lung Cancer: A Meta-Analysis of Randomized Controlled Trials. *J. Cancer* **2019**, *10*, 6261–6268. [CrossRef]
39. Shen, K.; Cui, J.; Wei, Y.; Chen, X.; Liu, G.; Gao, X.; Li, W.; Lu, H.; Zhan, P.; Lv, T.; et al. Effectiveness and safety of PD-1/PD-L1 or CTLA4 inhibitors combined with chemotherapy as a first-line treatment for lung cancer: A meta-analysis. *J. Thorac. Dis.* **2018**, *10*, 6636–6652. [CrossRef] [PubMed]
40. Addeo, A.; Banna, G.L.; Metro, G.; Di Maio, M. Chemotherapy in Combination with Immune Checkpoint Inhibitors for the First-Line Treatment of Patients With Advanced Non-small Cell Lung Cancer: A Systematic Review and Literature-Based Meta-Analysis. *Front. Oncol.* **2019**, *9*, 264. [CrossRef] [PubMed]
41. Cappuzzo, F.M.M.; Hussein, M.; Morabito, A.; Rittmeyer, A.; Conter, H.J.; Kopp, H.; Daniel, D.; McCune, S.; Mekhail, T.; Zer, A.; et al. IMpower130: Progression-free survival (PFS) and safety analysis from a randomised phase 3 study of carboplatin + nab-paclitaxel (CnP) with or without atezolizumab (atezo) as first-line (1L) therapy in advanced non-squamous NSCLC. *Ann. Oncol.* **2018**, *29*, mdy424-065. [CrossRef]
42. Barlesi, F.N.M.; Cobo, M.; Steele, N.; Paramonov, V.; Parente, B.; Dear, R.; Berard, H.; Peled, N.; Seneviratne, L.C.; Baldini, E.; et al. IMpower132: Efficacy of atezolizumab (atezo)+carboplatin (carbo)/cisplatin (cis)+pemetrexed (pem) as 1L treatment in key subgroups with stage IV non-squamous non-small cell lung cancer (NSCLC). *Ann. Oncol.* **2018**, *29*, mdy424-066. [CrossRef]
43. Garassino, M.C.; Gadgeel, S.; Esteban, E.; Felip, E.; Speranza, G.; Angelis, F.D.; Domine, M.; Clingan, P.; Hochmair, M.J.; Powell, S.F.; et al. Abstract CT043: Outcomes among patients (pts) with metastatic nonsquamous NSCLC with liver metastases or brain metastases treated with pembrolizumab (pembro) plus pemetrexed-platinum: Results from the KEYNOTE-189 study. *Cancer Res.* **2019**, *79*, CT043.

13

Concomitant *TP53* Mutation Confers Worse Prognosis in *EGFR*-Mutated Non-Small Cell Lung Cancer Patients Treated with TKIs

Matteo Canale [1], Elisabetta Petracci [2], Angelo Delmonte [3], Giuseppe Bronte [3], Elisa Chiadini [1], Vienna Ludovini [4], Alessandra Dubini [5], Maximilian Papi [6], Sara Baglivo [4], Nicoletta De Luigi [7], Alberto Verlicchi [3], Rita Chiari [8], Lorenza Landi [9], Giulio Metro [4], Marco Angelo Burgio [3], Lucio Crinò [3] and Paola Ulivi [1,*]

1. Biosciences Laboratory, Istituto Scientifico Romagnolo per lo Studio e la Cura dei Tumori (IRST) IRCCS, 47014 Meldola, Italy; matteo.canale@irst.emr.it (M.C.); elisa.chiadini@irst.emr.it (E.C.)
2. Biostatistics and Clinical Trials Unit, Istituto Scientifico Romagnolo per lo Studio e la Cura dei Tumori (IRST) IRCCS, 47014 Meldola, Italy; elisabetta.petracci@irst.emr.it
3. Department of Medical Oncology, Istituto Scientifico Romagnolo per lo Studio e la Cura dei Tumori (IRST) IRCCS, 47014 Meldola, Italy; angelo.delmonte@irst.emr.it (A.D.); giuseppe.bronte@irst.emr.it (G.B.); alberto.verlicchi@irst.emr.it (A.V.); marco.burgio@irst.emr.it (M.A.B.); lucio.crino@irst.emr.it (L.C.)
4. Department of Medical Oncology, Santa Maria della Misericordia Hospital, 06129 Perugia, Italy; oncolab@hotmail.com (V.L.); baglivosara@gmail.com (S.B.); giulio.metro@yahoo.com (G.M.)
5. Department of Pathology, Morgagni-Pierantoni Hospital, 47121 Forlì, Italy; alessandra.dubini@auslromagna.it
6. Department of Medical Oncology, Per gli Infermi Hospital, Rimini 47923, Italy; maximilianpapi@libero.it
7. UOS Oncology, Istituto per la Sicurezza Sociale, State Hospital, Cailungo 47893, San Marino, Italy; nicolettadeluigi@hotmail.com
8. Department of Medical Oncology, Ospedali Riuniti Padova Sud "M. Teresa di Calcutta", ULSS6 Euganea, 35131 Padova, Italy; rita.chiari@aulss6.veneto.it
9. Department of Medical Oncology, S. Maria delle Croci Hospital, 48121 Ravenna, Italy; landi.lorenza@gmail.com

* Correspondence: paola.ulivi@irst.emr.it

Abstract: Background: Non-small cell lung cancer (NSCLC) is the primary cause of cancer-related deaths worldwide. Epidermal Growth Factor Receptor (*EGFR*)-mutated patients usually benefit from TKIs treatment, but a significant portion show unresponsiveness due to primary resistance mechanisms. We investigated the role of *TP53* mutations in predicting survival and response to *EGFR*-TKIs in EGFR-mutated NSCLC patients, to confirm, on an independent case series, our previous results. Methods: An independent retrospective cohort study was conducted, on a case series of 136 *EGFR*-mutated NSCLC patients receiving first or second generation TKIs as a first line therapy, and a smaller fraction of patients who acquired the T790M resistance mutation and were treated with third generation TKIs in the second or further line of treatment. *TP53* mutations were evaluated in relation to disease control rate (DCR), objective response rate (ORR), progression-free survival (PFS) and overall survival (OS) of the patients. Results: Forty-two patients (30.9%) showed a *TP53* mutation. Considered together, *TP53* mutations had no significant impact on time-to-event endpoints. Considering the different *TP53* mutations separately, exon 8 mutations confirmed their negative effect on PFS (HR 3.16, 95% 1.59–6.28, $p = 0.001$). In patients who developed the T790M resistance mutation, treated with third generation TKIs, the *TP53* exon 8 mutations predicted worse PFS (even though not statistically significant), and OS (HR 4.86, 95% CI: 1.25–18.90, $p = 0.023$). Conclusions: *TP53* exon 8 mutations confirmed their negative prognostic impact in patients treated with first and second generation TKIs and demonstrated a role in affecting clinical outcome in patients treated with third generation TKIs.

Keywords: non-small-cell lung cancer; epidermal growth factor receptor; tyrosine kinase inhibitors; *TP53* mutations; responsiveness; prognosis

---

1. Introduction

Epidermal growth factor receptor (*EGFR*)-tyrosine kinase inhibitors (TKIs) have changed the natural history of non-small-cell lung cancer (NSCLC) patients harboring specific *EGFR* mutations at exons 18, 19 and 21. Randomized trials have demonstrated a median progression-free survival (PFS) of 9.7 and 9.5 months in patients harboring sensitizing *EGFR* mutations treated with first-generation *EGFR*-TKIs versus platinum-based chemotherapy [1,2], and 11.1 months for second generation TKIs [3]. Third generation TKI osimertinib, initially designed to overcome the arising of T790M resistance mutation in *EGFR* pre-treated patients [4], has recently become the gold standard for *EGFR*-mutated patients, reaching a median PFS of 18.9 months [5].

Despite the high sensitivity of *EGFR*-mutated patients to *EGFR*-TKIs, the objective response rate is of about 70–80% for 1st, 2nd and 3rd generation TKIs [2,3,5], meaning that a portion of patients do not respond to *EGFR*-TKI treatment, notwithstanding the presence of sensitizing *EGFR* mutation, suggesting the presence of primary resistance mechanisms.

Our previous study and several others showed that the concomitant presence of *TP53* mutation confers a worse prognosis in *EGFR*-mutated patients treated with first and second generation TKIs [6–8]. Subsequent studies performed using next generation sequencing methodologies showed that the presence of concomitant mutation in different genes is associated with a lower response to *EGFR*-TKIs and, however, *TP53* mutation confirms to be the most significant predictor of worse outcome. In particular, it seems that specific *TP53* mutations are more implicated in predicting the worse prognosis [6,9,10], confirming that different *TP53* mutations confer different p53 functions. Within the coding region of the *TP53* gene, several studies have reported that a higher frequency of mutations occurs in the exons 5–8, and that mutations in these exons are associated to differential functions of p53 protein [9,10]. As the different published studies have analyzed principally patients treated with first and second generation TKIs, few data are available with regard to the role of *TP53* mutation in relation to response to third generation TKIs.

The main purpose of this research was to confirm our previously published results on the role of *TP53* mutations, in an independent cohort of advanced *EGFR*-mutated patients treated with first or second generation TKIs in the first line setting, and to investigate the role of *TP53* mutations in predicting prognosis of patients with acquired T790M mutation treated with third generation TKIs.

2. Materials and Methods

To confirm our previous results on the role of *TP53* mutations in relation to the effectiveness of TKIs, an independent retrospective cohort study was conducted. All consecutive patients with advanced *EGFR*-mutated NSCLC receiving a first line TKI treatment (i.e., gefitinib, erlotinib, or afatinib) from July 2010 to May 2018 at the Medical Oncology Units of the Romagna catchment area (Area Vasta Romagna, AVR) and at the S. Maria della Misericordia Hospital of Perugia, Italy, were included in this study. Demographic and clinical characteristics of the patients were obtained using a medical and radiographic records review including age, gender, smoking history, histology, and information on death and response to treatment. *EGFR* status had been routinely determined at the Biosciences Laboratory of IRST-IRCCS and the Laboratory of Molecular Biology of the S. Maria della Misericordia Hospital, Perugia, by MassARRAY, pyrosequencing, direct sequencing or Next-Generation Sequencing (NGS) methodologies.

To evaluate the independent role of *TP53* mutations, that is, eventually adjusting for other covariates, and to obtain a more accurate estimate of their prognostic effect, an analysis combining the data of the present work with those from our previous one [6], was also performed, updating follow-ups of the previous case series to 30 June 2018.

Moreover, considering the two cohorts together, we identified a subgroup of 42 patients who developed the T790M resistance mutation and were treated with third generation TKI, osimertinib. All patients provided an informed consent, and the study was approved by the AVR Ethical Committee (study code IRST-B053).

2.1. *EGFR and TP53 Mutation Analysis*

EGFR mutation analyses were performed on both cytologic and histologic samples, accurately selected by a dedicated expert pathologist from each center at the time of diagnosis. The same DNA specimens were used for the determination of *TP53* mutation status, blindly to the clinical outcomes. Quality controls were periodically performed during the course of the study to ensure concordance of molecular results.

DNA was extracted by macro-dissection of an area comprising at least 50% of tumor cells. Cells were lysed in a digestion buffer of 50 mmol/L KCl, 10 mmol/L Tris-HCl pH 8.0, 2.5 mmol/L $MgCl_2$, and Tween-20 0.45%; proteinase K at 1.25 mg/mL were added to each specimen, with an overnight incubation at 56 °C. After proteinase K inactivation at 95 °C for 10 min, samples were centrifuged twice to eliminate debris and supernatant DNA quantity and quality was assessed by Nanodrop (Celbio) before molecular analyses.

Mutation status for exons 5–8 of *TP53* gene was performed by PCR amplification and Direct Sequencing using 3130 Genetic Analyzer (Applied Biosystems, Monza, Italy), or Next-Generation Sequencing by Ion S5 platform (Thermofisher, Monza, Italy), or MySeq platform (Illumina, San Diego, CA, USA).

2.2. *Response Evaluation*

Best clinical response to treatment with TKI was classified on the basis of interval CT scans as complete response (CR), partial response (PR), stable disease (SD), or progressive disease (PD) using standard Response Evaluation Criteria in Solid Tumors criteria (RECIST) version 1.1. Patients with both baseline imaging and at least one repeated evaluation after continuous *EGFR*-TKI monotherapy were evaluable for radiographic response. The same criteria for response evaluation and periodicity were used by all centers taking part in the study.

2.3. *Statistical Analyses*

Data were summarized by mean ± standard deviation (SD) for continuous variables and through natural frequencies and percentages for categorical ones.

Treatment responses were reported as objective response rate (ORR) and disease control rate (DCR). The time-to-event endpoints examined were progression-free survival (PFS) and overall survival (OS). PFS was defined as the time from start of first line treatment (or from start of osimertinib for the subgroup analysis) to disease progression or death for any cause, whichever occurred first. Patients who were alive and progression-free at 30 June 2018, the last follow-up update, were censored at that date.

OS was defined as the time from start of first line treatment to death for any cause. Alive patients were censored at the date of the last follow-up update. PFS and OS functions were estimated using the Kaplan–Meier method, and the log-rank test was used to assess differences between groups. Median PFS and OS were reported as point estimates and 95% confidence intervals (CI) in round brackets. The Cox proportional hazards regression model was used to quantify the association between specific covariates and the time-to-event endpoints. Results are reported as HR and 95% CI in round brackets. To assess the association between mutations and the duration of response to TKIs, patients were divided into short-term responders (PFS less than 6 months), intermediate-term responders (PFS ≥6 months and ≤24 months) or long-term responders (PFS >24 months). The association between categorical variables was tested by the Pearson's χ^2 test or Fisher exact test, when appropriate, whereas those between a continuous variable and a categorical one was tested by means of the Student *t*-test or *F* test for more than two categories. To evaluate the independent role of *TP53* mutations in a multivariate analysis and to obtain more accurate estimates of their prognostic effect, a combined analysis including data of the present work with those from our previous one, was performed. Follow-up of our previous cohort was updated on 30 June 2018. A multivariable model was obtained using backward stepwise variable selection, setting the significance level for variable removal from the model equal to 0.10. In a perspective of parsimonious modelling, when appropriate, categories of some study variables were grouped. The proportional hazards assumption was evaluated using a statistical test based on Schoenfeld residuals. In case of non-proportional hazards for a specific variable, a Cox model with time-dependent coefficient, $\beta(t)$, was fitted. To simplify model interpretation, a step function for $\beta(t)$ was used, dividing the follow-up period in three time periods since treatment started: the first 6 months, 6–12 months, and greater than 12 months.

Overall and when not otherwise specified, a two-sided *p*-value (p) <0.05 was considered statistically significant. All statistical analyses were performed using STATA 15.0 software (College Station, TX, USA) and R version 3.6.1.

3. Results

3.1. Clinico-Pathologic and Molecular Features of Patients

Patients characteristics, *EGFR* mutations, type of TKI received and *TP53* mutations are reported in Table 1. All 136 patients carried an *EGFR* mutation (exon 19 deletions 53.7%, exon 21 L858R 35.3%, other *EGFR* mutations 11.0%) and received a first line *EGFR*-TKI (36.7% Erlotinib, 5.1% Erlotinib plus bevacizumab, 30.9% gefitinib, 27.2% afatinib). Of the patients with available information on smoking habit, half were never smokers (50.8%), and half were former or current smokers (28.8% and 20.3%, respectively). We found *TP53* mutations in 42 (30.9%) of the 136 analyzed patients: 12 mutations were in exon 5 (28.6%), 6 in exon 6 (14.3%), 13 in exon 7 (31.0%) and 11 in exon 8 (26.2%). Following the classification of *TP53* mutations into disruptive and non-disruptive ones [6], 11 patients had a disruptive mutation whereas 31 had a non-disruptive one (26.2% and 73.8%, respectively).

Table 1. Demographic, clinicopathological and molecular characteristics of patients (n = 136).

Characteristic	*n*	(%)
Gender		
Female	86	(62.2)
Male	50	(36.8)
Age at first line TKI		
Mean ± SD	67.6 ± 11.2	
Smoking habit †		
Never smoker	60	(50.9)
Former smoker	34	(28.8)
Current smoker	24	(20.3)
Type of *EGFR* mutation		
Exon 19 deletion	73	(53.7)
Exon 21 L858R	48	(35.3)
Other uncommon mutations	15	(11.0)
Type of *EGFR* exon 19 deletion		
No exon 19 deletion	63	(46.3)
Deletion starts at codon 746	62	(45.6)
Deletion starts at codon 747	11	(8.1)
Type of TKI received in first line setting		
Erlotinib *	57	(41.9)
Gefitinib	42	(30.9)
Afatinib	37	(27.2)
***TP53* mutation**		
Wild type	94	(69.1)
Exon 5	12	(8.8)
Exon 6	6	(4.4)
Exon 7	13	(9.6)
Exon 8	11	(8.1)
Type of *TP53* mutation		
Wild type	94	(69.1)
Disruptive	11	(8.1)
Non-disruptive	31	(22.8)

† The sum does not add up to the total due to missing values. * Of these patients, 7 received Erlotinib plus Bevacizumab as a first line therapy, as provided in the Beverly clinical trial.

While for patients with exon 19 deletion the three different TKIs were used in an almost similar proportion (32.9% patients received erlotinib, 30.1% gefitinib, and 37.0% afatinib), patients with a mutation in exon 21 L858R were predominantly treated with erlotinib or gefitinib (52.1% and 39.6% of the patients, respectively), and those with uncommon mutations received predominantly erlotinib or afatinib (53.3% and 40.0%, respectively, Table S1).

No statistically significant associations were observed between type of *TP53* mutation, type of *EGFR* mutation and patient characteristics (Table S2).

3.2. Patients Outcome in Relation to EGFR Mutations

Overall, ORR and DCR were 67.4%, and 89.3%, respectively. Considering the clinical responses by type of *EGFR* mutation, ORR was considerably higher in the subgroup of patients with exon 19 deletion (77.5%), with respect to patients with L585R mutation (55.3%), and the subgroup with other mutations (54.6%), $p = 0.029$. A higher percentage of long responders was observed in patients carrying exon 19 deletion (12.3%), with respect to patients with L858R point mutation (7.3%), or patients with the other *EGFR* mutations (6.6%), Table 2.

Table 2. Best clinical response according to *EGFR* mutations.

	All *EGFR* Mutations (n = 136)		Exon 19 Deletion (n = 73)		Exon 21 L858R (n = 48)		Other *EGFR* Mutations (n = 15)		p
	n	(%)	n	(%)	n	(%)	n	(%)	
Best response †									0.026
CR	13	(9.9)	8	(11.3)	4	(8.5)	1	(7.1)	
PR	76	(57.6)	47	(66.2)	22	(46.8)	7	(50.0)	
SD	29	(22.0)	7	(9.9)	17	(36.2)	5	(35.7)	
PD	14	(10.6)	9	(12.7)	4	(8.5)	1	(7.1)	
ORR	89	(67.4)	55	(77.5)	26	(55.3)	6	(54.6)	0.029
DCR	118	(89.4)	62	(87.3)	43	(91.5)	11	(100.0)	0.844
Duration of response									0.260
Short-term responders	36	(26.4)	19	(26.0)	10	(20.8)	7	(46.7)	
Medium-term responders	87	(64.0)	45	(61.6)	35	(72.9)	7	(46.7)	
Long-term responders	13	(9.6)	9	(12.3)	2	(6.3)	1	(6.6)	

† The sum does not add up to the total due to missing values.

Median PFS and OS were 12.3 (95% CI: 9.9–13.8) and 27.3 (95% CI: 21.9–52.9) months, respectively. No statistically significant association between PFS, OS and type of *EGFR* mutations was found ($p = 0.282$ and $p = 0.207$, respectively).

3.3. Patients Outcome in Relation to TP53 Mutations

No statistically significant associations were found between *TP53* mutations and ORR and DCR (Table S3). When considering any type of *TP53* mutation with regard to PFS, no association was found; however, significant results were observed considering only *TP53* exon 8 mutations. As previously reported [6], patients with this gene mutation showed a shorter median PFS than non-exon 8 mutated and wild type *TP53* patients: 5.8 months (95% CI: 2.4–10.2) vs. 14.4 (95% CI: 6.7–21.8) and 12.4 (95% CI: 10.0–15.0), respectively (Figure 1A). These patients also showed a poorer OS as compared with the other groups, even though this result was not statistically significant: median OS were 18.53 months (95% CI: 7.3–NR), 34.8 (95% CI: 21.6–NR), 27.3 (95% CI: 20.2–52.9), respectively (Figure 1B).

The presence of *TP53* exon 8 mutation seemed to be associated with a worse prognosis in a similar way in the patients with the different *EGFR* mutations, both in terms of PFS and OS.

In particular, patients with wild type *TP53* exon 8 had a better clinical outcome independently by *EGFR* status: median PFS and OS were 12.9 (95% CI: 10.0–16.3) and 29.7 months (95% CI: 23.0–60.5) for patients with *EGFR* exon 19 deletion vs. 12.4 months (95% CI: 7.9–15.0) and 23.2 months (95% CI: 19.2–63.7) for those with other *EGFR* mutations, respectively; in the subgroup of patients with *TP53* exon 8 mutations, median PFS and OS were 5.8 months (95% CI: 2.5–NR) and 21.9 months (95% CI: 7.3–NR) for patients with *EGFR* exon 19 deletion vs. 6.4 (95% CI: 2.4–NR) and 18.5 months (95% CI: 7.6–NR) for those with other *EGFR* mutations. In Table S4, the univariate Cox analysis results are reported.

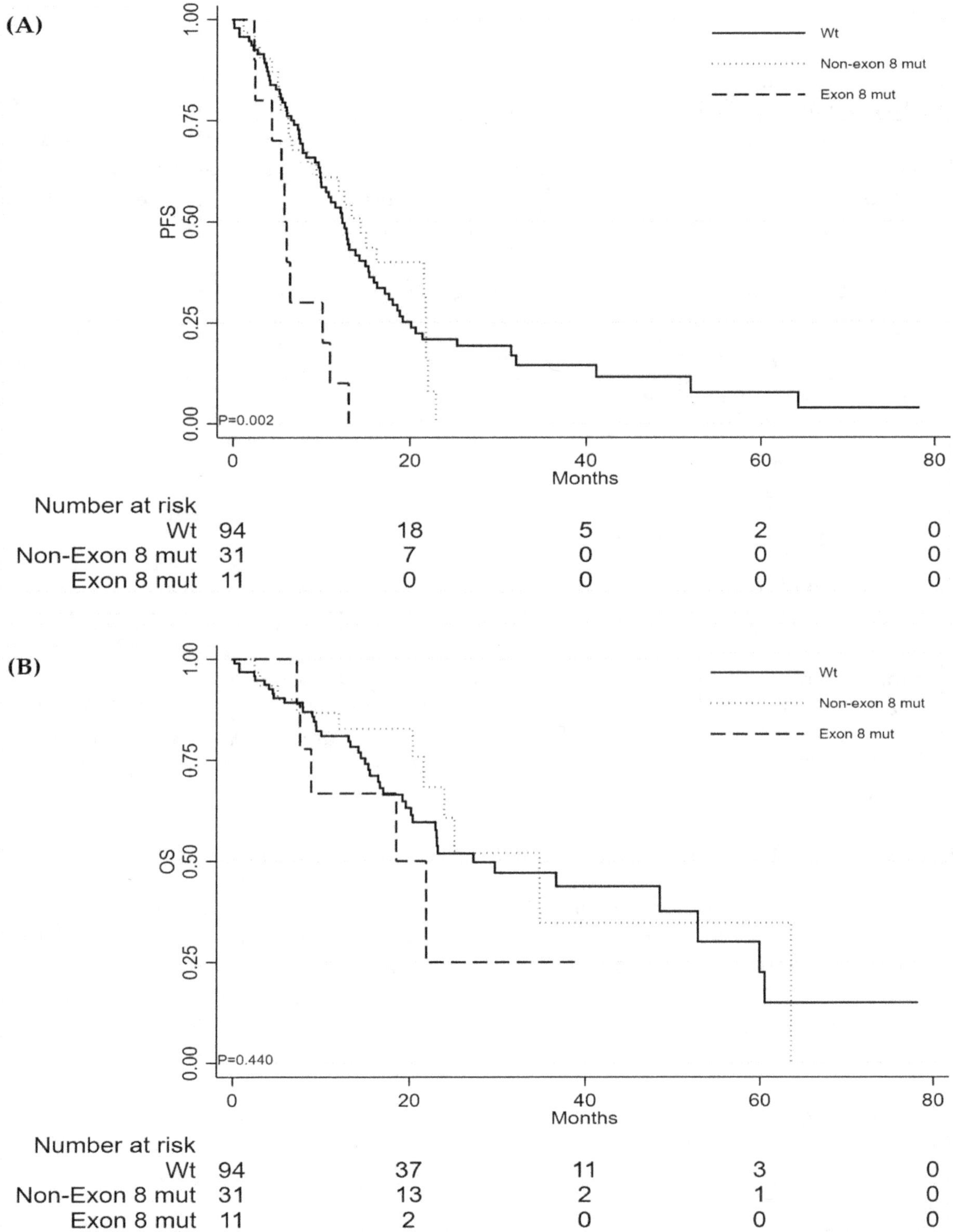

Figure 1. Progression-free survival (**A**) and Overall Survival (**B**) of patients according to *TP53*.

3.4. Multivariate Analysis of the Role of TP53 Mutation: Combined Cohorts of Patients

To obtain a more precise estimate of the effect of *TP53* exon 8 mutation on PFS and OS, and to determine its potential independent role considering other information, a pooled analysis considering either data from our previously analyzed cohort and the one described in the present study, was performed.

The final multivariate model for PFS included both *EGFR* exon 19 deletion as well as TP53 mutation. As soon as the effect of exon 19 deletion on the hazard of disease progression or death is not constant over time, that is, the proportional hazards assumption underlying the Cox model was violated, to obtain a better model fit, this variable was entered into the model with a time-dependent coefficient. Table 3 shows that the effect of exon 19 mutation changes over time, showing a strong protective effect over the first six months that vanishes afterward.

Table 3. Multivariate Cox analysis of progression-free survival (PFS) (n = 272).

	HR	PFS 95% CI	p
Exon 19 deletion			
No	1		
Yes			
0–6 months	0.56	(0.35–0.89)	0.014
6–12 months	0.67	(0.40–1.12)	0.123
>12 months	1.27	(0.80–2.03)	0.314
***TP53* exon 8 mutations**			
Wild-type *TP53*	1		
Non-Exon 8 mutations	1.02	0.73–1.42	0.905
Exon 8 mutations	1.81	1.13–2.92	0.014

Adjusting for presence of *EGFR* exon 19 deletion, *TP53* mutations affecting exon 8 demonstrated to be the unique independent negative prognostic factor for PFS (HR 1.81, 95% CI: 1.13–2.92, Table 3). With regard to OS, only deletion in *EGFR* Exon 19 resulted associated to OS, probably due to data from our previous cohort (HR 0.52 (95% CI: 0.26–1.03) for the first 6 months of follow-up, HR 0.44 (95% CI: 0.22–0.90), for successive 6 months, and HR 1.08 (95% CI: 0.72–1.61) after 12 months).

3.5. TP53 Mutations in Relation to Responsiveness to Third Generation TKIs: Combined Cohorts of Patients

Considering both patients' cohorts (n = 272 patients), we considered 42 patients who developed a T790M resistance mutation and were treated with third generation TKI osimertinib, in the second or further lines of therapy. Of these, 41 were evaluable for *TP53* mutation status; we found 10 *TP53* mutated patients (24.4%): 3 mutations in exon 5 (30%), 1 in exon 6 (10%), 2 in exon 7 (20%) and 4 in exon 8 (40%). Within the 41 patients with available clinical information, median PFS and OS were 13.86 (95% CI: 5.5–18.53) and 44.38 months (95% CI: 10.64–24.28), respectively. Median PFS of exon 8 *TP53* mutated patients was 2.83 (2.17–NR) months, with respect to a median PFS of 16.79 (5.55–22.31) and 15.28 (1.91–NR) months, for wt *TP53* and patients with mutations in other exons of the gene, respectively (Figure 2A). Even though a good separation, the difference among curves was not statistically significant (p = 0.304), due to small numbers of the exon 8 mutated patients. On the other hand, exon 8 *TP53* gene mutations significantly affected the survival of the patients, with a median OS for exon 8 *TP53* mutated patients of 18.53 (7.26–NR) months, with respect to 42.15 (29.43–NR) and 59.92 (29.73–NR) months of patients with mutations in other exons of *TP53* and wt *TP53*, respectively (p = 0.044) (Figure 2B). Table 4 shows the univariate hazard ratios for PFS and OS with respect to the presence of *TP53* exon 8 mutation.

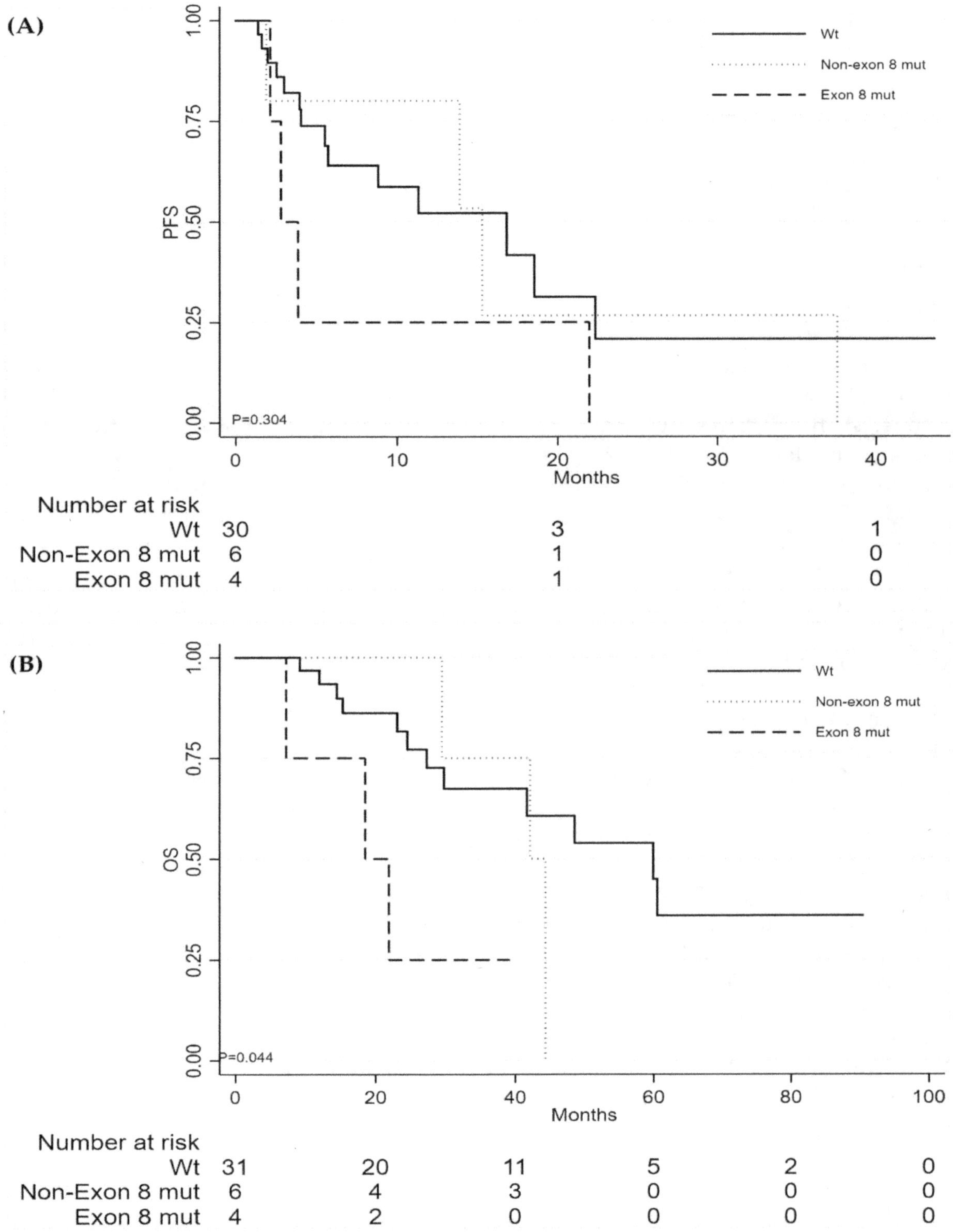

Figure 2. Progression-free survival (**A**) and Overall Survival (**B**) in relation to *TP53* mutations of patients with acquired T790M treated with third generation TKIs.

Table 4. *TP53* mutations in relation to progression-free survival (PFS) and overall survival (OS) of patients receiving osimertinib in second or further lines of treatment.

	PFS			OS		
	HR	**(95% CI)**	***p***	**HR**	**(95% CI)**	***p***
TP53 Exon 8						
Wild type	1			1		
Non-Exon 8 mutations	1.15	(0.37–3.59)	0.811	1.55	(0.42–5.76)	0.514
Exon 8 mutations	2.39	(0.77–7.45)	0.134	4.86	(1.25–18.90)	0.023

4. Discussion

In this study, we analyzed *TP53* mutations in relation to clinical outcome in a large cohort of *EGFR*-mutated NSCLC patients receiving first or second generation TKIs as a first line therapy. Our results confirm that exon 8 *TP53* mutations are associated with a shorter PFS, in all settings of treatment.

Moreover, such a negative effect was also observed in the subgroup of patients treated with third generation after the development of T790M mutation.

Numerous studies demonstrated the role of *TP53* mutations in predicting poor prognosis of advanced NSCLC patients [9,11–15], and this was confirmed also in the subgroup of NSCLC patients carrying *EGFR* mutations [8,9,16]. In particular, different recent studies showed that the concurrent presence of *TP53* mutations negatively affects response to TKIs in *EGFR*-mutated NSCLC patients, suggesting a role for these gene mutations in determining primary resistance to these drugs [6,7,17–20]. *TP53* is the most frequently mutated gene in lung adenocarcinoma, with mutation rates reported up to 55% [13,21–23], with a predominantly clonal expression [24]. In our case series, we found 30% of patients carrying a *TP53* mutation in the exons 5–8, the same percentage we previously reported in an independent case series. It is well known that different *TP53* mutations lead to changes in the P53 protein that may have diverse biological significance [9,10,25], and mutations in the DNA-binding domain (exons 5–8), are frequently associated with gain-of-function properties, resulting in pro-oncogenic features of the P53 protein [26]. In our previous work, we found that exon 8 *TP53* mutations were able to predict worse response to *EGFR* TKIs, especially in the subgroup of patients with *EGFR* exon 19 deletion. In the present study we confirmed the negative prognostic value of *TP53* exon 8 mutation in an independent cohort of *EGFR*-mutated NSCLC treated with both first and second generation TKIs in the first line setting. In the present study, the prognostic value of exon 8 *TP53* mutation was evident independently from the type of *EGFR* mutation. In a combined analysis, we showed that the effect was evident on overall survival in *EGFR*-mutated patients who developed T790M at progression after first line TKIs and osimertinib.

These results, in agreement with those reported by Kim et al. [7], suggest a negative predictive role of *TP53* mutation in all lines of therapy and in relation to all TKIs. Furthermore, our results are consistent with a recent study that found that *TP53* mutations in exon 8 are associated with shorter OS of patients receiving a TKI as a first line treatment [27].

In another study, missense mutations in *TP53* gene resulted in shorter PFS in *EGFR* mutated patients treated with TKIs but showed no associations with PFS and OS in patients undergoing surgical resection [28]. According to Xu et al., who reported *TP53* mutations in 88% of NSCLC *EGFR*-mutated patients that responded for <6 months to an *EGFR* TKIs, with respect to 13% of responders for >24 months [29], our results show a higher rate of *TP53* mutations in non-responders group, with no *TP53* mutated patients in the long responder group.

To investigate the role of *TP53* mutations in predicting clinical outcome of patients treated with third generation TKIs, we considered 42 patients' developed T790M mutation to first line treatment with first or second generation TKI and received a third generation drug in the second or further line of therapy. In this subgroup, we found a diminished PFS in patients carrying *TP53* mutations in exon 8, even though without statistical significance, probably due to the small number of analyzed patients; exon 8 *TP53* mutated patients had a significantly shorter OS, with respect to wt *TP53* patients and patients with mutations in other exons of *TP53*. This observation is consistent with previous observations, that identified *TP53* mutations (not only in exon 8) as a negative prognostic predictor [7,16]. This result was not confirmed by a study from Labbé et al., that found no differences in ORR of patients treated with third generation TKIs, based on *TP53* mutation status; this could be for the small size of the analyzed case series [28]. In the light of the paradigm shift brought by FLAURA trial [5], there is a need to identify which biomarkers could predict primary resistance to osimertinib as a first line therapy; if confirmed in a larger case series treated with third generation TKI in the first line, these results could help to better stratify patients, suggesting an *EGFR*-independent mechanism of resistance, as others have already highlighted [30].

5. Conclusions

In conclusion, we confirmed that *TP53* exon 8 mutations identify a subgroup of patients with primary resistance to *EGFR* TKIs, and that this is true also in relation to third generation TKIs such as osimertinib. These data suggest that patients with concomitant *EGFR* and exon 8 *TP53* mutations should be candidates for more aggressive therapeutic schemes and should be monitored with a stricter follow-up.

Author Contributions: Conceptualization, A.D. (Angelo Delmonte) , L.C. and P.U.; methodology, M.C., E.P., E.C., V.L. and S.B.; validation, M.C., E.C., V.L., S.B. and P.U.; formal analysis, M.C., E.P., A.D. (Angelo Delmonte), A.D. (Alessandra Dubini) R.C., L.C. and P.U.; investigation, all authors; resources, A.D. (Angelo Delmonte), V.L., R.C., L.C. and P.U.; data curation, A.D. (Angelo Delmonte), A.D. (Alessandra Dubini) G.B., M.P., N.D.L., A.V., R.C., L.L., G.M. and M.A.B.; writing—original draft preparation, M.C., E.P., L.C. and P.U.; writing—review and editing, all authors; visualization, M.C., E.P. A.D. (Angelo Delmonte), L.C. and P.U.; supervision, A.D. (Angelo Delmonte), L.C. and P.U. All authors have read and agreed to the published version of the manuscript.

References

1. Rosell, R.; Carcereny, E.; Gervais, R.; Vergnenègre, A.; Massuti, B.; Felip, E.; Palmero, R.; Garcia-Gomez, R.; Pallares, C.; Sanchez, J.M.; et al. Erlotinib versus standard chemotherapy as first-line treatment for European patients with advanced EGFR mutation-positive non-small-cell lung cancer (EURTAC): a multicentre, open-label, randomised phase 3 trial. *Lancet Oncol.* **2012**, *13*, 239–246. [CrossRef]
2. Mok, T.S.; Wu, Y.-L.; Thongprasert, S.; Yang, J.C.-H.; Chu, D.-T.; Saijo, N.; Sunpaweravong, P.; Han, B.; Margono, B.; Ichinose, Y.; et al. Gefitinib or Carboplatin–Paclitaxel in Pulmonary Adenocarcinoma. *N. Engl. J. Med.* **2009**, *361*, 947–957. [CrossRef]
3. Yang, J.C.-H.; Wu, Y.-L.; Schuler, M.; Sebastian, M.; Popat, S.; Yamamoto, N.; Zhou, C.; Hu, C.-P.; O'Byrne, K.; Feng, J.; et al. Afatinib versus cisplatin-based chemotherapy for EGFR mutation-positive lung adenocarcinoma (LUX-Lung 3 and LUX-Lung 6): analysis of overall survival data from two randomised, phase 3 trials. *Lancet Oncol.* **2015**, *16*, 141–151. [CrossRef]
4. Mok, T.S.; Wu, Y.-L.; Ahn, M.-J.; Garassino, M.C.; Kim, H.R.; Ramalingam, S.R.; Shepherd, F.A.; He, Y.; Akamatsu, H.; Theelen, W.S.; et al. Osimertinib or Platinum-Pemetrexed in EGFR T790M-Positive Lung Cancer. *N. Engl. J. Med.* **2016**, *376*, 629–640. [CrossRef]
5. Soria, J.-C.; Ohe, Y.; Vansteenkiste, J.; Reungwetwattana, T.; Chewaskulyong, B.; Lee, K.H.; Dechaphunkul, A.; Imamura, F.; Nogami, N.; Kurata, T.; et al. Osimertinib in UntreatedEGFR-Mutated Advanced Non–Small-Cell Lung Cancer. *N. Engl. J. Med.* **2018**, *378*, 113–125. [CrossRef]
6. Canale, M.; Petracci, E.; Delmonte, A.; Chiadini, E.; Dazzi, C.; Papi, M.; Capelli, L.; Casanova, C.; De Luigi, N.; Mariotti, M.; et al. Impact of TP53 Mutations on Outcome in EGFR-Mutated Patients Treated with First-Line Tyrosine Kinase Inhibitors. *Clin. Cancer Res.* **2016**, *23*, 2195–2202. [CrossRef]
7. Kim, Y.; Lee, B.; Shim, J.H.; Lee, S.-H.; Park, W.-Y.; Choi, Y.-L.; Sun, J.-M.; Ahn, J.S.; Ahn, M.-J.; Park, K. Concurrent Genetic Alterations Predict the Progression to Target Therapy in EGFR-Mutated Advanced NSCLC. *J. Thorac. Oncol.* **2019**, *14*, 193–202. [CrossRef]

8. VanderLaan, P.A.; Rangachari, D.; Mockus, S.M.; Spotlow, V.; Reddi, H.V.; Malcolm, J.; Costa, D.B. Mutations in TP53, PIK3CA, PTEN and other genes in EGFR mutated lung cancers: Correlation with clinical outcomes. *Lung Cancer* **2018**, *106*, 17–21. [CrossRef]
9. Molina-Vila, M.A.; Bertran-Alamillo, J.; Gascó, A.; Mayo-de-las-Casas, C.; Sánchez-Ronco, M.; Pujantell-Pastor, L.; Majem, M. Nondisruptive p53 Mutations Are Associated with Shorter Survival in Patients with Advanced Non–Small Cell Lung Cancer. *Clin. Cancer Res.* **2014**, *2*, 4647–4660. [CrossRef]
10. Poeta, M.L.; Manola, J.; Goldwasser, M.A.; Forastiere, A.; Benoit, N.; Califano, J.A.; Ridge, J.A.; Goodwin, J.; Kenady, D.; Saunders, J.; et al. TP53 mutations and survival in squamous-cell carcinoma of the head and neck. *N. Engl. J. Med.* **2007**, *357*, 2552–2561. [CrossRef]
11. La Fleur, L.; Falk-Sörqvist, E.; Smeds, P.; Berglund, A.; Sundström, M.; Mattsson, J.S.; Brandén, E.; Koyi, H.; Isaksson, J.; Brunnström, H.; et al. Mutation patterns in a population-based non-small cell lung cancer cohort and prognostic impact of concomitant mutations in KRAS and TP53 or STK11. *Lung Cancer* **2019**, *130*, 50–58. [CrossRef]
12. Zhao, J.; Han, Y.; Li, J.; Chai, R.; Bai, C. Prognostic value of KRAS/TP53/PIK3CA in non-small cell lung cancer. *Oncol Lett.* **2019**, *17*, 3233–3240. [CrossRef]
13. Volckmar, A.-L.; Leichsenring, J.; Kirchner, M.; Christopoulos, P.; Neumann, O.; Budczies, J.; De Oliveira, C.M.M.; Rempel, E.; Buchhalter, I.; Brandt, R.; et al. Combined targeted DNA and RNA sequencing of advanced NSCLC in routine molecular diagnostics: Analysis of the first 3,000 Heidelberg cases. *Int. J. Cancer* **2019**, *145*, 649–661. [CrossRef]
14. Jiao, X.-D.; Qin, B.-D.; You, P.; Cai, J.; Zang, Y.-S. The prognostic value of TP53 and its correlation with EGFR mutation in advanced non-small cell lung cancer, an analysis based on cBioPortal data base. *Lung Cancer* **2018**, *123*, 70–75. [CrossRef]
15. Gu, J.; Zhou, Y.; Huang, L.; Ou, W.; Wu, J.; Li, S.; Xu, J.; Feng, J.; Liu, B. TP53 mutation is associated with a poor clinical outcome for non-small cell lung cancer: Evidence from a meta-analysis. *Mol. Clin. Oncol.* **2016**, *5*, 705–713. [CrossRef]
16. Aggarwal, C.; Davis, C.W.; Mick, R.; Thompson, J.C.; Ahmed, S.; Jeffries, S.; Bagley, S.; Gabriel, P.; Evans, T.L.; Bauml, J.M.; et al. Influence of TP53 Mutation on Survival in Patients With Advanced EGFR-Mutant Non–Small-Cell Lung Cancer. *JCO Precis. Oncol.* **2018**, 1–29. [CrossRef]
17. Yu, H.A.; Arcila, M.E.; Rekhtman, N.; Sima, C.S.; Zakowski, M.F.; Pao, W.; Kris, M.; Miller, V.A.; Ladanyi, M.; Riely, G.J. Analysis of tumor specimens at the time of acquired resistance to EGFR-TKI therapy in 155 patients with EGFR-mutant lung cancers. *Clin. Cancer Res.* **2013**, *19*, 2240–2247. [CrossRef]
18. Hou, H.; Qin, K.; Liang, Y.; Zhang, C.; Liu, N.; Jiang, H.; Liu, K.; Zhu, J.; Lv, H.; Li, T.; et al. Concurrent TP53 mutations predict poor outcomes of EGFR-TKI treatments in Chinese patients with advanced NSCLC. *Cancer Manag. Res.* **2019**, *11*, 5665–5675. [CrossRef]
19. Jin, Y.; Shi, X.; Zhao, J.; He, Q.; Chen, M.; Yan, J.; Ou, Q.; Wu, X.; Shao, Y.W.; Yu, X. Mechanisms of primary resistance to EGFR targeted therapy in advanced lung adenocarcinomas. *Lung Cancer* **2018**, *124*, 110–116. [CrossRef]
20. Chen, M.; Xu, Y.; Zhao, J.; Zhong, W.; Zhang, L.; Bi, Y.; Wang, M. Concurrent Driver Gene Mutations as Negative Predictive Factors in Epidermal Growth Factor Receptor-Positive Non-Small Cell Lung Cancer. *EBioMedicine* **2019**, *42*, 304–310. [CrossRef]
21. Comprehensive molecular characterization of gastric adenocarcinoma. *Nature* **2014**, *513*, 202–209. [CrossRef] [PubMed]
22. Corrigendum: Comprehensive molecular profiling of lung adenocarcinoma. *Nature* **2014**, *514*, 262. [CrossRef]
23. Shi, J.; Hua, X.; Zhu, B.; Ravichandran, S.; Wang, M.; Nguyen, C.; Brodie, S.A.; Palleschi, A.; Alloisio, M.; Pariscenti, G.; et al. Somatic Genomics and Clinical Features of Lung Adenocarcinoma: A Retrospective Study. *PLoS Med.* **2016**, *13*, 1–24. [CrossRef] [PubMed]
24. Jamal-Hanjani, M.; Wilson, G.A.; McGranahan, N.; Birkbak, N.J.; Watkins, T.B.; Veeriah, S.; Shafi, S.; Johnson, D.H.; Mitter, R.; Rosenthal, R.; et al. Tracking the Evolution of Non-Small-Cell Lung Cancer. *N. Engl. J. Med.* **2017**, *376*, 2109–2121. [CrossRef]
25. Brosh, R.; Rotter, V. When mutants gain new powers: news from the mutant p53 field. *Nat. Rev. Cancer* **2009**, *9*, 701. [CrossRef]
26. Muller, P.A.J.; Vousden, K.H. P53 mutations in cancer. *Nat. Cell Biol.* **2013**, *15*, 2–8. [CrossRef]
27. Liu, Y.; Xu, F.; Wang, Y.; Wu, Q.; Wang, B.; Yao, Y.; Zhang, Y.; Han-Zhang, H.; Ye, J.; Zhang, L.; et al. Mutations

in exon 8 of TP53 are associated with shorter survival in patients with advanced lung cancer. *Oncol. Lett.* **2019**, *18*, 3159–3169. [CrossRef]

28. Labbé, C.; Cabanero, M.; Korpanty, G.J.; Tomasini, P.; Doherty, M.K.; Mascaux, C.; Leighl, N.B. Lung Cancer Prognostic and predictive e ff ects of TP53 co-mutation in patients with EGFR-mutated non-small cell lung cancer (NSCLC). *Lung Cancer* **2017**, *111*, 23–29. [CrossRef]
29. Xu, Y.; Tong, X.; Yan, J.; Wu, X.; Shao, Y.W.; Fan, Y. Short-Term Responders of Non–Small Cell Lung Cancer Patients to EGFR Tyrosine Kinase Inhibitors Display High Prevalence of TP53 Mutations and Primary Resistance Mechanisms. *Transl. Oncol.* **2018**, *11*, 1364–1369. [CrossRef]
30. Leonetti, A.; Sharma, S.; Minari, R.; Perego, P.; Giovannetti, E.; Tiseo, M. Resistance mechanisms to osimertinib in EGFR-mutated non-small cell lung cancer. *Br. J. Cancer* **2019**, *121*, 725–737. [CrossRef]

14

Clinicopathological Significance of *RUNX1* in Non-Small Cell Lung Cancer

Yujin Kim [1], Bo Bin Lee [1], Dongho Kim [1], Sangwon Um [2], Eun Yoon Cho [3], Joungho Han [3], Young Mog Shim [4] and Duk-Hwan Kim [1,*]

1. Department of Molecular Cell Biology, Sungkyunkwan University School of Medicine, Suwon 440-746, Korea; yujin0328@hanmail.net (Y.K.); whitebini@hanmail.net (B.B.L.); jindonghao2001@hotmail.com (D.K.)
2. Department of Internal Medicine, Samsung Medical Center, Sungkyunkwan University School of Medicine, Seoul 135-710, Korea; sangwon72.um@samsung.com
3. Department of Pathology, Samsung Medical Center, Sungkyunkwan University School of Medicine, Seoul 135-710, Korea; eunyoon.cho@samsung.com (E.Y.C.); joungho.han@samsung.com (J.H.)
4. Department of Thoracic and Cardiovascular Surgery, Samsung Medical Center, Sungkyunkwan University, School of Medicine, Seoul 135-710, Korea; youngmog.shim@samsung.com

* Correspondence: dukhwan.kim@samsung.com

Abstract: This study aimed to understand the clinicopathological significance of runt-related transcription factor 1 (*RUNX1*) in non-small cell lung cancer (NSCLC). The methylation and mRNA levels of *RUNX1* in NSCLC were determined using the Infinium HumanMethylation450 BeadChip and the HumanHT-12 expression BeadChip. RUNX1 protein levels were analyzed using immunohistochemistry of formalin-fixed paraffin-embedded tissues from 409 NSCLC patients. Three CpGs (cg04228935, cg11498607, and cg05000748) in the CpG island of *RUNX1* showed significantly different methylation levels (Bonferroni corrected $p < 0.05$) between tumor and matched normal tissues obtained from 42 NSCLC patients. Methylation levels of the CpGs in the tumor tissues were inversely related to mRNA levels of *RUNX1*. A logistic regression model based on cg04228935 showed the best performance in predicting NSCLCs in a test dataset (N = 28) with the area under the receiver operating characteristic (ROC) curve (AUC) of 0.96 (95% confidence interval (CI) = 0.81–0.99). The expression of RUNX1 was reduced in 125 (31%) of 409 patients. Adenocarcinoma patients with reduced RUNX1 expression showed 1.97-fold (95% confidence interval = 1.16–3.44, $p = 0.01$) higher hazard ratio for death than those without. In conclusion, the present study suggests that abnormal methylation of *RUNX1* may be a valuable biomarker for detection of NSCLC regardless of race. And, reduced RUNX1 expression may be a prognostic indicator of poor overall survival in lung adenocarcinoma.

Keywords: lung cancer; RUNX1; methylation; biomarker; survival

---

1. Introduction

Lung cancer is the leading cause of cancer-related death in the world. Despite significant advances in the diagnosis and treatment of the disease over the past 20 years, its prognosis is still very poor, with the overall 5-year survival rate staying at 15%–20% [1]. The prognosis of cancer patients is mostly determined by disease stage. The occult metastatic spread of cancer cells to surrounding tissues in more than 50% of lung cancer patients at the time of diagnosis affects a poor prognosis. The majority of patients undergoing curative surgical resection at an early stage and, if necessary, adjuvant chemotherapy have achieved favorable long-term survival. Patients with surgically resected stage IA, stage IB, and stage II non-small cell lung cancers (NSCLCs) had an overall five-year survival rate of 83%, 69%, and 48%, respectively [2]. Targeted therapy has a great effect on the prognosis of specific patients; however, it is applicable to only about 10%–20% of patients. Accordingly, it is important to identify novel diagnostic and therapeutic biomarkers for the detection of early-stage lung cancer and for the development of new molecular-targeted therapies for NSCLC.

Runt-related transcription factor 1 (RUNX1) is one of the RUNX family proteins (RUNX1, RUNX2, and RUNX3), which forms a heterodimeric complex with the core binding factor β (CBFβ), resulting in enhanced transcription of the RUNX gene family by stimulating the DNA binding ability and stability of the family proteins [3,4]. RUNX1 is essential for hematopoiesis and is involved in the generation of hematopoietic stem cells. Mutations and translocations in *RUNX1* are well established as causes of myelodysplastic syndrome or acute myelogenous leukemia [5–7]. Gain- or loss-of-function mutations of *RUNX1* have also been reported in various solid tumors. Missense mutations of *RUNX1* were reported in luminal-type breast cancer [8], and loss-of-function somatic mutations or deletion of *RUNX1* have been reported in breast cancer and lung cancer [9,10].

To understand the clinicopathological significance of *RUNX1* in NSCLC, we analyzed the methylation status of *RUNX1* in different types of samples from a total of 118 NSCLC patients and 60 healthy individuals. The prediction performance of classifiers was validated in The Cancer Genome Atlas (TCGA) lung cancer. Expression levels of RUNX1 were also analyzed using HT-12 array and immunohistochemistry in tissue specimens from 42 and 409 NSCLC patients, respectively.

2. Materials and Methods

2.1. Study Population

Formalin-fixed paraffin-embedded tumor tissues were obtained from 409 NSCLC patients who underwent curative surgical resection at the Department of Thoracic and Cardiovascular Surgery, Samsung Medical Center, Seoul, Korea, between August 1994 and May 2014. All samples were obtained from operative patients. Follow-up of patients for the detection of recurrence or death following curative resection was conducted by a nurse specialized in oncology as described previously [11]. The pathological stage of NSCLC was determined using the tumor/node/metastasis (TNM) system provided by the American Joint Committee on Cancer (AJCC) [12]. This study was conducted in accordance with the ethical principles stated in the Declaration of Helsinki and approved by the Institutional Review Board (IRB#: 2010-07-204) of the Samsung Medical Center. Written informed consent to use pathological specimens for research was obtained from all patients prior to surgery. All data are not publicly available due to privacy and ethical restriction.

2.2. Analysis of RUNX1 Methylation and mRNA Levels

We previously analyzed the DNA methylation and mRNA expression at the level of genome using the Infinium HumanMethylation450 BeadChip and the HumanHT-12 expression BeadChips (Illumina, San Diego, CA, USA), respectively, in 42 surgically resected tumor and matched normal tissues, 136 bronchial washings, 12 sputums, or 6 bronchial biopsy specimens obtained from a total of 118 NSCLC patients and 60 cancer-free patients [13]. We used the reported data for the analysis of methylation and mRNA levels of *RUNX1*. Preprocessing such as background or batch effect correction, probe filtering, and adjustment of the background signal difference between types I and II probes was conducted using the R software package called wateRmelon [14]. Methylation level (β-value), ranging from 0 (no methylation) to 1 (100% methylation), was estimated as the ratio of fluorescence signal intensity between methylated alleles and the sum of methylated and unmethylated alleles at each CpG locus. The levels of mRNA expression from HT-12 chips were normalized using the R lumi package (https://bioconductor.org/biocLite.R).

2.3. Feature Selection for Prediction of Lung Cancer

To select candidate CpGs for lung cancer prediction among differentially methylated CpGs and to build models for lung cancer prediction, we divided the normal and tumor tissues from 42 patients into training and test datasets, according to a 7:3 ratio. Supervised machine learning algorithms were applied to select features in the training dataset. Age-related CpGs or any CpGs that were significantly correlated in the normal or tumor tissues were removed during the model building. Supervised machine learning algorithms for feature selection and model building were applied using RapidMiner Studio version 8.2 (RapidMiner Inc, Boston, MA, USA).

2.4. Evaluation of Prediction Performance of Models in The Cancer Genome Atlas (TCGA) Lung Cancer

Prediction performance of selected models was further tested using 899 TCGA lung cancers, including 75 normal and 824 tumor tissues. The performance was tested without distinction between adenocarcinoma and squamous cell carcinoma. The prediction performance of models was evaluated using receiver operating characteristic (ROC) curves, plotted using the MedCalc statistical Software version 19.0.5 (MedCalc Softward bvba, Ostend, Belgium).

2.5. Immunohistochemistry

The expression of RUNX1, Ki-67, phospho-pRb (Ser-807/811) proteins in the 409 NSCLC patients was determined using immunohistochemistry of tissue microarrays (TMAs). In brief, the 4-mm–thick TMA tissue sections on glass slide were deparaffinized in xylene and rehydrated in a series of decreasing concentrations of alcohol. Antigens were recovered by putting sections into 10 mmol/L citrate buffer solution (pH 6.0) and by heating in a microwave oven for 10 min. The sections were then incubated overnight at 4 °C with a mouse monoclonal antibody to RUNX1 (AML1/RUNX1 Antibody (clone 3A1) IHC-plus™ LS-B5382, LifeSpan BioSciences, Seattle, WA, USA), a polyclonal anti-phospho-pRb (Ser-807/811) antibody (Cell Signaling, Danvers, MA, USA), and a mouse monoclonal anti-Ki-67 (DAKO; clone MIB-1) antibody. Immunoreactivity of the proteins was detected using the Envision-Plus/horseradish peroxidase system (Dako, Carpinteria, CA, USA), and the antibody-bound peroxidase activity was visualized by incubating in 0.05% 3,3′-diaminobenzidine tetrahydrochloride (DAB) for 3 min at room temperature. All sections were counterstained with Mayer's hematoxylin and a negative control was included by excluding the primary antibody each time. Three samples with RUNX1 expression in normal bronchial epithelial cells were used as a positive control for RUNX1 staining, and IHC was performed in duplicate.

2.6. Interpretation of Immunohistochemical Staining

The immunohistochemical stainings were interpreted by two authors (EY Cho and D-H Kim) in a double-blinded fashion, and samples showing poor inter-rater reliability ($\kappa < 0.20$) were removed from data analysis. RUNX1 expression was considered positive when nuclear staining was present, and the intensity and proportion of positive nuclear staining was assessed for scoring. A composite score of RUNX1 protein expression was semi-quantitatively calculated by multiplying the proportion score of positive cells (0, absent; 1, 0%–10%; 2, 10%–50%; 3, 50%–80%; and 4, >80%) with the staining intensity score (0, none; 1, weak; 2, moderate; and 3, strong). A cutoff for the reduced expression of RUNX1 protein was determined by taking into account the distribution of the composite scores between normal and tumor tissues and by comparing both false-negative and false-positive rates at different cutoffs. RUNX1 expression was considered reduced in a tumor with a composite score less than two. To score for phospho-pRb (Ser-807/811) and Ki-67, positive staining was determined according to the percentage of positively stained nuclei.

2.7. *Statistical Analysis*

Univariate analysis was performed using the *t*-test (or Wilcoxon rank sum test) and the chi-square test (or Fisher's exact test) for continuous and categorical variables, respectively. The correlation between methylation levels of CpGs in the *RUNX1* gene was analyzed using Spearman's rank correlation coefficient. The effect of reduced RUNX1 expression on survival was estimated using the Kaplan–Meier survival curves, and the difference between the survival curves of any two groups was evaluated by the log-rank test. Cox proportional hazards analysis was conducted to estimate the hazard ratios of reduced RUNX1 expression for survival after controlling for potential confounding factors. Statistical analysis was conducted using R software version 3.3.3. (R Foundation for Statistical Computing, Vienna, Austria).

3. Results

3.1. *RUNX1 Hypermethylation Is Inversely Associated with Its Expression*

Data reported previously were used to identify differentially methylated CpGs in *RUNX1* gene in tumor and matched normal tissues from 42 NSCLC patients. The Wilcoxon rank-sum test was applied because the distribution of β-values obtained from tumor tissues using a 450 K array was negatively skewed and did not follow a normal distribution (Shapiro-Wilk test, $p < 0.05$). Three CpGs with a p-value less than or equal to 1.03×10^{-7} (Bonferroni significance threshold) were identified from the 450K array: three CpGs (cg11498607, cg04228935, cg05000748) at the CpG island of *RUNX1* showed hypermethylation in tumor tissues compared with normal tissues (Figure 1A). The methylation levels of the three CpGs did not vary significantly with histology (Figure 1B). Altered methylation of three CpGs was not significantly correlated with a patient's age (Figure 1C).The methylation levels were not also associated with smoking status (Figure 1D) and recurrence (Figure 1E). However, the methylation levels were found to be higher in the poorly differentiated type of NSCLC than in the well differentiated type (Figure S1). The *RUNX1* mRNA levels were analyzed using the HT-12 array to determine the association between methylation changes and changes in *RUNX1* gene expression. The methylation levels of individual CpGs were negatively associated with the mRNA levels of *RUNX1* ($p < 0.05$; Figure 1F).

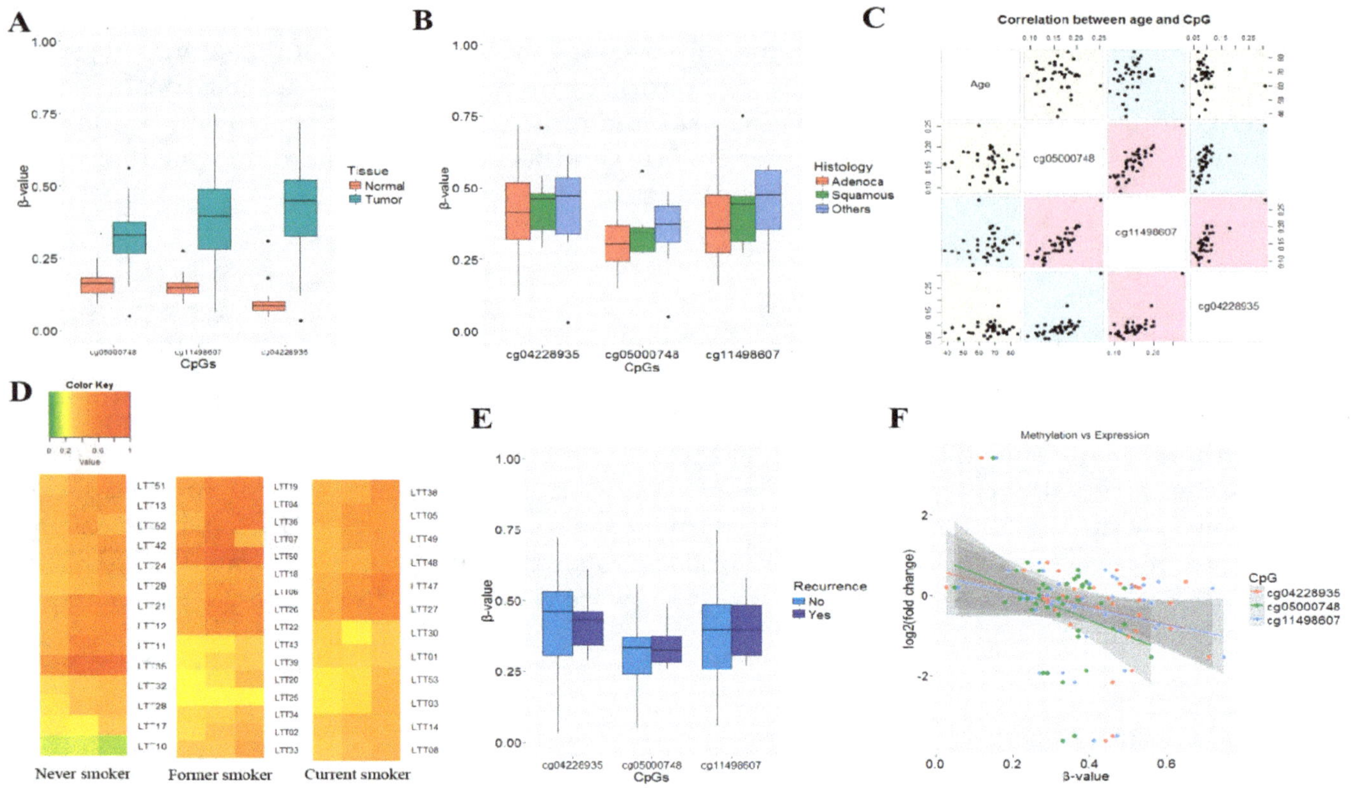

Figure 1. Relationship between methylation and mRNA levels of runt-related transcription factor 1 (*RUNX1*) in 42 lung tumor and matched normal tissues. (**A**) Methylation levels of three CpGs at the CpG island of *RUNX1* gene were compared between the tumor and matched normal tissues obtained from 42 NSCLC patients. Y-axis indicates β-values. (**B**) Methylation levels of the three CpGs were compared according to histologic subtypes. (**C**) Correlations between the patient's age and the methylation levels of the three CpGs were analyzed in 42 tumor tissues. Spearman's correlation coefficient was used to calculate *p*-values. Magenta color indicates $p < 0.05$. (**D**) Methylation levels of three CpGs at a CpG island of *RUNX1* were compared in never-smokers, former smokers, and current smokers. Y-axis indicates sample identification numbers. Methylation levels are represented using gradient-based colors from green (0%–20%) to yellow (21%–50%) to red (51%–100%). (**E**) The association between recurrence and the methylation levels at three CpGs were analyzed in 42 NSCLCs. (**F**) The correlation between methylation levels of three CpGs and the mRNA expression of *RUNX1* was analyzed in 42 tumor tissues from patients with NSCLC. Y-axis indicates the log2 fold change (= log2(tumor/normal)) between tumor and matched normal tissues. X-axis indicates β-values in tumor tissues.

3.2. Prediction of Non-Small Cell Lung Cancer (NSCLC) Using Abnormal Methylation Levels of RUNX1

Features for prediction of NSCLC were selected in 42 tumors and matched normal tissues. Lung tumor and matched normal tissues were divided into training and test datasets at a ratio of 7:3, respectively. We built models using the training dataset and tested the performance of the models using the test dataset. Supervised machine learning algorithms such as k-nearest neighbor (kNN), support vector machine (SVM), neural network, logistic regression, and decision tree were applied for feature selection. Since individual CpGs were correlated with each other, only one CpG was included in the models. Among the applied algorithms, a logistic regression model based on cg04228935 showed the best performance in classifying NSCLCs in a test dataset (N = 28) with a sensitivity of 92.9% and a specificity of 92.9% (area under the curve (AUC) = 0.96; 95% confidence interval (CI) = 0.81–0.99, $p < 0.0001$; Figure 2A).

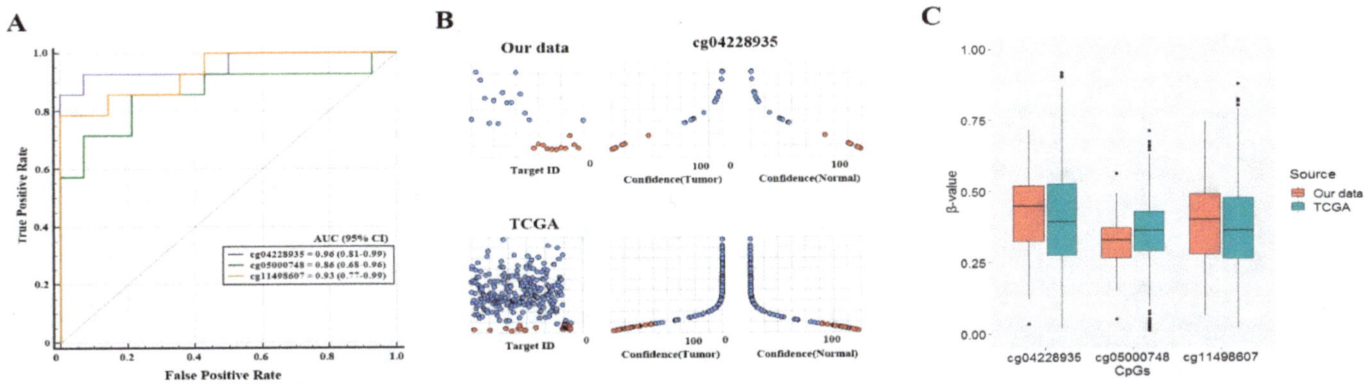

Figure 2. Evaluation of prediction performance of five supervised machine learning algorithms in non-small cell lung cancer (NSCLC). (**A**) The true and false positive rates of logistic regression model based on three CpGs were evaluated in a test dataset (N = 28) of 42 NSCLCs, and the receiver operating characteristic (ROC) curves were plotted using the MedCalc software. (**B**) The prediction certainty of the support vector machine model was evaluated in the test dataset of our data and TCGA lung cancer. The X-axis indicates the degree (0% to 100%) of certainty for prediction of our and TCGA tissues as normal or tumor for each β-value on the Y-axis. The sky blue and red orange circles indicate tumor and normal tissues, respectively. (**C**) The β-values of the three CpGs in our and TCGA data were compared to understand the difference of *RUNX1* hypermethylation among other ethnic groups or populations.

To determine if *RUNX1* hypermethylation may be a biomarker for the detection of NSCLC in other races, we tested *RUNX1* hypermethylation in the 899 TCGA primary lung cancers (75 normal tissues and 824 tumor tissues). As with our data, the TCGA data was divided into a training dataset (N = 630) and a test dataset (N = 269), and the performance of logistic regression model based on three CpGs was evaluated on the test dataset (Table S1). The sensitivity and specificity of the model based on cg04228935 in a test dataset (N = 269) were 91.8% and 96.4%, respectively. AUC was 0.95 (95% confidence interval = 0.93–0.98, $p < 0.0001$). The degree of prediction certainty of NSCLC in the test datasets was high in our data and TCGA lung cancer data (Figure 2B). We finally compared the methylation levels of three CpGs at a CpG island of *RUNX1* between our data and TCGA lung cancer data. No significant difference was found between the two data (Figure 2C).

3.3. Methylation Pattern of RUNX1 in Tumor Tissue Is Similar to that in Bronchial Biopsy Specimen

To test if bronchial washing, sputum, and bronchial biopsy specimens could be used as surrogate samples for analyzing *RUNX1* methylation in the lung, we compared the methylation levels of the CpG (cg04228935) in 42 tumors and matched normal tissues, 136 bronchial washings, 12 sputum samples, and 6 bronchial biopsy specimens. The clinical and pathological characteristics of the NSCLC patients were previously reported [13]. The methylation levels of the CpG in lung tumor tissues were not significantly different from those in bronchial biopsy specimens from lung cancer patients ($p > 0.05$, Wilcoxon rank sum test), unlike bronchial washings and sputum samples (Figure 3A). The CpG methylation levels were further compared between paired bronchial washing and sputum samples from 12 NSCLC patients (Figure 3B) and between bronchial washing and paired bronchial biopsies from 6 NSCLC patients (Figure 3C). The methylation levels of the CpG were found to be similar between bronchial washings and sputum samples but significantly higher in bronchial biopsy than in bronchial washing ($p < 0.05$, Wilcoxon signed-rank test). These findings suggest that a detection model for NSCLC using abnormal methylation of *RUNX1* is applicable to bronchial biopsy specimens.

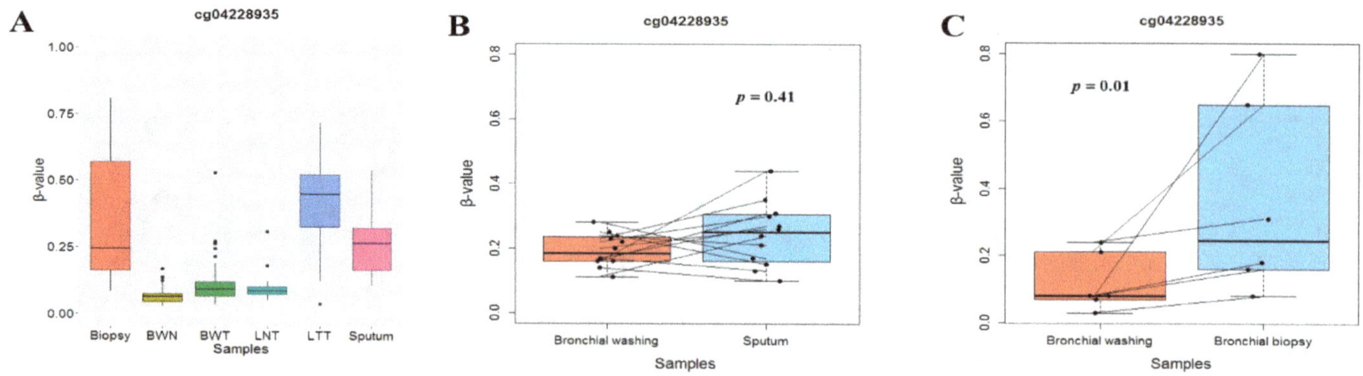

Figure 3. Comparison of *RUNX1* methylation levels among different types of specimens. (**A**) The methylation levels of a CpG (cg04228935) selected for NSCLC prediction were compared among bronchial biopsies from 6 lung cancer patients (biopsy), bronchial washing samples from 60 healthy individuals (bronchial washing normal, BWN) and 76 lung cancer patients (bronchial washing tumor, BWT), tumor (lung tumor tissue, LTT) and matched normal (lung normal tissue, LNT) tissues from 42 NSCLC patients, and sputum specimens from 12 lung cancer patients (sputum). (**B**,**C**) Methylation levels of a CpG (cg04228935) were compared using parallel coordinate plots between paired bronchial washing and sputum specimens from 12 NSCLC patients (**B**) and between paired bronchial washing and biopsy samples from six NSCLC patients (**C**). Methylation levels in bronchial washings were similar to those in sputum samples but were significantly low compared with those in bronchial biopsy (Wilcoxon signed-rank test). Y-axis indicates β-values from the 450 K array.

3.4. *RUNX1 Affects Overall Survival in Adenocarcinoma*

To elucidate the effect of RUNX1 expression on survival of NSCLC patient, we analyzed the expression of RUNX1 using immunohistochemistry of formalin-fixed paraffin-embedded tumor tissues from 409 NSCLCs. Representative positive staining patterns of RUNX1 are shown in adenocarcinoma and squamous cell carcinoma (Figure 4A). Clinicopathological characteristics of 409 non-small cell lung cancer patients are listed in Table S2. The median follow-up period of patients was 5.2 years. RUNX1 expression was reduced in 31% of the samples. Reduced RUNX1 expression was not related to pathologic stage (Figure S2), but was found more frequently in woman (Figure 4B) and in adenocarcinoma (Figure 4C) and was significantly associated with poor overall survival in adenocarcinoma ($p = 0.005$; Figure 4D) but not in squamous cell carcinoma ($p = 0.87$). The median survival of adenocarcinoma patients with and without reduced RUNX1 expression was 41 and 81 months, respectively. Cox proportional hazards analysis also showed that overall survival of adenocarcinoma patients with reduced RUNX1 expression was approximately 1.97 (95% CI = 1.16–3.44; $p = 0.01$) times poorer than in those without, after controlling for age, recurrence, and pathologic stage (Table 1). However, RUNX1 expression was not associated with recurrence-free survival irrespective of histology in NSCLC ($p = 0.21$).

Table 1. Cox proportional hazards analysis of overall survival according to RUNX1 expression.

Histology	RUNX1 Expression	HR	95% CI	*p*-Value
Adeno (N = 189)	Normal	1.00		
	Reduced	1.97	1.16–3.44	0.01
Squamous (N = 192)	Normal	1.00		
	Reduced	1.46	0.78–5.32	0.21

Abbreviations: Adeno, adenocarcinoma; squamous, squamous cell carcinoma; HR, hazard ratio; CI, confidence interval; RUNX1, runt-related transcription factor 1.

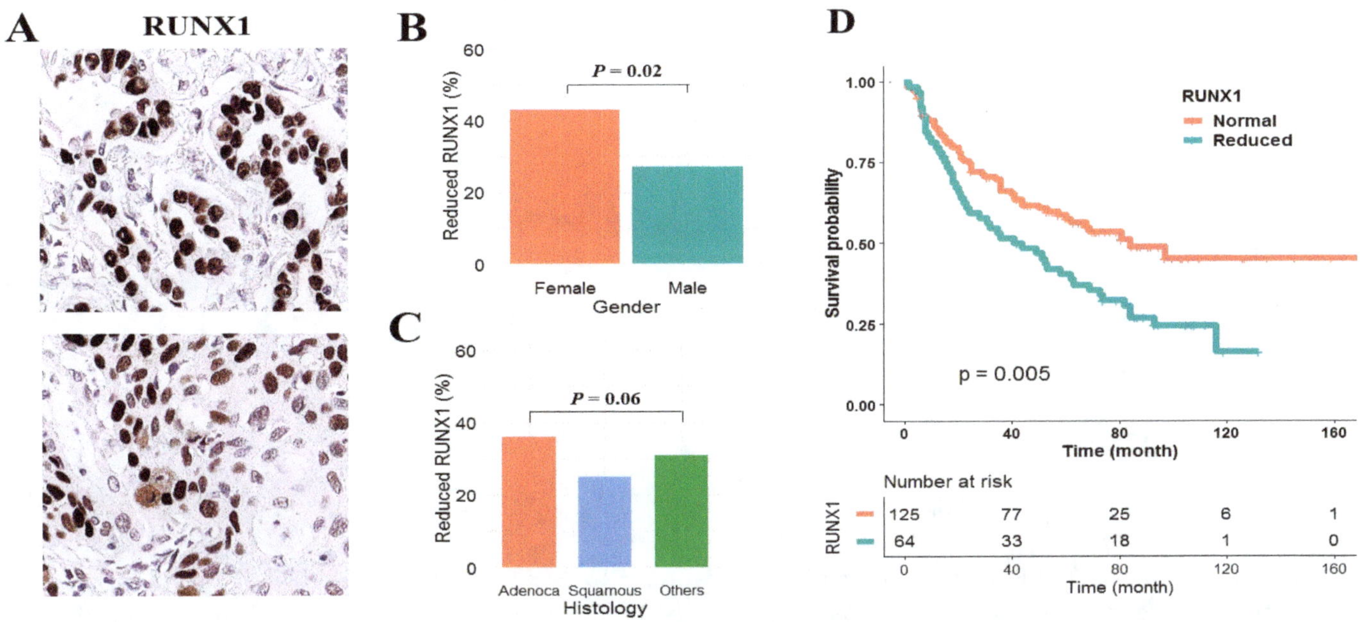

Figure 4. The effect of RUNX1 expression on overall survival in NSCLC. (**A**) RUNX1 expression was analyzed using immunohistochemistry in 409 NSCLC patients. Positive staining occurred in the nucleus of adenocarcinoma (upper) and squamous cell carcinoma. (X200). (**B**,**C**) Reduced expression levels were compared according to gender (**B**) and histologic subtypes (**C**). *p*-values are based on Student *t*-test. (**D**) The effect of reduced RUNX1 expression on overall survival of patients with adenocarcinoma was analyzed using Kaplan-Meier survival curve. *p*-value was calculated using log-rank test.

3.5. No Correlation between Reduced RUNX1 Expression and Expression Levels of Phospho-Rb and Ki67 Proliferation Index

RUNX proteins are implicated in diverse signaling pathways and cellular processes, including the cell cycle and stress response. In order to elucidate the effect of RUNX1 on the cell cycle and cell proliferation in NSCLC, we analyzed the phospho-pRb (Ser-807/811) levels and Ki-67 proliferation index according to the expression status of RUNX1. The average phospho-pRb (Ser-807/811) levels were 2.7% in tumor tissues with reduced RUNX1 expression and 2.1% in tumor tissues without reduced RUNX1 expression. The difference was not statistically significant ($p = 0.18$), irrespective of histology (Figure 5A). The Ki-67 proliferation index in tumor tissues with reduced RUNX1 expression was slightly higher than in tumor tissues without reduced RUNX1 expression, but the difference was also not statistically significant (28.8% vs. 22.3%, $p = 0.18$), irrespective of histology (Figure 5B).

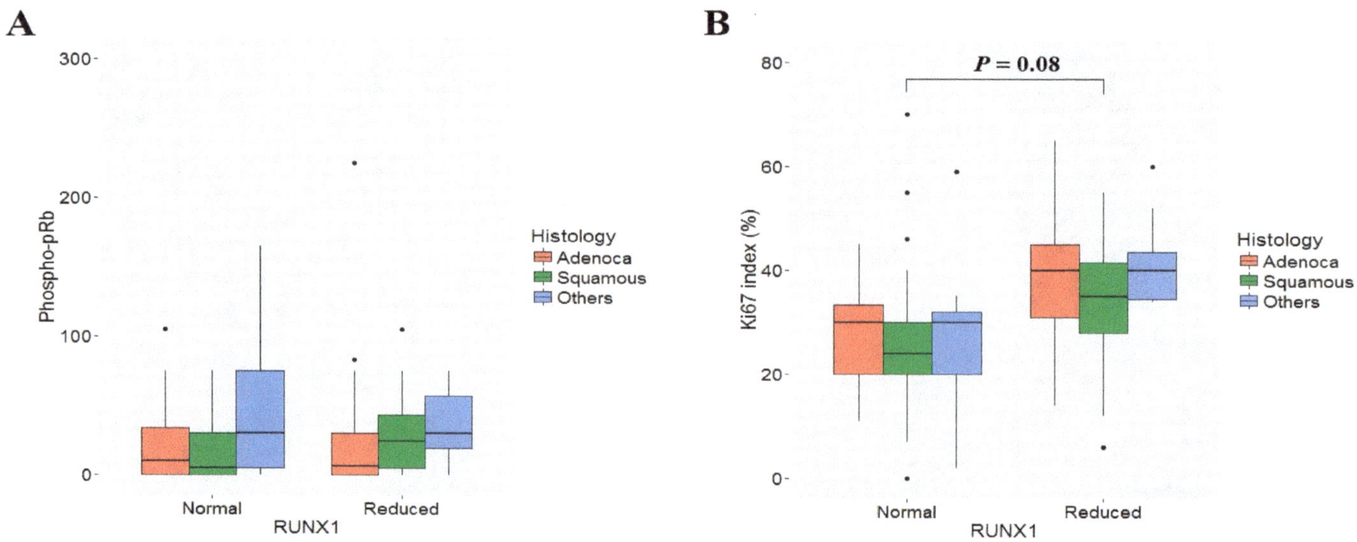

Figure 5. The effect of RUNX1 expression on phospho-pRb (Ser-807/811) level and Ki-67 proliferation index. The expression levels of phosphorylated pRb stained using polyclonal anti-phospho-pRb (Ser-807/811) antibody (Cell Signaling, Danvers, MA, USA) (**A**) and Ki-67 proliferation index (**B**) were compared according to the expression status of RUNX1 using Student *t*-test. The phospho-pRb levels and Ki-67 proliferation index were not significantly different between tumor tissues with normal or reduced RUNX1 expression irrespective of histologic subgroup.

4. Discussion

RUNX1 causes a wide range of leukemias through translocation with genes such as eight-twenty-one (ETO) [7] and acts as an oncogene in various solid tumors such as ovarian cancer [15], and endometrial cancer [16], as well as in the mouse mammary tumor virus-polyoma middle tumor-antigen (MMTV-PyMT) transgenic mouse model of breast cancer [17], and in the transgenic adenocarcinoma of mouse prostate (TRAMP) model of prostate cancer [18]. RUNX1 is also known to function as a tumor suppressor in different types of cancer. For example, the ectopic expression of RUNX1 in esophageal adenocarcinoma cells reduced the anchorage-independent growth [19], and the knockdown of *RUNX1* by siRNAs enhanced androgen-independent proliferation of prostate cancer cells [20]. In addition, the inhibition of endogenous *RUNX1* using short-hairpin RNA targeting RUNX1 (shRunx1) in breast cancer cells resulted in loss of epithelial morphology and promotion of epithelial-mesenchymal transition [9], and the ectopic expression of RUNX1 reduced the population of breast cancer stem cells [21]. RUNX1 also inhibited the migration and stemness of mammary epithelial cells [22]. Ramsay et al. [10] reported that lentiviral-mediated RNAi knockdown of *RUNX1* increased the proliferation and migration of lung cancer cells. In the present study, *RUNX1* showed abnormal methylation in primary NSCLCs, and the reduced expression of RUNX1 was associated with poor overall survival, suggesting that RUNX1 may play a role as a tumor suppressor in normal bronchial epithelial cells.

Functional disruption of RUNX1 usually occurs by chromosomal translocation, point mutation, or deletion in leukemia and some solid tumors. *RUNX1* mutation has been reported rarely in lung cancer [23], although changes in its methylation have been reported by a couple of studies [24,25]. In this study, *RUNX1* was found to be abnormally methylated at the CpG island of *RUNX1* in NSCLC tumor tissues, and the methylation and mRNA levels of *RUNX1* showed a linear negative correlation. Unlike most genes whose transcription is regulated by a single promoter, *RUNX1* is regulated by two promoters in the upstream region of 5′ UTR [26]. The three hypermethylated CpGs in this study might affect the transcription of *RUNX1*, which may also be affected by tissue-specific control factors. Further studies are needed to understand the mechanisms underlying transcriptional repression mediated by abnormal methylation of *RUNX1* in NSCLC.

A CpG (cg04228935) for the prediction of NSCLC was identified using tumor and matched normal tissues obtained from 42 NSCLC patients. Although the number of normal samples in the TCGA lung cancer data is small and the prevalence of lung cancer is not the exact same between Koreans and Americans, the present study suggests that RUNX1 hypermethylation may be a useful biomarker for the early detection of NSLC in other populations worldwide. Screening of lung cancer using low-dose computed tomography (LDCT) reduces mortality; however, approximately 20% of pulmonary nodules were found to be false positive [27,28]. A biopsy is needed for a more accurate diagnosis of lung cancer, but it is very difficult to obtain tissue in some patients. Methylation levels of a CpG (cg04228935) from bronchial biopsy were comparable to those from surgically resected lung tumor tissues. Accordingly, bronchial biopsy specimens may be used for the molecular analysis of *RUNX1*, and advances in technology such as electromagnetic navigation bronchoscopy (ENB) and endobronchial ultrasonography using a guided sheath (EBUS-GS) may provide more adequate specimens with fewer complications.

The association of *RUNX1* mutations or changes in expression with the prognosis of patients has been reported in various carcinomas, and the effect of RUNX1 on prognosis varies considerably depending on the type of cancer. *RUNX1* mutations are associated with poor overall survival in adult acute myelogenous leukemia (AML) as well as in pediatric AML [29,30]. The RUNX1 expression in prostate cancer tissues was negatively associated with poor prognosis [20]. The low RUNX1 expression in breast cancers is associated with metastasis to lymph nodes and poor survival [9,21]. In addition, the RUNX1-RUNX3 expression showed a significant effect on the survival of breast cancer patients with high YAP-signature expression levels [22]. Lung adenocarcinomas with low RUNX1 expression were associated with poor overall survival compared to tumors with high RUNX1 expression [10]. Our data also showed that reduced RUNX1 expression was associated with poor overall survival in adenocarcinomas. Based on these observations, it is likely that the reduced expression of RUNX1 may serve as an indicator of poor prognosis in patients with lung adenocarcinoma.

RUNX proteins are known to regulate a wide range of biological processes via various interacting proteins in human cancer and to be implicated in carcinogenesis mediated via TGF-β and Wnt signaling pathways, and in cell cycle or stress response. For example, RUNX1 promoter is regulated by EZH2 (enhancer of zeste homolog 2)-dependent histone H3 lysine 27 (K27) trimethylation in prostate cancer cells [20]. RUNX1 directly regulates E-cadherin, and rescues TGFβ-induced EMT phenotype in breast cancer cells [9]. RUNX1 suppresses breast cancer growth by repressing the activity of breast cancer stem cells and inhibiting ZEB1 expression directly [21]. RUNX1 acts as a negative regulator of oncogenic function of YAP that is involved in solid tumor progression [22]. The effect of RUNX1 on cell cycle in lung cancer differs between study groups. RUNX1 stimulated G1 to S progression in hematopoietic cells, partly via transcriptional induction of cyclin D2 promoter [31], whereas RUNX1 depletion resulted in an increased E2F1 mRNA levels in lung cancer cells [10]. In this study, tumor tissues with reduced RUNX1 expression did not show high levels of pRb phosphorylation (Ser-807/811) or the Ki67 proliferation index, suggesting that the reduced expression of RUNX1 may be involved in lung carcinogenesis through other mechanisms rather than cell-cycle regulation and growth control.

This study was limited by several factors. First, the effect of the two promoters on abnormal methylation of three CpGs in *RUNX1* gene and the tissue-specific factors affecting the expression of RUNX1 were not fully elucidated. Second, we failed to analyze *RUNX1* methylation in circulating cell-free DNA and to evaluate the prediction performance of the model due to assay failure. Third, the present study was a retrospective case-control study, which can result in a biased estimate of the population prevalence of NSCLC. In addition, sputum analysis was limited to the very few specimens from NSCLC patients only. Accordingly, the prediction performance of the model needs to be validated using several molecular techniques such as droplet digital polymerase chain reaction (ddPCR) in sputums and cell-free DNAs from a large cohort. Fourth, it is unclear the abnormal methylation of RUNX1 as a predictive biomarker can also be applied to tissue samples from metastatic lesions because the data from the present study and TCGA was from surgical specimens of early stage tumors. Fifth, methylation levels from benign lung tumors such as localized organizing pneumonia and hamartoma were not analyzed due to lack of samples.

In conclusion, the present study suggests that abnormal methylation at the CpG island of the *RUNX1* gene may be a valuable biomarker for the detection of NSCLC regardless of races. Reduced expression of RUNX1 may be associated with poor overall survival in patients with lung adenicarcinoma.

Author Contributions: Conceptualization, Y.K. and D.-H.K.; Data curation, Y.K., B.B.L., and D.K.; Formal analysis, B.B.L., E.Y.C., J.H., and D.K.; Methodology, Y.K. and D.-H.K.; Software, Y.K. and D.-H.K.; Supervision, D.-H.K.; Validation, Y.K., B.B.L., and D.K.; Resources, S.U., E.Y.C., J.H., and Y.M.S.; Visualization, Y.K.; Writing—original draft preparation, Y.K. and D.-H.K.; Writing—review and editing, Y.K., B.B.L., D.K., S.U., E.Y.C., J.H., Y.M.K., and D.-H.K.; Funding acquisition, D.-H.K. All authors have read and agreed to the published version of the manuscript.

Acknowledgments: The authors thank Eunkyung Kim and Jin-Hee Lee for data collection and management, and Hoon Suh for sample collection.

References

1. Siegel, R.L.; Miller, K.D.; Jemal, A. Cancer statistics, 2016. *CA Cancer J. Clin.* **2016**, *66*, 7–30. [CrossRef] [PubMed]
2. Yamamoto, K.; Ohsumi, A.; Kojima, F.; Imanishi, N.; Matsuoka, K.; Ueda, M.; Miyamoto, Y. Long-term survival after video-assisted thoracic surgery lobectomy for primary lung cancer. *Ann. Thorac. Surg.* **2010**, *89*, 353–359. [CrossRef]
3. Warren, A.J.; Bravo, J.; Williams, R.L.; Rabbitts, T.H. Structural basis for the heterodimeric interaction between the acute leukaemia-associated transcription factors AML1 and CBFbeta. *EMBO J.* **2000**, *19*, 3004–3015. [CrossRef] [PubMed]
4. Yan, J.; Liu, Y.; Lukasik, S.M.; Speck, N.A.; Bushweller, J.H. CBFbeta allosterically regulates the Runx1 Runt domain via a dynamic conformational equilibrium. *Nat. Struct. Mol. Biol.* **2004**, *11*, 901–906. [CrossRef] [PubMed]
5. Langabeer, S.E.; Gale, R.E.; Rollinson, S.J.; Morgan, G.J.; Linch, D.C. Mutations of the AML1 gene in acute myeloid leukemia of FAB types M0 and M7. *Genes Chromosomes Cancer* **2002**, *34*, 24–32. [CrossRef]
6. Harada, H.; Harada, Y.; Niimi, H.; Kyo, T.; Kimura, A.; Inaba, T. High incidence of somatic mutations in the AML1/RUNX1 gene in myelodysplastic syndrome and low blast percentage myeloid leukemia with myelodysplasia. *Blood* **2004**, *103*, 2316–2324. [CrossRef]
7. Lam, K.; Zhang, D.E. RUNX1 and RUNX1-ETO: Roles in hematopoiesis and leukemogenesis. *Front Biosci.* **2012**, *17*, 1120–1139. [CrossRef]
8. Ellis, M.J.; Ding, L.; Shen, D.; Luo, J.; Suman, V.J.; Wallis, J.W.; Van Tine, B.A.; Hoog, J.; Goiffon, R.J.; Goldstein, T.C.; et al. Whole-genome analysis informs breast cancer response to aromatase inhibition. *Nature* **2012**, *486*, 353–360. [CrossRef]
9. Hong, D.; Messier, T.L.; Tye, C.E.; Dobson, J.R.; Fritz, A.J.; Sikora, K.R.; Browne, G.; Stein, J.L.; Lian, J.B.; Stein, G.S. Runx1 stabilizes the mammary epithelial cell phenotype and prevents epithelial to mesenchymal transition. *Oncotarget* **2017**, *8*, 17610–17627. [CrossRef]
10. Ramsey, J.; Butnor, K.; Peng, Z.; Leclair, T.; van der Velden, J.; Stein, G.; Lian, J.; Kinsey, C.M. Loss of RUNX1 is associated with aggressive lung adenocarcinoma. *J. Cell Physiol.* **2018**, *233*, 3487–3497. [CrossRef]
11. Kim, J.S.; Han, J.; Shim, Y.M.; Park, J.; Kim, D.H. Aberrant methylation of H-cadherin (CDH13) promoter is associated with tumor progression in primary nonsmall cell lung carcinoma. *Cancer* **2005**, *104*, 1825–1833. [PubMed]
12. Edge, S.B.; Byrd, D.R.; Compton, C.C.; Fritz, A.G.; Greene, F.L.; Troth, A. American Joint Committee on Cancer. In *AJCC Cancer Staging Manual*, 7th ed.; Springer: New York, NY, USA, 2010; pp. 253–270.
13. Um, S.W.; Kim, H.K.; Kim, Y.; Lee, B.B.; Kim, D.; Han, J.; Kim, H.; Shim, Y.M.; Kim, D.H. Bronchial biopsy specimen as a surrogate for DNA methylation analysis in inoperable lung cancer. *Clin. Epigenetics* **2017**, *9*, 131. [CrossRef] [PubMed]

14. Pidsley, R.; Y Wong, C.C.; Volta, M.; Lunnon, K.; Mill, J.; Schalkwyk, L.C. A data-driven approach to preprocessing Illumina 450K methylation array data. *BMC. Genomics* **2013**, *14*, 293. [CrossRef] [PubMed]
15. Ketia, M.; Bachvarova, M.; Morin, C.; Plante, M.; Gregoire, J.; Renaud, M.C.; Sebastianelli, A.; Trinh, X.B.; Bachvarov, D. The RUNX1 transcription factor is expressed in serous epithelial ovarian carcinoma and contributes to cell proliferation, migration and invasion. *Cell Cycle* **2013**, *12*, 972–986.
16. Planagumà, J.; Díaz-Fuertes, M.; Gil-Moreno, A.; Abal, M.; Monge, M.; García, A.; Baró, T.; Thomson, T.M.; Xercavins, J.; Alameda, F.; et al. A differential gene expression profile reveals overexpression of RUNX1/AML1 in invasive endometrioid carcinoma. *Cancer Res.* **2004**, *64*, 8846–8853. [CrossRef] [PubMed]
17. Browne, G.; Taipaleenmaki, H.; Bishop, N.M.; Madasu, S.C.; Shaw, L.M.; van Wijnen, A.J.; Stein, J.L.; Stein, G.S.; Lian, J.B. Runx1 is associated with breast cancer progression in MMTV-PyMT transgenic mice and its depletion in vitro inhibits migration and invasion. *J. Cell Physiol.* **2015**, *230*, 2522–2532. [CrossRef]
18. Farina, N.H.; Zingiryan, A.; Akech, J.A.; Callahan, C.J.; Lu, H.; Stein, J.L.; Languino, L.R.; Stein, G.S.; Lian, J.B. A microRNA/Runx1/Runx2 network regulates prostate tumor progression from onset to adenocarcinoma in TRAMP mice. *Oncotarget* **2016**, *7*, 70462–70474. [CrossRef]
19. Dulak, A.M.; Schumacher, S.; van Lieshout, J.; Imamura, Y.; Fox, C.; Shim, B.; Ramos, A.H.; Saksena, G.; Baca, S.C.; Baselga, J.; et al. Gastrointestinal adenocarcinomas of the esophagus, stomach and colon exhibit distinct patterns of genome instability and oncogenesis. *Cancer Res.* **2012**, *72*, 4383–4393. [CrossRef]
20. Takayama, K.; Suzuki, T.; Tsutsumi, S.; Fujimura, T.; Urano, T.; Takahashi, S.; Homma, Y.; Aburatani, H.; Inoue, S. RUNX1, an androgen- and EZH2-regulated gene, has differential roles in AR-dependent and -independent prostate cancer. *Oncotarget* **2015**, *6*, 2263–2276. [CrossRef]
21. Hong, D.; Fritz, A.J.; Finstad, K.H.; Fitzgerald, M.P.; Weinheimer, A.; Viens, A.L.; Ramsey, J.; Stein, J.L.; Lian, J.B.; Stein, G.S. Suppression of breast cancer stem cells and tumor growth by the RUNX1 transcription factor. *Mol. Cancer Res.* **2018**, *16*, 1952–1964. [CrossRef]
22. Kulkarni, M.; Tan, T.Z.; Syed Sulaiman, N.B.; Lamar, J.M.; Bansal, P.; Cui, J.; Qiao, Y.; Ito, Y. RUNX1 and RUNX3 protect against YAP-mediated EMT, stem-ness and shorter survival outcomes in breast cancer. *Oncotarget* **2018**, *9*, 14175–14192. [CrossRef] [PubMed]
23. Hao, C.; Wang, L.; Peng, S.; Cao, M.; Li, H.; Hu, J.; Huang, X.; Liu, W.; Zhang, H.; Wu, S.; et al. Gene mutations in primary tumors and corresponding patient-derived xenografts derived from non-small cell lung cancer. *Cancer Lett.* **2015**, *357*, 179–185. [CrossRef]
24. Feng, Q.; Hawes, S.E.; Stern, J.E.; Wiens, L.; Lu, H.; Dong, Z.M.; Jordan, C.D.; Kiviat, N.B.; Vesselle, H. DNA methylation in tumor and matched normal tissues from non-small cell lung cancer patients. *Cancer Epidemiol. Biomarkers Prev.* **2008**, *17*, 645–654. [CrossRef] [PubMed]
25. Rauch, T.A.; Wang, Z.; Wu, X.; Kernstine, K.H.; Riggs, A.D.; Pfeifer, G.P. DNA methylation biomarkers for lung cancer. *Tumour Biol.* **2012**, *33*, 287–296. [CrossRef] [PubMed]
26. Ghozi, M.C.; Bernstein, Y.; Negreanu, V.; Levanon, D.; Groner, Y. Expression of the human acute myeloid leukemia gene AML1 is regulated by two promoter regions. *Proc. Natl. Acad. Sci. USA* **1996**, *93*, 1935–1940. [CrossRef]
27. National Lung Screening Trial Research Team; Aberle, D.R.; Adams, A.M.; Berg, C.D.; Black, W.C.; Clapp, J.D.; Fagerstrom, R.M.; Gareen, I.F.; Gatsonis, C.; Marcus, P.M.; et al. Reduced lung-cancer mortality with low-dose computed tomographic screening. *N. Engl. J. Med.* **2011**, *365*, 395–409.
28. Bach, P.B.; Mirkin, J.N.; Oliver, T.K.; Azzoli, C.G.; Berry, D.A.; Brawley, O.W.; Byers, T.; Colditz, G.A.; Gould, M.K.; Jett, J.R.; et al. Benefits and harms of CT screening for lung cancer: A systematic review. *JAMA* **2012**, *307*, 2418–2429. [CrossRef]
29. Jalili, M.; Yaghmaie, M.; Ahmadvand, M.; Alimoghaddam, K.; Mousavi, S.A.; Vaezi, M.; Ghavamzadeh, A. Prognostic Value of RUNX1 Mutations in AML: A Meta-Analysis. *Asian Pac. J. Cancer Prev.* **2018**, *19*, 325–332.
30. Yamato, G.; Shiba, N.; Yoshida, K.; Hara, Y.; Shiraishi, Y.; Ohki, K.; Okubo, J.; Park, M.J.; Sotomatsu, M.; Arakawa, H.; et al. RUNX1 mutations in pediatric acute myeloid leukemia are associated with distinct genetic features and an inferior prognosis. *Blood* **2018**, *131*, 2266–2270. [CrossRef]
31. Strom, D.K.; NiP, J.; Westendorf, J.J.; Linggi, B.; Lutterbach, B.; Downing, J.R.; Lenny, N.; Hiebert, S.W. Expression of the AML-1 oncogene shortens the G(1) phase of the cell cycle. *J. Biol. Chem.* **2002**, *275*, 3438–3445. [CrossRef]

15

Potential of FDG-PET as Prognostic Significance After Anti-PD-1 Antibody against Patients with Previously Treated Non-Small Cell Lung Cancer

Kosuke Hashimoto [1], Kyoichi Kaira [1,*], Ou Yamaguchi [1], Atsuto Mouri [1], Ayako Shiono [1], Yu Miura [1], Yoshitake Murayama [1], Kunihiko Kobayashi [1], Hiroshi Kagamu [1] and Ichiei Kuji [2]

1 Department of Respiratory Medicine, Comprehensive Cancer Center, International Medical Center, Saitama Medical University, 1397-1 Yamane, Hidaka-City, Saitama 350-1298, Japan; hkosuke@saitama-med.ac.jp (K.H.); ouyamagu@saitama-med.ac.jp (O.Y.); mouria@saitama-med.ac.jp (A.M.); respiratory@hotmail.co.jp (A.S.); you_mi@saitama-med.ac.jp (Y.M.); ymura114@saitama-med.ac.jp (Y.M.); kobakuni@saitama-med.ac.jp (K.K.); kagamu19@saitama-med.ac.jp (H.K.)

2 Department of Nuclear Medicine, Comprehensive Cancer Center, International Medical Center, Saitama Medical University, 1397-1 Yamane, Hidaka-City, Saitama 350-1298, Japan; kuji@saitama-med.ac.jp

* Correspondence: kkaira1970@yahoo.co.jp

Abstract: It remains unclear whether the accumulation of 2-deoxy-2-[^{18}F]fluoro-D-glucose (^{18}F-FDG) before the initiation of anti-programmed death-1 (PD-1) antibody can predict the outcome after its treatment. The aim of this study is to retrospectively examine the prognostic significance of ^{18}F-FDG uptake as a predictive marker of anti-PD-1 antibody. Eighty-five patients with previously treated non-small cell lung cancer (NSCLC) who underwent ^{18}F-FDG-positron emission tomography (PET) just before administration of nivolumab or pembrolizumab monotherapy were eligible in our study, and metabolic tumor volume (MTV), total lesion glycolysis (TLG) and the maximum of standardized under value (SUV_{max}) on ^{18}F-FDG uptake were assessed. Objective response rate, median progression-free survival and median overall survival were 36.6%, 161 days and 716 days, respectively. The frequency of any immune-related adverse events was significantly higher in patients with low ^{18}F-FDG uptake on PET than in those with high uptake. By multivariate analysis, the tumor metabolic activity by TLG and MTV was identified as an independent prognostic factor for predicting outcome after anti-PD-1 antibody therapy, but not SUV_{max}, predominantly in patients with adenocarcinoma. Metabolic tumor indices as TLG and MTV on ^{18}F-FDG uptake could predict the prognosis after anti-PD-1 antibodies in patients with previously treated NSCLC.

Keywords: FDG-PET; immune checkpoint inhibitor; PD-1; lung cancer; prognosis

---

1. Introduction

Non-small cell lung cancer (NSCLC) is the leading cause of cancer-related deaths worldwide. Recent studies have proven that anti-programmed death-1 (PD-1)/programmed death ligand-1 (PD-L1) antibodies provide significant survival benefits in patients with advanced NSCLC, when compared with standard chemotherapy [1–4]. Although the efficacy of the anti-PD-1 antibody varies according to the immunohistochemical degree of PD-L1 expression within tumor cells, there are no established biomarkers to predict the outcome after the administration of the anti-PD-1 antibody and the expression of PD-L1. If a useful biomarker is obtained from common modalities, this discovery can be easily adopted into daily practice.

Notably, 2-deoxy-2-[^{18}F]fluoro-D-glucose (^{18}F-FDG) positron emission tomography (PET) is a distinguished radiological modality to distinguish benign lesions from malignant tumors [5]. The uptake of ^{18}F-FDG is observed in non-malignant lesions such as sarcoidosis, granuloma, pneumonia, and tuberculosis, but it can closely resemble the metabolic activity of malignant tumors [5]. Previous reports demonstrated that the accumulation of ^{18}F-FDG within tumor cells was significantly linked to the presence of glucose transporter 1 (Glut1), hypoxia-inducible factor 1α (HIF-1α), and vascular endothelial growth factor (VEGF)b [6]. Several researchers have described that the accumulation of ^{18}F-FDG exhibited a significant correlation with the expression of PD-L1 in patients with NSCLC [7–9]. Although little is known about the close association between immune environment and glucose metabolism, it is important to discover how metabolic tumor activity can affect the upregulation of PD-L1 expression. Moreover, it has been reported that ^{18}F-FDG-PET is useful for assessing the therapeutic monitoring of anti-PD-1 antibody with regard to the prognosis and overall response rate [10]. Little is known as to whether the uptake of ^{18}F-FDG before the administration of anti-PD-1 antibody can predict the efficacy and prognosis of immune checkpoint inhibitors (ICI) in patients with advanced NSCLC.

The maximum standardized uptake value (SUVmax) is extensively used to evaluate the metabolic degree of ^{18}F-FDG within tumor cells. Since SUVmax reflects the maximal point of glucose metabolism within tumor specimens, it remains unclear whether it can indicate the total metabolic tumor volume (MTV). Recently, total lesion glycolysis (TLG) and MTV—indicators of ^{18}F-FDG accumulation within tumor cells—have been identified as significant prognostic markers for predicting the treatment outcome in patients with NSCLC. A meta-analysis described TLG and MTV as better predictive markers than SUVmax [11]. Moreover, an exploratory study documented that the tumor metabolic activity assessed by TLG and MTV is better than SUVmax in evaluating the therapeutic monitoring of anti-PD-1 antibody in patients with previously treated NSCLC [10]. Recent reports suggested that baseline tumor size could predict adverse outcomes in patients with NSCLC who received ICI [12–14]. However, the detailed mechanism behind tumor burden (TB), determined by baseline tumor size and causing poor efficacy of ICI, is unclear. Tumors possibly suppress the immune response by different mechanisms other than the PD-1/PD-L1 pathway. Tumor hypoxia, determined by HIF-1, induces VEGF, which induces immunosuppressive T-lymphocytes such as regulatory T-cells (Tregs) and myeloid-derived suppressor cells [15,16]. These evidences suggest that the high HIF-1 expression caused by an increased tumor size creates an immunosuppressive environment regardless of ICI treatment and contributes to the poor outcome for patients with NSCLC [15,16]. However, whether morphological assessment, based on baseline tumor size, can accurately reflect the volume of tumor hypoxia or tumor metabolic activity is debatable. Therefore, ^{18}F-FDG uptake is expected to assess tumor activity more accurately than TB on computed tomography (CT).

We conducted this study to investigate whether the degree of ^{18}F-FDG uptake before the administration of anti-PD-1 antibody can predict the prognosis in patients with previously treated advanced NSCLC, by evaluating the correlation between TB and SUVmax, TLG, and MTV.

2. Materials and methods

2.1. Patients

We retrospectively examined the medical records at Saitama Medical University International Medical Center, Saitama, Japan (ethical approval code: 19-225; date of approval: 13 November 2019) and selected patients with previously treated NSCLC who received anti-PD-1 antibody monotherapy, such as nivolumab and pembrolizumab, and underwent ^{18}F-FDG-PET after previous treatment and before the initiation of anti-PD-1 antibody as a recurrent survey. From February 2016 through April 2019, 97 patients with pretreated NSCLC were administered nivolumab and pembrolizumab. Twelve patients were excluded because of inadequate medical information and absence of an evaluable target lesion. Therefore, the final cohort consisted of 85 patients.

This study was approved by the institutional ethics committee of the Saitama Medical University International Medical Center. All procedures performed in studies involving human participants were in accordance with the ethical standards of the institutional and/or national research committee and with the 1964 Helsinki declaration and its later amendments or comparable ethical standards. The requirement for written informed consent was waived because of the retrospective nature of the study.

2.2. Treatment, Efficacy Evaluation, and Assessment of Baseline Tumor Burden

Nivolumab and pembrolizumab were intravenously administered at 3 mg/kg every 2 weeks and at 200 mg/day every 3 weeks, respectively. Complete blood cell count, differential count, routine chemistry measurements, physical examination, and toxicity assessment were performed weekly. Acute toxicity was graded using the Common Terminology Criteria for Adverse Events version 4.0. Tumor response was evaluated using the Response Evaluation Criteria in Solid Tumors version 1.1 [17]. Baseline TB was evaluated using CT for target lesions [13,14]. TB was defined as the sum of the longest diameter for a maximum of five target lesions and up to two lesions per organ [13,14].

2.3. PET Imaging and Data Analysis

Patients fasted for at least 6 hours before PET imaging, performed using a PET/CT scanner (Biograph 6 or 16, Siemens Healthineers K.K., Japan) with a 585 mm field of view. Three-dimensional data acquisition was initiated 60 minutes after injecting 3.7 MBq/kg of FDG. We acquired eight bed positions (2-minute acquisition per bed position) according to the range of imaging. Attenuation-corrected transverse images obtained with ^{18}F-FDG were reconstructed with the ordered-subsets expectation-maximization algorithm, based on the point spread function into 168×168 matrices with a slice thickness of 2.00 mm.

For the semiquantitative analysis, functional images of SUV were produced using attenuation-corrected transaxial images, injected dosage of ^{18}F-FDG, patient's body weight, and he cross-calibration factor between PET and the dose calibrator. SUV was defined as follows:

SUV = Radioactive concentration in the region of interest (ROI) (MBq/g)/Injected dose (MBq)/Patient's body weight (g).

A nuclear physician conducted the volume of interest (VOI) analysis using CT scans, eliminating the physiological uptake in the heart, urinary tracts, and gastrointestinal tracts. We used GI-PET software (Nihon Medi-physics Co. Ltd., Tokyo, Japan) on a Windows workstation to semi-automatically calculate the MTV and TLG (= $SUV_{mean} \times$ MTV), of each lesion using SUV thresholds in the liver VOI (= $SUV_{mean} + [1.5 \times SUV_{Standard\_Deviation}]$). These SUV thresholds were the optimum values to generate VOIs in which the whole tumor mass is completely enclosed in all cases, with the CT image as the reference. SUV_{max} and SUV_{mean} within the generated VOI were also calculated automatically. VOIs over all measurable lesions on pretreatment PET/CT were automatically registered. In case of multiple lesions in the same organ, a maximum of 100 lesions were measured.

2.4. Statistical Analysis

Statistical significance was indicated by $p < 0.05$. Fisher's exact tests were used to examine the association between two categorical variables. Correlations between SUVmax, MTV, and TLG on ^{18}F-FDG uptake were analyzed using the Pearson rank test. The Kaplan–Meier method was used to estimate survival as a function of time, and survival differences were analyzed by log-rank tests. Progression-free survival (PFS) was defined as the time from the initiation of anti-PD-1 antibody to tumor recurrence or death from any cause, while overall survival (OS) was defined as the time from the initiation of anti-PD-1 antibody to death from any cause. Statistical analyses were performed using GraphPad Prism 7 (Graph Pad Software, San Diego, CA, USA) and JMP 14.0 (SAS Institute Inc., Cary, NC, USA).

3. Results

3.1. Assessment of SUV_{max}, MTV, and TLG on ^{18}F-FDG Uptake

In all 85 patients, the median values of SUVmax, MTV, and TLG on ^{18}F-FDG and TB were 6.0 (range, 3.1–21.0), 17.8 cm^3 (range, 1.1–379 cm^3), 75.4 gcm^3/mL (range, 3.9–2550 $g{\cdot}cm^3/mL$), and 65 cm (range, 6.6–230.6 cm), respectively. According to histological types, the median values of SUVmax, MTV, and TLG on ^{18}F-FDG and TB in adenocarcinoma were 6.7 (range, 3.1–21.3), 11.3 cm^3 (range, 1.1–276 cm^3), 58.3 $g{\cdot}cm^3/mL$ (range, 3.9–1398 $g{\cdot}cm^3/mL$), and 53 cm (range, 6.6–230.6 cm), respectively, and those in non-adenocarcinoma displayed 8.4 (range, 3.2–20.4) 24.8 cm^3 (range, 1.1–379 cm^3), 105.6 $g{\cdot}cm^3/mL$ (range, 4.0–2550 $g{\cdot}cm^3/mL$), and 75 cm (range, 18.2–228.3 cm), respectively. The difference of each parameter for SUVmax, MTV, and TLG on ^{18}F-FDG and TB was not significant between adenocarcinoma and non- adenocarcinoma. The SUVmax correlated significantly with MTV ($r = 0.49$, $p < 0.01$), TLG ($r = 0.56$, $p < 0.01$), and TB ($r = 0.33$, $p < 0.01$). Figure 1 is a representative PET image showing the assessment of SUVmax, MTV, and TLG on ^{18}F-FDG.

The discriminative value of various SUVmax, MTV, and TLG cutoffs for ^{18}F-FDG uptake were explored in the context of OS and PFS (Figure 2) [13]. For prognosis in OS and PFS analyses, the most discriminative cutoffs based on log-rank test for SUVmax, MTV, and TLG were 6.0, 5.0, and 20, respectively. The TLG cutoff of 20 was significant in the OS analysis, but not in the PFS analysis, although it was the most favorable TLG cutoff. The SUVmax cutoff of 6 was not significant in either OS or PFS analysis, but still seemed better considering the results of the log-rank test. The 12 cm cutoff for TB was based on a previous study [13].

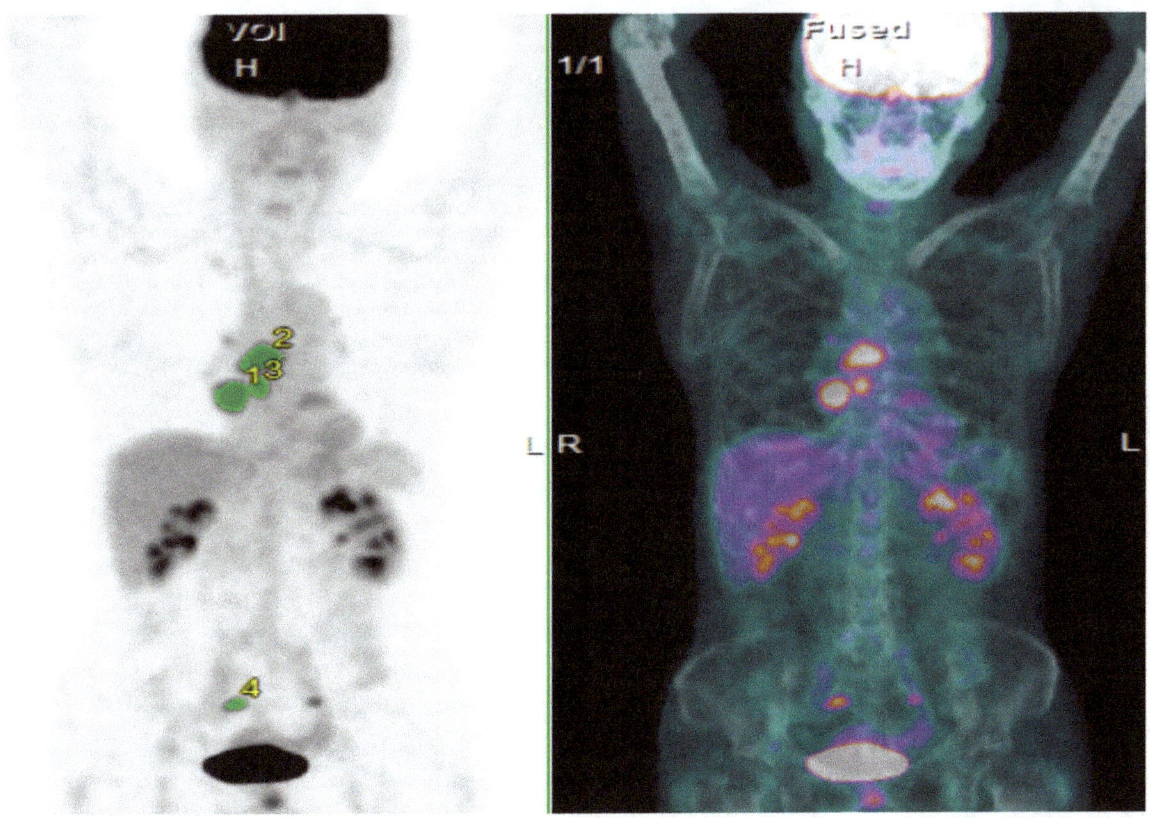

Figure 1. Imaging from a positron emission tomography (PET) scan of non-small cell lung cancer (NSCLC), indicating the measurement of SUVmax, metabolic tumor volume (MTV) and total lesion glycolysis (TLG) on 2-deoxy-2-[^{18}F]fluoro-D-glucose (^{18}F-FDG).

3.2. Patient Demographics

Patient demographics according to the cutoff values of SUVmax, MTV, and TLG on ^{18}F-FDG uptake are listed in Table 1. In the 17 patients harboring epidermal growth factor receptor (*EGFR)* mutation, deletion 19 and L858R were observed in 11 and 6 patients, respectively. High TLG and SUVmax on ^{18}F-FDG uptake were significantly associated with smoking history. The objective response rate and disease control rate were 36.6% [95% confidence internal (CI); 26.2%–47.0%] and 65.9% [95%CI; 55.6%–76.1%]. No significant difference in the response to ICI was observed according to the degree of SUVmax, MTV, and TLG on ^{18}F-FDG uptake. The median time from the date of ^{18}F-FDG-PET scan to the initiation of anti-PD-1 antibodies was 18 days (range, 1–107 days). Next, we analyzed different incidences of immune-related adverse events (irAEs) according to the degree of SUVmax, MTV, and TLG on ^{18}F-FDG uptake and TB. The frequency of any irAE was significantly higher in patients with low values of SUVmax, MTV, and TLG on PET than in those with high values, but not for TB (Table S1, online only). The incidence of grade 3 or 4 irAEs exhibited no close correlation with the degree of ^{18}F-FDG uptake on PET and TB.

Table 1. Patient's demographics according to the assessment of FDG uptake.

Variables	Total (n = 85)	TLG			MTV			SUVmax		
		High (n = 59)	Low (n = 26)	p-Value	High (n = 58)	Low (n = 27)	p-Value	High (n =5 2)	Low (n = 33)	p-Value
Age **≤ 70/>70** **(range: 38–86 years)**	42/43	29/30	13/13	>0.99	25/33	17/10	0.11	26/26	16/17	>099
Gender Male/Female	65/20	47/12	18/8	0.41	46/12	19/8	0.42	42/10	23/10	0.29
Smoking history Yes/No	71/14	51/8	10/16	**<0.01**	50/8	21/6	0.35	47/5	24/9	**0.04**
Performance status 0 or 1/2 or 3	79/6	53/6	26/0	0.17	52/6	27/0	0.17	46/6	33/0	0.07
Histological type AC/Non-AC	51/34	33/26	18/8	0.34	32/26	19/8	0.24	27/25	24/9	0.07
EGFR mutation Yes/No	17/68	12/47	5/21	>0.99	12/47	5/22	>0.99	10/42	7/26	>0.99
Response to ICI # CR or PR/SD or PD CR, PR or SD/PD	29/51 53/27	20/35 34/21	9/16 19/6	>0.99 0.31	20/34 36/18	9/17 17/9	>0.99 >0.99	21/27 34/15	8/24 19/12	0.10 0.47

Abbreviations: TLG, total lesion glycolysis; MTV, metabolic tumor volume; SUVmax, the maximum of standardized uptake value; AC, adenocarcinoma; Non-AC, non-adenocarcinoma; EGFR, epidermal growth factor receptor; CR, complete response; PR, partial response; SD, stable disease; PD, progressive disease; ICI, immune checkpoint inhibitor. #, because of 6 patients with no measurable lesion, 82 patients were analyzed according to the uptake of FDG; Bold character shows statistically significance.

3.3. Survival and ^{18}F-FDG-PET:

The median OS and PFS were 716 and 161 days, respectively, and the 2-year OS rate was 44.8%. Among all patients, those with a low TLG exhibited significantly better OS than those with a high TLG. Similarly, the survival analysis of MTV on ^{18}F-FDG uptake demonstrated a significantly worse OS and PFS for patients with a high MTV (Figure 2). No statistically significant difference in the OS and PFS was observed between patients with a low and high SUVmax (Figure 2). However, in 70 patients without an EGFR mutation, a statistically significant difference in OS and PFS was recognized between patients with low and high TLG or low and high MTV, but not between those with low and high SUVmax and low and high TB (Figure 3). Survival analysis results are listed in Table 2. Univariate analysis in all patients identified performance status (PS), TLG, and MTV as significant prognostic markers for OS; the significant predictors for PFS were PS and MTV. Subsequently, we performed a multivariate analysis according to TLG and MTV and confirmed that PS, TLG, and MTV were independent prognostic factors for poor OS and PFS; the significant prognostic marker for PFS was PS (Table 3). In patients without EGFR mutation, a multivariate analysis identified TLG and MTV as independent prognostic factors for predicting poor OS. Histological typing confirmed TLG and MTV as significant prognostic factors in patients with adenocarcinoma, but not in those with non-adenocarcinoma.

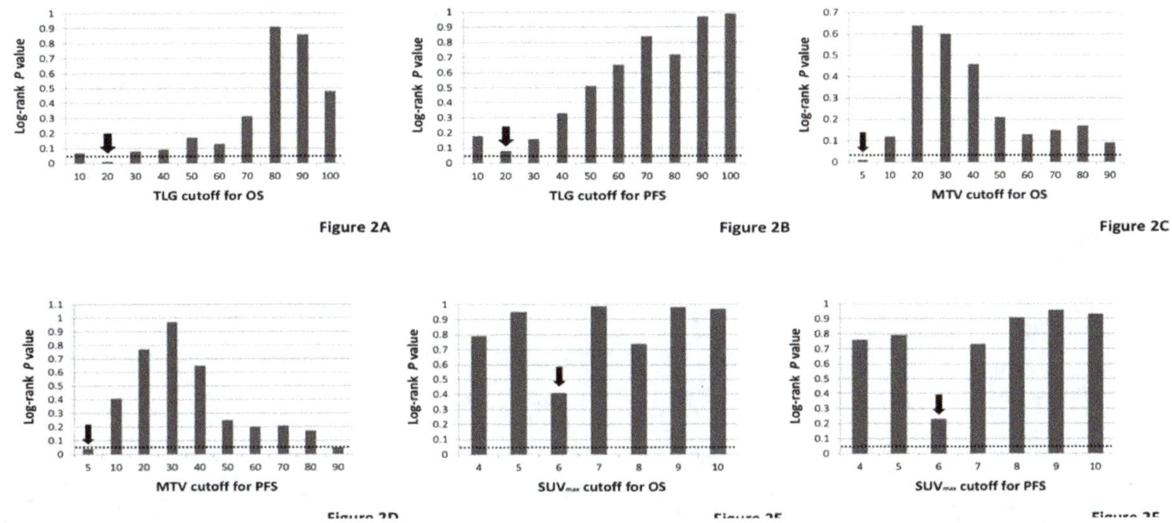

Figure 2. Discriminative value by log-rank test according to various TLG (**A**), MTV (**C**) and SUVmax (**E**) cutoff for OS and TLG (**B**), MTV (**D**) and SUVmax (**F**) cutoff for PFS in 18F-FDG-PET.

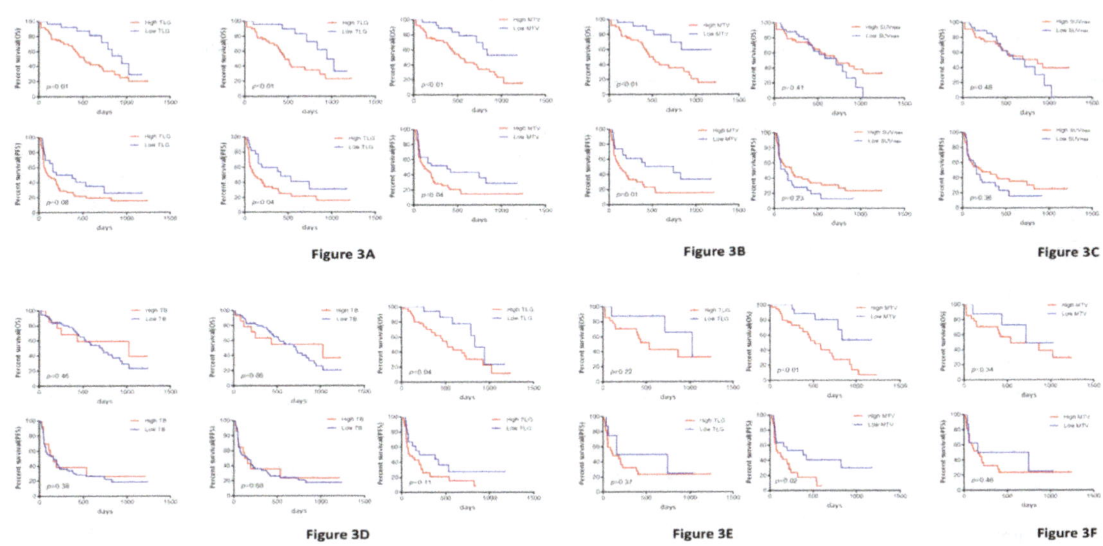

Figure 3. Kaplan–Meier curves according to various TLG (**A**), MTV (**B**), SUVmax (**C**) and TB (**D**) for OS and PFS. (**A**); OS (upper left) and PFS (lower left) in all patients and OS (upper right) and PFS (lower right) in those without EGFR mutation according to TLG. (**B**); OS (upper left) and PFS (lower left) in all patients and OS (upper right) and PFS (lower right) in those without EGFR mutation according to MTV. (**C**); OS (upper left) and PFS (lower left) in all patients and OS (upper right) and PFS (lower right) in those without EGFR mutation according to SUVmax. (**D**); OS (upper left) and PFS (lower left) in all patients and OS (upper right) and PFS (lower right) in those without EGFR mutation according to TB. (**E**); OS (upper left) and PFS (lower left) in patients with AC patients and OS (upper right) and PFS (lower right) in those with non-AC according to TLG. (**F**); OS (upper left) and PFS (lower left) in patients with non-AC patients and OS (upper right) and PFS (lower right) in those with non-AC according to MTV. Abbreviation: TLG, total lesion glycolysis; MTV, metabolic tumor volume; SUVmax: maximal standardized under value; TB, tumor burden; OS, overall survival; PFS, progression-free survival; AC, adenocarcinoma; non-AC, non-adenocarcinoma.

Table 2. Univariate analysis in overall survival and progression-free survival.

Variables	Overall Survival				Progression-Free Survival			
	All Patients (n = 85)		Patients without EGFR Mutation (n = 70)		All Patients (n = 85)		Patients without EGFR Mutation (n = 70)	
	MST (days)	p-Value	MST (days)	p-Value	MST (days)	p-Value	MST (days)	p-Value
Age (≤70/>70)	737/693	0.73	865/693	0.85	164/161	0.88	181/180	0.92
Gender (Male/Female)	716/737	0.85	693/837	0.59	181/75	0.67	172/420	0.23
Smoking (Yes/No)	716/737	0.53	716/637	0.74	181/72	0.09	181/272	0.85
PS (0 or 1/2 or 3)	724/115	**<0.01**	716/74	**<0.01**	172/40	**<0.01**	200/25	0.10
Histological type (AC/Non-AC)	724/716	0.84	693/716	0.66	146/161	0.76	220/161	0.39
TLG (High/Low)	516/945	**0.01**	465/945	**<0.01**	114/291	0.08	114/420	**0.04**
MTV (High/Low)	536/NR	**<0.01**	465/NR	**<0.01**	125/382	**0.04**	127/382	**0.02**
SUVmax (High/Low)	724/716	0.41	865/716	0.48	201/125	0.23	204/161	0.36
TB (High/Low)	793/693	0.46	837/693	0.86	204/137	0.38	182/181	0.68

Abbreviations: TLG, total lesion glycolysis; MTV, metabolic tumor volume; SUVmax, the maximum of standardized uptake value; AC, adenocarcinoma; Non-AC, non-adenocarcinoma; PS, performance status; HR, hazard ratio; 95% CI, 95% confidence interval; NR, not reached; EGFR, epidermal growth factor receptor; TB, tumor burden; Bold character shows statistically significance.

Table 3. Multivariate analysis of overall survival and progression-free survival.

Variables	Overall Survival				Progression-Free Survival			
	All Patients (n = 85)		Patients without EGFR Mutation (n = 70)		All Patients (n = 85)		Patients without EGFR Mutation (n = 70)	
	HR 95% CI	p-Value	HR 95% CI	p-Value	HR 95% CI	p-Value	HR 95% CI	p-Value
Survival Analysis Including TLG								
Age (≤ 70/> 70)	1.02 0.74–1.39	0.91	1.02 0.72–1.44	0.90	0.95 0.74–1.23	0.74	0.98 0.73–1.31	0.89
Gender (Male/Female)	1.11 0.76–1.55	0.55	0.95 0.55–1.48	0.85	1.07 0.79–1.41	0.61	0.81 0.49–1.19	0.31
PS (0 or 1/2 or 3)	1.68 1.05–2.51	**0.03**	2.22 1.06–3.93	**0.03**	1.63 1.02–2.36	**0.04**	1.41 0.68–2.43	0.31
TLG (High/Low)	1.47 1.03–2.21	**0.03**	1.63 1.10–2.60	**0.01**	1.21 0.92–1.63	0.16	1.32 0.97–1.86	0.07
Survival Analysis Including MTV								
Age (≤ 70/> 70)	0.92 0.68–1.26	0.64	0.87 0.61–1.25	0.46	0.91 0.71–1.18	0.51	0.91 0.67–1.21	0.51
Gender (Male/Female)	1.09 0.75–1.52	0.61	0.97 0.56–1.51	0.91	1.06 0.78–1.40	0.66	0.80 0.49–1.18	0.28
PS (0 or 1/2 or 3)	1.69 1.06–2.51	**0.02**	2.23 1.06–3.94	**0.03**	1.59 1.02–2.33	**0.04**	1.41 0.68–2.41	0.31
MTV (High/Low)	1.59 1.09–2.45	**0.01**	1.83 1.19–3.04	**<0.01**	1.28 0.97–1.73	0.07	1.45 1.05–2.05	**0.02**

Abbreviations: TLG, total lesion glycolysis; MTV, metabolic tumor volume; PS, performance status; HR, hazard ratio; 95% CI, 95% confidence interval; EGFR, epidermal growth factor receptor.

4. Discussion

To the best of our knowledge, this is the first study to evaluate the prognostic significance of metabolic parameters measured by ^{18}F-FDG-PET for predicting outcomes after the initiation of anti-PD-1 antibodies in patients with previously treated NSCLC. We found that the tumor metabolic volume assessed by TLG and MTV was an independent prognostic factor, but not SUVmax and TB. The roles of TLG and MTV as significant predictive markers after anti-PD-1 antibody therapy may be closely associated with patients with a histology of adenocarcinoma and without EGFR mutation.

Although the value of SUVmax on ^{18}F-FDG uptake within tumor cells was closely correlated with that of TLG and MTV, SUVmax on ^{18}F-FDG uptake before anti-PD-1 antibody could not accurately predict the outcome after the initiation of treatment. Furthermore, we found that low uptake of ^{18}F-FDG was closely associated with the occurrence of irAEs and the incidence of grade 3 or 4 irAEs exhibited no close correlation with the degree of ^{18}F-FDG uptake on PET. In addition, there was no significant correlation between the response to the anti-PD-1 antibody and the degree of ^{18}F-FDG uptake. However, we discovered that MTV of pretreatment ^{18}F-FDG-PET plays a crucial role in the prognostic significance of anti-PD-1 antibody treatment. Unlike previous studies [12,13], our study indicated that TB determined by baseline tumor size was not a significant predictor of ICI or irAEs. Further studies are warranted to investigate whether pretreatment of MTV can predict the outcome of ICI plus ICI or the combination of ICI plus cytotoxic chemotherapy as first-line treatment.

A recent study reported that the metabolic response to ^{18}F-FDG uptake measured by TLG or MTV was a stronger biomarker for the prediction of efficacy and survival at one month after the initiation of nivolumab than SUV_{max} [10]. The predictive probability of partial response (100% versus 29%, $p = 0.021$) and progressive disease (100% versus 22.2%, $p = 0.002$) at one month after nivolumab treatment was significantly higher in ^{18}F-FDG-PET than in CT. Moreover, multivariate analysis confirmed the ^{18}F-FDG uptake measurement by TLG or MTV as an independent prognostic factor. Thus, ^{18}F-FDG-PET may be a useful radiographic modality for immune monitoring to predict the efficacy of ICI. However, a large-scale prospective study is required to confirm these results [10,18]. A recent meta-analysis suggested that in lung cancer, metabolic parameters such as TLG and MTV are better prognostic predictors after any treatment when compared with SUV_{max} [11].

Recently, Jreige et al. described that the metabolic-to-morphological volume ratio (MMVR)—calculated by dividing MTV by morphological tumor volume (MoTV)—was able to predict the radiological response to anti-PD-1/PD-L1 blockade and was negatively correlated with tumor PD-L1 expression and tumor necrosis [18]. Although their study analyzed only 17 patients who received anti-PD-1 therapy, they suggested that anti-PD-1 therapy is effective for tumor tissues with a low ratio of MTV, and the presence of a low MTV contributes to the upregulation of PD-L1 expression by the hypoxic environment in the tumor arising from necrosis and inflammation. However, it remained unclear whether MMVR could predict the outcome after anti-PD-1 therapy. Our study, however, indicated that patients with a low MTV exhibited a favorable prognosis after anti-PD-1 therapy. Several studies have demonstrated that tumor necrosis triggers inflammation, which facilitates the influx of lymphocytes and the upregulation of PD-L1, related to tumor necrosis factor-α, and that necrosis or inflammation was closely linked to tumor recurrence and worse survival [19,20]. Our study could not investigate the relationship between necrosis or inflammation and tumor metabolic volume; therefore, it remains unclear whether low MTV and TLG are associated with necrosis, inflammation, and hypoxic environment in the tumor. Further investigation is warranted to elucidate the prognostic significance of MTV and TLG as predictive markers of anti-PD-1 therapy based on the biological aspect.

The mechanism by which tumor cells uptake ^{18}F-FDG requires glucose metabolism, hypoxia, and angiogenesis, and ^{18}F-FDG is closely associated with the expression of these markers [6]. The expression of PD-L1 is significantly related to Glut1, HIF-1α and SUV_{max} on ^{18}F-FDG uptake in lung cancer [7–9]. However, it is reported that TLG and MTV on ^{18}F-FDG uptake were not closely correlated with PD-L1 expression levels [18], but Foxp3-Tregs are described to be positively associated with TLG and MTV [21]. Considering these evidences, the active environment with high MTV may form an immunosuppressive state, contributing to the resistant situation to ant-PD-1 blockage.

Our study has several limitations. First, we employed a retrospective approach and a small cohort, which may have introduced bias in our results. More than half of the patients with previously treated NSCLC had not undergone ^{18}F-FDG-PET just before the initiation of anti-PD-1 antibody treatment. Therefore, we think that the number of eligible patients was slightly limited. However, the current study is meaningful for the prediction of anti-PD-1 therapy. Second, our study suggests that MTV could be a predictive marker for ICI treatment compared to the morphological tumor volume. However, the appropriateness of morphological assessment used for calculating the optimal tumor volume of all metastatic lesions using CT scan is debatable. Thus, it may be difficult to perform a concise comparison between metabolic and morphological tumor volumes. Moreover, we had no information about the calculation of MMVR in our study, thus, there were some limitations in discussing the prognostic significance of metabolic tumor volume compared to MMVR. Lastly, an the immunohistochemical analysis of PD-L1, expression within tumor cells using tumor specimens was not performed before anti-PD1 antibody treatment. At our institution, re-biopsy was not done routinely before ICI treatment except for the initial diagnosis. Further study is warranted to investigate the relationship between MTV and the immune environment.

In conclusion, TLG and MTV on ^{18}F-FDG uptake may predict the prognosis after anti-PD-1 antibodies in patients with previously treated NSCLC, but not SUVmax on ^{18}F-FDG uptake. Although MTV may indirectly reflect the presence of morphological tumor volume with active tumor cells, the assessment of TLG and MTV on ^{18}F-FDG uptake is easily executable in daily practice. A prospective study is needed to confirm these results.

Author Contributions: K.H., A.S., K.K. (Kunihiko Kobayashi) and H.K.: conception and preparation of the manuscript. A.M., A.S., O.Y., K.H., Y.M. (Yu Miura), and Y.M. (Yoshitake Murayama): management of the patient. O.Y.: statistical analysis and patient's data collection. A.S., A.M., O.Y., K.K. (Kyoichi Kaira), I.K. and H.K.: revising the manuscript. All authors contributed and agreed with the content of the manuscript. All authors have read and agreed to the published version of the manuscript.

References

1. Borghaei, H.; Paz-Ares, L.; Horn, L.; Spigel, D.R.; Steins, M.; Ready, N.E.; Chow, L.Q.; Vokes, E.E.; Felip, E.; Holgado, E.; et al. Nivolumab versus Docetaxel in Advanced Nonsquamous Non-Small-Cell Lung Cancer. *N. Engl. J. Med.* **2015**, *373*, 1627–1639. [CrossRef] [PubMed]
2. Robert, C.; Long, G.V.; Brady, B.; Dutriaux, C.; Maio, M.; Mortier, L.; Hassel, J.C.; Rutkowski, P.; McNeil, C.; Kalinka-Warzocha, E.; et al. Nivolumab in previously untreated melanoma without BRAF mutation. *N. Engl. J. Med.* **2015**, *372*, 320–330. [CrossRef] [PubMed]
3. Reck, M.; Rodríguez-Abreu, D.; Robinson, A.G.; Hui, R.; Csőszi, T.; Fülöp, A.; Gottfried, M.; Peled, N.; Tafreshi, A.; Cuffe, S.; et al. Pembrolizumab versus Chemotherapy for PD-L1-Positive Non-Small-Cell Lung Cancer. *N. Engl. J. Med.* **2016**, *375*, 1823–1833. [CrossRef] [PubMed]
4. Rittmeyer, A.; Barlesi, F.; Waterkamp, D.; Park, K.; Ciardiello, F.; von Pawel, J.; Gadgeel, S.M.; Hida, T.; Kowalski, D.M.; Dols, M.C.; et al. Atezolizumab versus docetaxel in patients with previously treated non-small-cell lung cancer (OAK): A phase 3, open-label, multicentre randomised controlled trial. *Lancet* **2017**, *389*, 255–265. [CrossRef]
5. Kaira, K.; Oriuchi, N.; Otani, Y.; Yanagitani, N.; Sunaga, N.; Hisada, T.; Ishizuka, T.; Endo, K.; Mori, M. Diagnostic usefulness of fluorine-18-alpha-methyltyrosine positron emission tomography in combination with 18F-fluorodeoxyglucose in sarcoidosis patients. *Chest* **2007**, *131*, 1019–1027. [CrossRef]
6. Kaira, K.; Endo, M.; Abe, M.; Nakagawa, K.; Ohde, Y.; Okumura, T.; Takahashi, T.; Murakami, H.; Tsuya, A.; Nakamura, Y.; et al. Biologic correlation of 2-[^{18}F]-fluoro-2-deoxy-D-glucose uptake on positron emission tomography in thymic epithelial tumors. *J. Clin. Oncol.* **2010**, *28*, 3746–3753. [CrossRef]
7. Takada, K.; Toyokawa, G.; Okamoto, T.; Baba, S.; Kozuma, Y.; Matsubara, T.; Haratake, N.; Akamine, T.; Takamori, S.; Katsura, M.; et al. Metabolic characteristics of programmed cell death-ligand 1-expressing lung cancer on ^{18}F-fluorodeoxyglucose positron emission tomography/computed tomography. *Cancer Med.* **2017**, *6*, 2552–2561. [CrossRef]
8. Kasahara, N.; Kaira, K.; Yamaguchi, K.; Masubuchi, H.; Tsurumaki, H.; Hara, K.; Koga, Y.; Sakurai, R.; Higuchi, T.; Handa, T.; et al. Fluorodeoxyglucose uptake is associated with low tumor-infiltrating lymphocyte levels in patients with small cell lung cancer. *Lung Cancer* **2019**, *134*, 180–186. [CrossRef]
9. Kaira, K.; Shimizu, K.; Kitahara, S.; Yajima, T.; Atsumi, J.; Kosaka, T.; Ohtaki, Y.; Higuchi, T.; Oyama, T.; Asao, T.; et al. 2-Deoxy-2-[fluorine-18] fluoro-d-glucose uptake on positron emission tomography is associated with programmed death ligand-1 expression in patients with pulmonary adenocarcinoma. *Eur. J. Cancer* **2018** *101*, 181–190. [CrossRef]

10. Kaira, K.; Higuchi, T.; Naruse, I.; Arisaka, Y.; Tokue, A.; Altan, B.; Suda, S.; Mogi, A.; Shimizu, K.; Sunaga, N.; et al. Metabolic activity by ^{18}F-FDG-PET/CT is predictive of early response after nivolumab in previously treated NSCLC. *Eur. J. Nucl. Med. Mol. Imaging* **2018**, *45*, 56–66. [CrossRef]
11. Im, H.J.; Pak, K.; Cheon, G.J.; Kang, K.W.; Kim, S.J.; Kim, I.J.; Chung, J.K.; Kim, E.E.; Lee, D.S. Prognostic value of volumetric parameters of ^{18}F-FDG PET in non-small-cell lung cancer: A meta-analysis. *Eur. J. Nucl. Med. Mol. Imaging* **2015**, *42*, 241–251. [CrossRef] [PubMed]
12. Katsurada, M.; Nagano, T.; Tachihara, M.; Kiriu, T.; Furukawa, K.; Koyama, K.; Otoshi, T.; Sekiya, R.; Hazama, D.; Tamura, D.; et al. Baseline tumor size as predictive and prognostic factor of immune checkpoint inhibitor therapy for non-small cell lung cancer. *Anticancer Res.* **2019**, *39*, 815–825. [CrossRef] [PubMed]
13. Sakata, Y.; Kawamura, K.; Ichikado, K.; Shingu, N.; Yasuda, Y.; Eguchi, Y.; Hisanaga, J.; Nitawaki, T.; Iio, M.; Sekido, Y.; et al. Comparisons between tumor burden and other prognostic factors that influence survival of patients with non-small cell lung cancer treated with immune checkpoint inhibitors. *Thorac. Cancer* **2019**, *10*, 2259–2266. [CrossRef] [PubMed]
14. Dercle, L.; Ammari, S.; Champiat, S.; Massard, C.; Ferté, C.; Taihi, L.; Seban, R.D.; Aspeslagh, S.; Mahjoubi, L.; Kamsu-Kom, N.; et al. Rapid and objective CT scan prognostic scoring identifies metastatic patients with long-term clinical benefit on anti-PD-1/L1 therapy. *Eur. J. Cancer* **2016**, *65*, 33–42. [CrossRef]
15. Fukumura, D.; Kloepper, J.; Amoozgar, Z.; Duda, D.G.; Jain, R.K. Enhancing cancer immunotherapy using antiangiogenics; opportunities and challenges. *Nat. Rev. Clin. Oncol.* **2018**, *29*, 325–340. [CrossRef]
16. Schaaf, M.B.; Garg, A.D.; Agostinis, P. Defining the role of the tumor vasculature in antitumor immunity and immunotherapy. *Cell Death Dis.* **2018**, *1*, 115. [CrossRef]
17. Eisenhauer, E.A.; Therasse, P.; Bogaerts, J.; Schwart, L.H.; Sargent, D.; Ford, R.; Dancey, J.; Arbuck, S.; Gwyther, S.; Mooney, M.; et al. New response evaluation criteria in solid tumour: Revised RECIST guideline (version 1.1). *Eur. J. Cancer* **2009**, *45*, 228–247. [CrossRef]
18. Jreige, M.; Letovanec, I.; Chaba, K.; Renaud, S.; Rusakiewicz, S.; Cristina, V.; Peters, S.; Krueger, T.; de Leval, L.; Kandalaft, L.E.; et al. ^{18}F-FDG PET metabolic-to-morphological volume ratio predicts PD-L1 tumour expression and response to PD-1 blockade in non-small-cell lung cancer. *Eur. J. Nucl. Med. Mol. Imaging* **2019**, *46*, 1859–1868. [CrossRef]
19. Garg, A.D.; Agostinis, P. Cell death and immunity in cancer from danger signals to mimicry of pathogen defense responses. *Immmunol. Rev.* **2017**, *280*, 126–148. [CrossRef]
20. Gkogkou, C.; Frangia, K.; Saif, M.W.; Trigidou, R.; Syrigos, K. Necrosis and apoptotic index as prognostic factors in non-small cell lung cancer: A review. *Springerplus* **2014**, *3*, 120. [CrossRef]
21. Wang, Y.; Zhao, N.; Wu, Z.; Pan, N.; Shen, X.; Liu, T.; Wei, F.; You, J.; Xu, W.; Ren, X. New insight on the correlation of metabolic status on ^{18}F-FDG PET/CT with immune marker expression in patients with non-small cell lung cancer. *Eur. J. Nucl. Med. Mol. Imaging* **2019**, in press. [CrossRef] [PubMed]

16

Predicting the Role of DNA Polymerase β Alone or with *KRAS* Mutations in Advanced NSCLC Patients Receiving Platinum-Based Chemotherapy

Maria Francesca Alvisi [1,†], Monica Ganzinelli [2,†], Helena Linardou [3,†], Elisa Caiola [4,†], Giuseppe Lo Russo [2], Fabiana Letizia Cecere [5], Anna Cecilia Bettini [6], Amanda Psyrri [7], Michele Milella [8], Eliana Rulli [1], Alessandra Fabbri [9], Marcella De Maglie [10,11], Pierpaolo Romanelli [10,11], Samuel Murray [12], Gloriana Ndembe [4], Massimo Broggini [4,*], Marina Chiara Garassino [2,‡] and Mirko Marabese [4,*,‡]

1 Laboratory of Methodology for Clinical Research, Department of Oncology, Istituto di Ricerche Farmacologiche Mario Negri IRCCS, 20156 Milan, Italy; mariafrancesca.alvisi@marionegri.it (M.F.A.); eliana.rulli@marionegri.it (E.R.)
2 Unit of Thoracic Oncology, Medical Oncology Department 1, Fondazione IRCCS Istituto Nazionale dei Tumori, 20133 Milan, Italy; monica.ganzinelli@istitutotumori.mi.it (M.G.); Giuseppe.LoRusso@istitutotumori.mi.it (G.L.R.); marina.garassino@istitutotumori.mi.it (M.C.G.)
3 4th Oncology Department, Metropolitan Hospital, 18547 Athens, Greece; elinardou@otenet.gr
4 Laboratory of Molecular Pharmacology, Department of Oncology, Istituto di Ricerche Farmacologiche Mario Negri IRCCS, 20156 Milan, Italy; elisa.caiola@marionegri.it (E.C.); gloriana.ndembe@marionegri.it (G.N.)
5 Division of Medical Oncology 1, IRCCS Regina Elena National Cancer Institute, 00144 Rome, Italy; fabianacecere@gmail.com
6 UO Oncologia Medica, ASST Papa Giovanni XXIII, 24127 Bergamo, Italy; abettini@asst-pg23.it
7 Section of Oncology, Department of Internal Medicine, Attikon Hospital, National Kapodistrian University of Athens, 12462 Athens, Greece; psyrri237@yahoo.com
8 Department of Medicine, Section of Medical Oncology, University and Hospital Trust of Verona, 37126 Verona, Italy; michele.milella@aovr.veneto.it
9 Department of Pathology and Laboratory Medicine, Fondazione IRCCS Istituto Nazionale dei Tumori, 20133 Milan, Italy; Alessandra.fabbri@istitutotumori.mi.it
10 Mouse & Animal Pathology Lab, Fondazione Filarete, 20139 Milan, Italy; marcellademaglie@libero.it (M.D.M.); pierpaolo.romanelli.medvet@gmail.com (P.R.)
11 Department of Veterinary Medicine, University of Milan, 20122 Milan, Italy
12 Biomarker Solutions Ltd., London EC1V 2NX, UK; smgenedb@gmail.com
* Correspondence: massimo.broggini@marionegri.it (M.B.); mirko.marabese@marionegri.it (M.M.)

† Shared first authors.
‡ Shared last authors.

Abstract: Clinical data suggest that only a subgroup of non-small cell lung cancer (NSCLC) patients has long-term benefits after front-line platinum-based therapy. We prospectively investigate whether KRAS status and DNA polymerase β expression could help identify patients responding to platinum compounds. Prospectively enrolled, advanced NSCLC patients treated with a first-line regimen containing platinum were genotyped for KRAS and centrally evaluated for DNA polymerase β expression. Overall survival (OS), progression-free survival (PFS), and the objective response rate (ORR) were recorded. Patients with KRAS mutations had worse OS (hazard ratio (HR): 1.37, 95% confidence interval (95% CI): 0.70–2.27). Negative DNA polymerase β staining identified a subgroup with worse OS than patients expressing the protein (HR: 1.43, 95% CI: 0.57–3.57). The addition of KRAS to the analyses further worsened the prognosis of patients with negative DNA polymerase β staining (HR: 1.67, 95% CI: 0.52–5.56). DNA polymerase β did not influence PFS and ORR. KRAS may have a negative role in platinum-based therapy responses in NSCLC, but its impact is limited.

DNA polymerase β, when not expressed, might indicate a group of patients with poor outcomes. KRAS mutations in tumors not expressing DNA polymerase β further worsens survival. Therefore, these two biomarkers together might well identify patients for whom alternatives to platinum-based chemotherapy should be used.

Keywords: NSCLC; KRAS; DNA polymerase beta; platinum-based first-line

---

1. Introduction

Over the last 40 years, several million lung cancer patients have received platinum-based regimens, and despite the clinical use of an impressive variety of targeted agents, these drugs are still one of the main therapeutic options for certain patients [1]. Platinum compounds are also the best choice in first-line immunotherapy combinations [2]. However, despite the good impact of platinum-based therapies, only a small proportion of patients have durable benefits [3]. Therefore, biomarkers to explain the resistance mechanisms to platinum compounds are urgently needed.

KRAS mutations have long been considered potential biomarkers to predict the outcome of platinum-based chemotherapy in NSCLC [4]. The TAILOR trial data shed light on the possibility that there was a small negative prognostic effect of *KRAS* mutations in advanced NSCLC patients treated with a platinum-based doublet when EGFR-mutant patients were excluded from the analysis [5].

Platinum adducts are repaired by different DNA repair systems. The Fanconi anemia (FA) pathway is thought to coordinate these systems, including homologous recombination (HR), nucleotide excision repair (NER), and translesion synthesis (TLS) repair [6,7]. Other DNA repair systems, such as base excision repair (BER), are involved in cisplatin-induced DNA damage, but so far, they have been assigned only a marginal role in repairing this damage [8].

Our group recently reported in a preclinical study that DNA polymerase β, an important component of the BER pathway, could be involved in platinum-based chemotherapy responses. Our results suggested a different pattern of sensitivity/resistance to cisplatin, dependent on *KRAS* mutational status [9].

The present work explores whether DNA polymerase β, alone or in combination with *KRAS* mutational status, can identify tumors with different abilities to respond to platinum compounds. This is the first study to prospectively assess the combined role of the selected biomarkers to identify patients who could benefit from platinum-based therapy.

2. Material and Methods

2.1. Study Population and Samples

The Fondazione IRCCS Istituto Nazionale dei Tumori (Milan, Italy), the Regina Elena National Cancer Institute (Rome, Italy), the Hospital Papa Giovanni XXIII (Bergamo, Italy), and the Metropolitan and Attikon Hospitals (Athens, Greece) were the centers involved. Consecutive patients with metastatic NSCLC who received platinum-based chemotherapy in combination with either vinorelbine, gemcitabine, or pemetrexed, according to the physician's choice, as first-line therapy between February 2014 and April 2017 were included in the BioRaRe prospective multicenter trial.

All patients had an Eastern Cooperative Oncology Group (ECOG) Performance Status (PS) between 0 and 2 and were at least 18 years of age. Exclusion criteria included any evidence of serious comorbidities that the investigator judged as a contraindication to the participation in the study, pregnancy, and breast-feeding.

Patients evaluable for tumor response according to the RECIST 1.1 criteria were examined, and their demographics and clinical and pathological characteristics were retrieved. E-CRF and medical records were used to collect data.

The study was approved by the Fondazione IRCCS Istituto Nazionale dei Tumori Institutional Review Board (INT18/13) and conducted according to the Declaration of Helsinki ethical principles for medical research involving human subjects. All patients gave signed written informed consent.

2.2. Mutational Analysis

KRAS mutational status was determined by Sanger sequencing at each center, following the protocol already used in a clinical trial by our group [10]. Briefly, DNA extraction was performed on histological tumor specimens by using standard phenol–chloroform procedure after macro/microdissection in order to recovery most of the cancer cells and to reduce contamination by normal ones. DNA preparations were verified for their concentration and quality by spectrophotometric measurement. Genomic DNAs were amplified by polymerase chain reaction (PCR) using high-fidelity Taq polymerase and specific primers encompassing intronic regions for KRAS exons 2–4. PCR products were then analyzed electrophoretically on agarose gel, and automated bidirectional sequencing was performed using BigDye Terminator chemistry. Sequences were then automatically compared with wild-type KRAS gene profiles by software analysis to assess the presence of possible mutations.

2.3. Immunohistochemical Analysis (IHC)

IHC was done centrally on single slides at the Fondazione Filarete, as previously reported [11]. Sections were immune-stained with anti-DNA polymerase β antibody ab26343 (Abcam, Cambridge, UK), and incubated with biotinylated secondary goat anti-rabbit antibody (VC-BA-1000-MM15, Vector Laboratories, Burlingame, CA, USA). Sections were labeled by the avidin–biotin–peroxidase (ABC) procedure with a commercial immunoperoxidase kit (VECTASTAIN Elite ABC-Peroxidase Kit Standard, VC-PK-6100-KI01, Vector Laboratories, Burlingame, CA, USA). The immune reaction was visualized with 3,3′-diaminobenzidine peroxidase DAB substrate kit (VC-SK-4100-KI01, Vector Laboratories, Burlingame, CA, USA) substrate and sections were counterstained with Mayer's hematoxylin. Figure S1 shows representative images of negative and positive DNA polymerase β staining.

A semiquantitative H-score (percentage of positive tumoral cells x intensity: 0 = negative, 1 = slight, 2 = moderate, 3 = strong) was calculated independently by two pathologists. In case of disagreement, a third opinion was requested.

2.4. Outcomes

The primary outcome of the study was progression-free survival (PFS). Secondary outcomes were objective response rate (ORR) and overall survival (OS). PFS was defined as the time from the start of the platinum-based first-line therapy to the date of progression or death from any cause, whichever came first. ORR was defined as the proportion of patients with a complete or partial response to treatment. OS was defined as the time from the platinum-based first-line therapy to the date of death from any cause.

2.5. Statistical Methods

Chi-squared and Kruskal–Wallis tests were used to analyze the relations between the DNA polymerase β H-score (Polβ) and categorical clinical variables. The Spearman correlation coefficient was used to measure the correlation between Polβ and continuous clinical variables. Polβ was analyzed as a continuous and dichotomous variable (Polβ = 0 as negative and Polβ > 0 as positive).

Patients who had not died or had no disease progression were censored at their last available information on status. Survival curves were calculated with the Kaplan–Meier method and tested by the log-rank test. Cox proportional hazard models were used to analyze the impact of DNA polymerase β on PFS and OS, adjusting for clinical and pathological characteristics such as ECOG-PS, age, histology, smoking, therapy, and, only for OS, immunotherapy. Results were expressed as hazard ratios (HRs) with their 95% confidence intervals (95% CIs).

The impact of DNA polymerase β on ORR was analyzed with logistic regression models and expressed as odds ratios (ORs) with their 95% CIs, while for dichotomized analysis, the chi-square test was used. A subgroup analysis was done for patients with both Polβ and KRAS mutational status available.

All statistical tests were two-sided, and $p < 0.05$ was considered statistically significant. Statistical analyses were done using SAS version 9.4 (SAS Institute, Cary, NC, USA).

3. Results

Of the 120 patients registered in the trial with material available, 109 had a DNA polymerase β H-score (Polβ) and 74 had both Polβ and *KRAS* mutational status. Figure 1 reports the flowchart of the study.

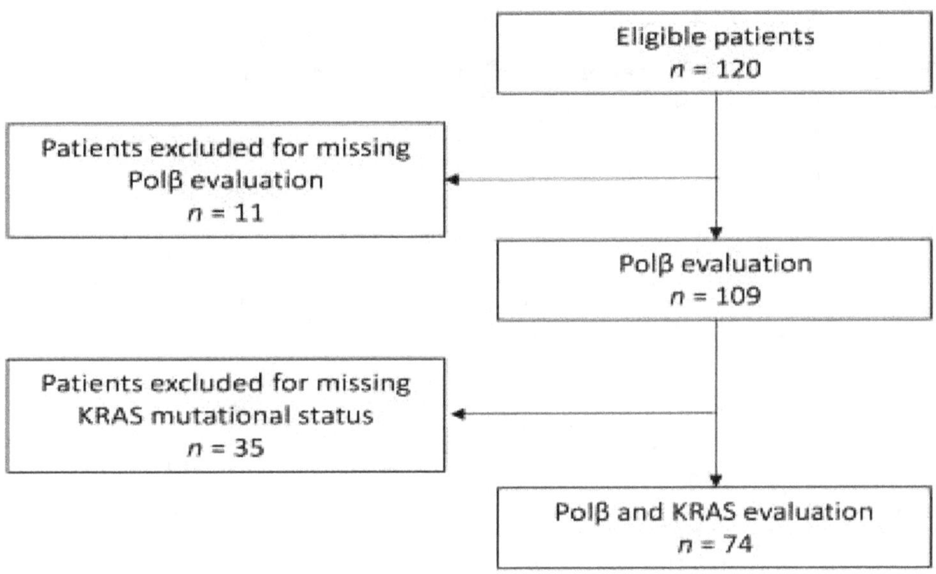

Figure 1. CONSORT diagram showing the flow of participants.

The main demographic characteristics of the population ($n = 109$) and the relationships between characteristics and Polβ are reported in Table 1.

3.1. Progression-Free Survival

The median PFS was, respectively, 5.9 and 7.2 months in the mutated (mut) and wild-type (wt) KRAS groups (adjusted HR mut vs. wt: 1.09, 95% CI: 0.56–2.08, $p = 0.815$).

Polβ, considered a continuous variable, did not have any significant impact on PFS in a multivariable Cox model. HR was 0.99 for each 10-unit increment of the score, with 95% CI 0.97–1.02 and $p = 0.579$. The inclusion of KRAS mutational status in the statistical model did not modify the impact of Polβ on progression or death risk (HR: 0.99, 95% CI: 0.96–1.02, $p = 0.501$). Considering Polβ as a dichotomous variable, median PFS were, respectively, 4 and 6.3 months for negative (neg) and positive (pos) staining. The absence or presence of DNA polymerase β had no impact on the risk of PFS, considering the multivariable models, either including KRAS status or not in the analysis (HR pos vs. neg: 1.10, 95% CI: 0.44–2.70, $p = 0.847$; HR pos vs. neg: 1.08, 95% CI: 0.49–2.38, $p = 0.857$). Detailed results of the multivariable analysis for PFS are reported in Table 2, and the Kaplan–Meier curves for PFS are shown in Figure 2A. The forest plot in Figure 2B graphically shows the effect of KRAS status on the relationship between Polβ and PFS.

3.2. Overall Survival

The median OS was, respectively, 12.4 and 20.5 months in the mutated and wild-type KRAS groups (adjusted HR mut vs. wt: 1.27, 95% CI: 0.70–2.27, $p = 0.441$).

Polβ, analyzed as a continuous variable, had no impact on survival in the multivariable models including KRAS status or not (HR: 0.99, 95% CI: 0.96–1.01, $p = 0.39$; HR = 0.99, 95% CI: 0.95–1.02, p-value = 0.388).

Patients who were negative for DNA polymerase β staining had a median OS of 11.6 months compared to 20.6 months in the positive group. The absence of DNA polymerase β caused a worse but not statistically significant OS compared to DNA polymerase β-expressing patients (HR pos vs. neg: 1.43, 95% CI: 0.57–3.57, $p = 0.439$). With the inclusion of KRAS mutational status in the statistical model, the effect on survival with Polβ was stronger (HR pos vs. neg: 1.67, 95% CI: 0.52–5.56, $p = 0.386$). The results of the multivariate analyses for OS are reported in Table 3. Kaplan–Meier curves for OS, reported in Figure 3A,B, show the effect of KRAS status on the relationship between Polβ and OS.

Table 1. Baseline characteristics of patients ($n = 109$) and their relation with Polβ as a continuous or dichotomous variable. Pos, positive; neg, negative.

		n (%)		*p* Polβ Continuous	*p* Polβ pos vs. neg
Age of diagnosis	Median(Q1–Q3)	66.8 (60.0–71.4)		0.448 *	0.788 †
	Missing	3			
Gender	Male	70	65.4	0.717 †	0.366 **
	Female	37	34.6		
	Missing	2			
ECOG-PS	0	78	81.3	0.157 †	0.443 **
	1	17	17.7		
	2	1	1		
	Missing	13			
Smoking	Never	21	20	0.618 †	1.000 **
	Former smokers	42	40		
	Smokers	42	40		
	Missing	4			
Stage at diagnosis	*IIIB*	28	26.2	0.038 †	0.507 **
	IV	79	73.8		
	Missing	2			
Histotype	Adenocarcinoma	90	82.6	0.291 †	0.184 **
	Squamous	17	15.6		
	Other	2	1.8		
Platinum-based therapy	Cisplatin	33	34.7	0.726 †	0.486 **
	Carboplatin	62	65.3		
	Missing	14			
Immunotherapy	No	62	58.5	0.248 †	0.352 **
	Yes	44	41.5		
	Missing	3			
Polβ	Median(Q1-Q3)	160.0 (60.0–200.0)		-	-
	negative	13	11.9	-	-
	positive	96	88.1		
KRAS	Mutated	35	47.3	0.053 †	0.125 **
	Wild-Type	39	52.7		
	Missing	35			

At a median follow-up of 18.8 months (Q1–Q3: 8.3–48.9), there were 90 progressions, 62 deaths, and 100 deaths or progressions. Q1–Q3: first–third quartile, pos: positive, neg: negative, †: Kruskal–Wallis test, *: Spearman correlation, **: Fisher test.

Table 2. Multivariable Cox models adjusted for ECOG-PS, age, histology, smoking, and therapy for progression-free survival, considering Polβ continuous or Polβ positive vs. negative. Pos, positive; neg, negative.

	Polβ Continuous		**Polβ pos vs. neg**	
	HR (95% CI)	***p***	**HR (95% CI)**	***p***
Polβ (10-unit increment)	0.99 (0.97–1.02)	0.579	-	-
Polβ				
Positive	-	-	reference	
Negative	-	-	1.07 (0.49–2.38)	0.857
Age at metastasis diagnosis (5 years increment)	0.82 (0.72–0.94)	0.005	0.82 (0.72–0.95)	0.006
Histology				
Adenocarcinoma	reference		reference	
Squamous	1.10 (0.60–2.03)	0.755	1.12 (0.60–2.10)	0.728
Nos or other	2.26 (0.27–18.6)	0.449	2.34 (0.28–19.5)	0.432
Smoke				
Never	reference		reference	
Previous	1.25 (0.69–2.26)	0.463	1.27 (0.70–2.29)	0.434
Current	0.79 (0.40–1.56)	0.495	0.81 (0.41–1.59)	0.543
ECOG-PS	1.51 (0.78–2.94)	0.223	1.51 (0.76–3.00)	0.244
Therapy				
Cisplatin	reference		reference	
Carboplatin	1.73 (1.02–2.92)	0.041	1.69 (1.01–2.85)	0.046

Table 3. Multivariable Cox models adjusted for ECOG-PS, age, histology, smoking, therapy, and immunotherapy for OS, considering Polβ continuous and Polβ positive or negative. Pos: positive, neg: negative.

	Polβ Continuous		**Polβ pos vs. neg**	
	HR (95% CI)	***p***	**HR (95% CI)**	***p***
Polβ (10-unit increment)	0.99 (0.96–1.01)	0.390	-	-
Polβ				
Positive	-	-	reference	
Negative	-	-	1.43 (0.57–3.57)	0.439
Age at metastasis diagnosis (5 years increments)	0.87 (0.75–1.01)	0.066	0.87 (0.75–1.01)	0.065
Histology				
Adenocarcinoma	reference		reference	
Squamous	0.94 (0.46–1.95)	0.877	0.98 (0.47–2.06)	0.960
Nos or other	7.67 (0.83–70.6)	0.072	8.86 (0.94–83.3)	0.056
Smoke				
Never	reference		reference	
Previous	2.65 (1.15–6.12)	0.022	2.76 (1.21–6.30)	0.016
Current	1.58 (0.61–4.11)	0.350	1.63 (0.63–4.26)	0.316
ECOG-PS	1.18 (0.48–2.90)	0.724	1.12 (0.44–2.87)	0.812
Therapy				
Cisplatin	reference		reference	
Carboplatin	1.74 (0.94–3.21)	0.075	1.70 (0.93–3.12)	0.084
Immunotherapy				
No	reference		reference	
Yes	0.57 (0.32–1.03)	0.063	0.55 (0.31–0.98)	0.041

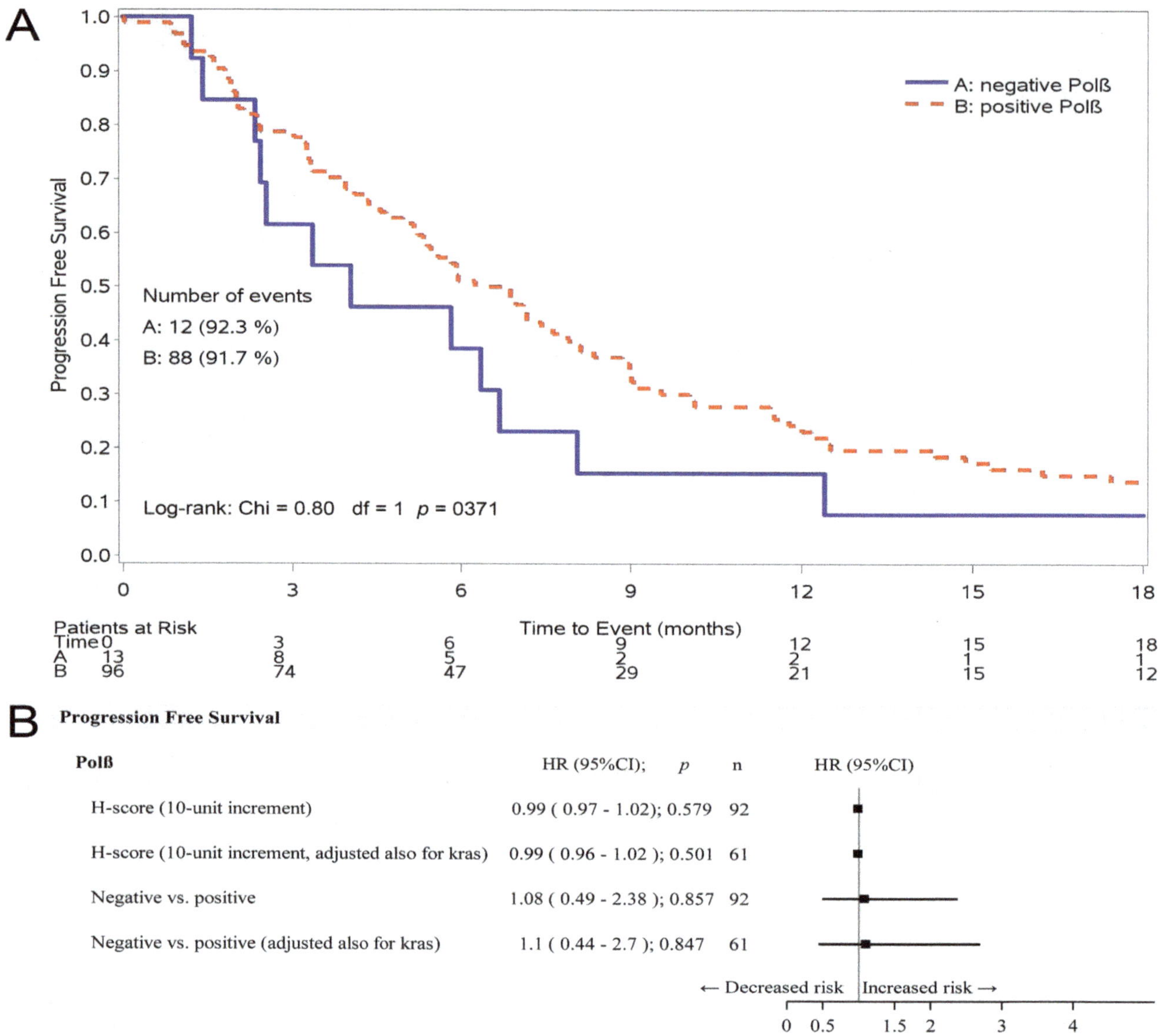

Figure 2. (**A**) Kaplan–Meier curves for PFS according to the positive or negative DNA polymerase β staining. (**B**) Effect of KRAS status on the relationship between Polβ and PFS adjusted for ECOG-PS, age, histology, smoking, and therapy.

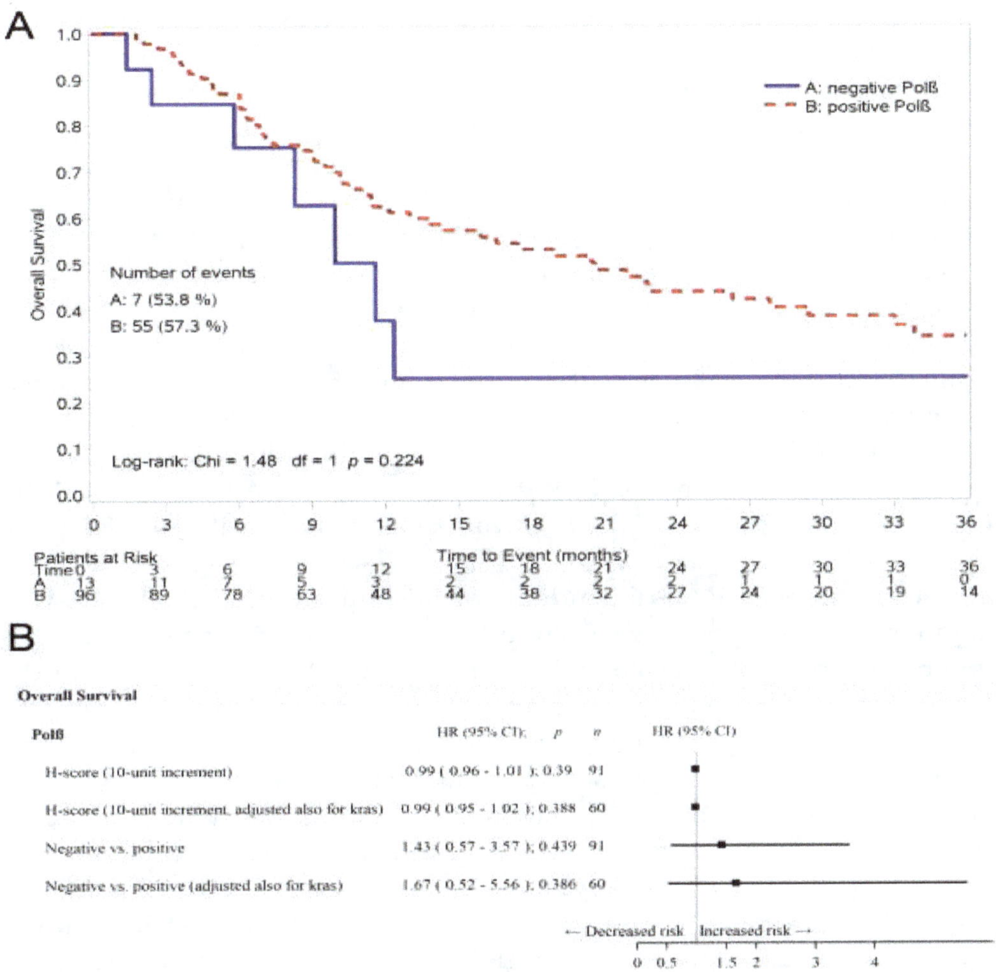

Figure 3. (**A**) Kaplan–Meier curves for OS, according to the positive or negative DNA polymerase β staining. (**B**) Effect of KRAS status on the relationship between Polβ and PFS adjusted for ECOG-PS, age, histology, smoking, therapy, and immunotherapy.

3.3. Overall Response Rate

There were no differences between the DNA polymerase β negative and positive staining groups, or among different Polβ as a continuous variable in ORR to platinum-based first-line therapy (Table 4).

Table 4. Objective response rates by DNA Polymerase β H-score (Polβ). CR, complete response; PR, partial response; SD, stable disease; PD, progressive disease.

	Polβ neg $n = 12$	**Polβ pos** $n = 64$	**Chi-Squared Test**	**Logistic Regression Model**
CR + PR −n (%)	4 (33.3)	23 (35.9)	Chi = 0.03	OR = 1.002
95% CI	34.9–90.1	51.1–75.7	Df = 1	95%CI = 0.997–1.006
SD + PD −n (%)	8 (66.7)	41 (64.1)	$p = 0.864$	$p = 0.505$
95% CI	9.9–65.1	24.3–48.9		

4. Discussion

KRAS mutations have often been investigated as possible biomarkers for selecting chemotherapy, but results have varied, casting doubt on the true utility of this protein. In a previously published randomized prospective trial from our group, an analysis of 247 patients showed that those carrying KRAS mutations and treated with a first-line platinum-based regimen had worse PFS than patients with wild-type KRAS [5]. The present study detected a not-statistically-significant effect for OS,

KRAS-mutated patients having a worse prognosis than KRAS wild-type patients. A possible explanation, although the trend is in line with previous observations, is that the statistical power of this cohort of patients was half that in our earlier study, where KRAS status was significantly associated with survival. On the other hand, the LACE-Bio pooled analysis, including data of 1543 patients participating in four clinical trials, showed that there is no difference in terms of outcomes in early-stage lung cancer patients with either wild-type or mutated KRAS [12]. Our different result may suggest that KRAS mutations could play different roles in early and advanced disease. In advanced stages, KRAS could be a condition necessary, but not sufficient, to explain a more aggressive phenotype.

There is preclinical evidence that KRAS and its mutated versions modulate DNA repair, hence the cellular response to genotoxic agents. Oncogenic RAS can inactivate BRCA-1 dependent homologous recombination (HR) by favoring the dissociation of BRCA-1 from chromatin [13]. Moreover, activated KRAS can suppress the expression of DNA repair genes (including BRCA1, BRCA2, EXO-1, and TP53) [14]. In leukemic cells, mutant KRAS promoted the upregulation of components of the alternative nonhomologous end-joining (NHEJ) pathway, such as DNA ligase IIIα, PARP1, and XRCC1, and the inhibition of the alternative NHEJ pathway selectively sensitized KRAS-mutated cells to chemotherapy [15].

Our group also suggested KRAS-dependent specific alterations in the BER system, where we found DNA polymerase β as a possible selection factor. We demonstrated at the preclinical level that DNA polymerase β could play a role in the response to cisplatin-based chemotherapy, and the data indicated a pattern of sensitivity or resistance depending on the KRAS mutational status [9]. These findings support the hypothesis that the combination of mutant-KRAS status with DNA repair could be a predictive biomarker for response to platinum-based therapy.

On the basis of these assumptions, we planned a translational study to clinically validate KRAS and DNA polymerase β as "biomarkers" for poor response and outcome to platinum-based first-line chemotherapy. We investigated DNA polymerase β as a possible selection marker, alone or in combination with KRAS status. DNA polymerase β expression, summarized in the H-score and considered as a continuous variable, was meaningless to both PFS and OS, alone or with KRAS.

When we compared negative or positive DNA polymerase β staining patients, we detected an interesting, though not statistically significant, difference: OS patients negative for DNA polymerase β staining had worse outcomes than the positive staining group. This result was confirmed even when KRAS status was considered in the analysis.

These data, although interesting and calling for further analysis, are not supported by the literature, where DNA polymerase β upregulation was described as causing resistance to cisplatin in an ovarian cancer model [16]. In a colorectal cancer model expressing high levels of DNA polymerase β, cisplatin was ineffective compared to the same model in which DNA polymerase β was downregulated. In the same paper, 5-year OS curves showed that patients with high DNA polymerase β expression had a significantly poorer prognosis than those with low expression [17]. However, DNA polymerase β has been investigated as a selection marker in very few, only retrospective studies, and our is the first attempt to investigate it, prospectively, in NSCLC.

A recent report suggests that if cells are not able to repair DNA single-strand break lesions through BER (as should be the case here for cells negative for DNA polymerase β), these lesions are channeled to the HR system [18]. We do not know whether this is also true for cisplatin-induced DNA lesions and whether these patients have HR alterations, but it does suggest an intriguing explanation for the worse outcome observed in DNA polymerase β-negative patients.

To our knowledge, this is the first investigation of the role and value of DNA polymerase β, alone or in combination with KRAS status, as a marker of response to platinum-based therapy in NSCLC. Besides the results, this paper also stimulates the idea to further investigate the combination of biomarkers that indicate how different biological pathways coexist or work together in those scenarios, where no single biomarker has been shown to have strong value.

In conclusion, KRAS may have a negative role in platinum-based therapy responses in NSCLC, but its impact is limited. The absence of DNA polymerase β might indicate a group of patients with poor outcomes compared to patients positively staining for this protein. In addition, a mutated form of KRAS in tumors not expressing DNA polymerase β further worsens survival. Therefore, these two biomarkers together might well identify patients for whom alternatives to platinum-based chemotherapy should be used.

Author Contributions: Conceptualization, H.L., M.B., M.C.G., and M.M. (Mirko Marabese); data curation, S.M.; formal analysis, M.F.A. and E.R.; funding acquisition, M.C.G. and M.M. (Mirko Marabese); investigation, M.G., H.L., E.C., G.L.R., F.L.C., A.C.B., A.P., M.M. (Michele Milella), A.F., M.D.M., P.R., and G.N.; writing—original draft, M.M. (Mirko Marabese); writing—review and editing, M.F.A., M.G., H.L., E.C., G.L.R., F.L.C., A.C.B., A.P., M.M. (Michele Milella), E.R., A.F., M.D.M., P.R., S.M., G.N., M.B., M.C.G., and M.M. (Mirko Marabese). All authors have read and agreed to the published version of the manuscript.

References

1. Schirrmacher, V. From chemotherapy to biological therapy: A review of novel concepts to reduce the side effects of systemic cancer treatment (Review). *Int. J. Oncol.* **2018**, *54*, 407–419. [PubMed]
2. Gandhi, L.; Rodriguez-Abreu, D.; Gadgeel, S.; Esteban, E.; Felip, E.; De Angelis, F.; Dómine, M.; Clingan, P.; Hochmair, M.J.; Powell, S.F.; et al. Pembrolizumab plus Chemotherapy in Metastatic Non–Small-Cell Lung Cancer. *N. Engl. J. Med.* **2018**, *378*, 2078–2092. [CrossRef] [PubMed]
3. Schmidt, E.V. Developing combination strategies using PD-1 checkpoint inhibitors to treat cancer. *Semin. Immunopathol.* **2019**, *41*, 21–30. [CrossRef] [PubMed]
4. Piva, S.; Ganzinelli, M.; Garassino, M.C.; Caiola, E.; Farina, G.; Broggini, M.; Marabese, M. Across the universe of K-RAS mutations in non-small-cell-lung cancer. *Curr. Pharm. Des.* **2014**, *20*, 3933–3943. [CrossRef] [PubMed]
5. Marabese, M.; Ganzinelli, M.; Garassino, M.C.; Shepherd, F.A.; Piva, S.; Caiola, E.; Macerelli, M.; Bettini, A.; Lauricella, C.; Floriani, I.; et al. KRAS mutations affect prognosis of non-small-cell lung cancer patients treated with first-line platinum containing chemotherapy. *Oncotarget* **2015**, *6*, 34014–34022. [CrossRef] [PubMed]
6. Deans, A.J.; West, S.C. DNA interstrand crosslink repair and cancer. *Nat. Rev. Cancer* **2011**, *11*, 467–480. [CrossRef] [PubMed]
7. Haynes, B.; Saadat, N.; Myung, B.; Shekhar, M.P. Crosstalk between translesion synthesis, Fanconi anemia network, and homologous recombination repair pathways in interstrand DNA crosslink repair and development of chemoresistance. *Mutat. Res.-Rev. Mutat. Res.* **2015**, *763*, 258–266. [CrossRef] [PubMed]
8. Jung, Y.; Lippard, S.J. Direct cellular responses to platinum-induced DNA damage. *Chem. Rev.* **2007**, *107*, 1387–1407. [CrossRef] [PubMed]
9. Caiola, E.; Salles, D.; Frapolli, R.; Lupi, M.; Rotella, G.; Ronchi, A.; Garassino, M.C.; Mattschas, N.; Colavecchio, S.; Broggini, M.; et al. Base excision repair-mediated resistance to cisplatin in KRAS(G12C) mutant NSCLC cells. *Oncotarget* **2015**, *6*, 30072–30087. [CrossRef] [PubMed]
10. Garassino, M.C.; Martelli, O.; Broggini, M.; Farina, G.; Veronese, S.M.; Rulli, E.; Bianchi, F.; Bettini, A.; Longo, F.; Moscetti, L.; et al. Erlotinib versus docetaxel as second-line treatment of patients with advanced non-small-cell lung cancer and wild-type EGFR tumours (TAILOR): A randomised controlled trial. *Lancet Oncol.* **2013**, *14*, 981–988. [CrossRef]
11. Marabese, M.; Marchini, S.; A Sabatino, M.; Polato, F.; Vikhanskaya, F.; Marrazzo, E.; Riccardi, E.; Scanziani, E.; Broggini, M. Effects of inducible overexpression of DNp73α on cancer cell growth and response to treatment in vitro and in vivo. *Cell Death Differ.* **2005**, *12*, 805–814. [CrossRef] [PubMed]
12. Shepherd, F.A.; Domerg, C.; Hainaut, P.; Jänne, P.A.; Pignon, J.-P.; Graziano, S.; Douillard, J.-Y.; Brambilla, E.; Le Chevalier, T.; Seymour, L.; et al. Pooled analysis of the prognostic and predictive effects of KRAS mutation status and KRAS mutation subtype in early-stage resected non–small-cell lung cancer in four trials of adjuvant chemotherapy. *J. Clin. Oncol.* **2013**, *31*, 2173–2181. [CrossRef] [PubMed]
13. Tu, Z.; Aird, K.M.; Bitler, B.G.; Nicodemus, J.P.; Beeharry, N.; Xia, B.; Yen, T.J.; Zhang, R. Oncogenic RAS regulates BRIP1 expression to induce dissociation of BRCA1 from Chromatin, Inhibit DNA repair, and promote senescence. *Dev. Cell* **2011** *21*, 1077–1091. [CrossRef] [PubMed]

14. Tsunoda, T.; Takashima, Y.; Fujimoto, T.; Koyanagi, M.; Yoshida, Y.; Doi, K.; Tanaka, Y.; Kuroki, M.; Sasazuki, T.; Shirasawa, S. Three-dimensionally specific inhibition of DNA repair-related genes by activated KRAS in colon crypt model. *Neoplasia* **2010**, *12*, 397–404. [CrossRef] [PubMed]
15. Hahnel, P.S.; Enders, B.; Sasca, D.; Roos, W.P.; Kaina, B.; Bullinger, L.; Theobald, M.; Kindler, T. Targeting components of the alternative NHEJ pathway sensitizes KRAS mutant leukemic cells to chemotherapy. *Blood* **2014**, *123*, 2355–2366. [CrossRef] [PubMed]
16. Bergoglio, V.; Canitrot, Y.; Hogarth, L.; Minto, L.; Howell, S.B.; Cazaux, C.; Hoffmann, J.-S. Enhanced expression and activity of DNA polymerase beta in human ovarian tumor cells: Impact on sensitivity towards antitumor agents. *Oncogene* **2001**, *20*, 6181–6187. [CrossRef] [PubMed]
17. Iwatsuki, M.; Mimori, K.; Yokobori, T.; Tanaka, F.; Tahara, K.; Inoue, H.; Baba, H.; Mori, M. A platinum agent resistance gene, POLB, is a prognostic indicator in colorectal cancer. *J. Surg. Oncol.* **2009**, *100*, 261–266. [CrossRef] [PubMed]
18. Giovannini, S.; Weller, M.C.; Repmann, S.; Moch, H.; Jiricny, J. Synthetic lethality between BRCA1 deficiency and poly(ADP-ribose) polymerase inhibition is modulated by processing of endogenous oxidative DNA damage. *Nucleic Acids Res.* **2019**, *47*, 9132–9143. [CrossRef] [PubMed]

17

Phase I/II Study of Docetaxel and S-1 in Previously-Treated Patients with Advanced Non-Small Cell Lung Cancer: LOGIK0408

Koichi Takayama [1,2], Junji Uchino [2,*], Masaki Fujita [3], Shoji Tokunaga [4], Tomotoshi Imanaga [5], Ryotaro Morinaga [6], Noriyuki Ebi [7], Sho Saeki [8], Kazuya Matsukizono [9], Hiroshi Wataya [10], Tadaaki Yamada [2] and Yoichi Nakanishi [1]

1 Research Institute for Diseases of the Chest, Graduate School of Medical Sciences, Kyushu University, Fukuoka 8190395, Japan; takayama@koto.kpu-m.ac.jp (K.T.); naka24@e-mail.jp (Y.N.)
2 Department of Respiratory Medicine, Kyoto Prefectural University of Medicine, Kyoto 6020841, Japan; tayamada@koto.kpu-m.ac.jp
3 Department of Respiratory Medicine, Fukuoka University Hospital, Fukuoka 8140133, Japan; mfujita@fukuoka-u.ac.jp
4 Medical Information Center, Kyushu University Hospital, Fukuoka 8190395, Japan; toksan@med.kyushu-u.ac.jp
5 Department of respiratory disease, Nippon Steel Yawata Memorial Hospital, Kitakyushu 8058508, Japan; imanaga.t@ns.yawata-mhp.or.jp
6 Department of Medical Oncology, Oita University Faculty of Medicine, Yuhu 8795593, Japan; r-morinaga@oitapref-hosp.jp
7 Department of Respiratory Medicine, Iizuka Hospital, Iizuka, 8208505 Japan; nebi1@aih-net.com
8 Department of Respiratory Medicine, Kumamoto University Hospital, Kumamoto 8608556, Japan; saeshow@wg7.so-net.ne.jp
9 Department of Internal Medicine, Kagoshima City Hospital, Kagoshima 8908544, Japan; kmatsukiz@yahoo.co.jp
10 Department of Internal Medicine, Saiseikai Fukuoka General Hospital, Fukuoka 8100001, Japan; h-wataya@saiseikai-hp.chuo.fukuoka.jp
* Correspondence: uchino@koto.kpu-m.ac.jp

Abstract: Background: As docetaxel plus S-1 may be feasible for cancer treatment, we conducted a phase I/II trial to determine the recommended docetaxel dose and the fixed S-1 dose (phase I), as well as confirm the regimen's efficacy and safety (phase II) for previously-treated patients with advanced non-small cell lung cancer. Methods: Patients ≤75 years with performance status ≤1 and adequate organ function were treated at three-week intervals with docetaxel on day 1 and 80 mg/m^2 oral S-1 from days 1–14. The starting docetaxel dose was 45 mg/m^2 and this was escalated to a maximum of 70 mg/m^2. In phase II, response rate, progression-free survival (PFS), overall survival (OS), and safety were assessed. Results: The recommended doses were 50 mg/m^2 docetaxel (day 1) and 80 mg/m^2 S-1 (days 1–14). Grades 3 and 4 leukocytopenia and neutropenia occurred in 44% and 67% of patients, respectively. Nonhematologic toxicities were generally mild. Overall response to chemotherapy was 7.7% (95% confidence interval (CI), 1.6–20.9%), and median PFS and OS were 18.0 weeks (95% CI; 11.3–22.9 weeks) and 53.0 weeks, respectively. Conclusion: Fifty mg/m^2 docetaxel plus 80 mg/m^2 oral S-1 had a lower response rate than anticipated; however, the survival data were encouraging. A further investigation is warranted to select the optimal patient population.

Keywords: non-small cell lung cancer; previously treated patients; phase I/II trial; chemotherapy; docetaxel; S-1

1. Introduction

Previous clinical trials confirmed that docetaxel alone displays good anticancer effects when used to treat non-small cell lung cancer. Treatment with docetaxel is associated with significant prolongation of survival [1]. Docetaxel is an antineoplastic taxoid prepared by partial chemical modification of the non-cytotoxic precursor 10-deacetyl baccatin III, which is extracted from the needles of the European pine. Its mechanism of action is to promote the polymerization and depolymerization of microtubule proteins, resulting in microtubule stabilization and microtubule hyperplasia, which prevent chromosome migration and arrest cell division in the M phase of the cell cycle [2]. Docetaxel is useful as a second-line chemotherapy for patients that are refractory to conventional platinum-based chemotherapy [3]. When combined with platinum, docetaxel displays better responses and survival rates than other platinum-containing regimens [4,5]. S-1 is a novel oral anticancer drug composed of the 5-fluorouracil (5-FU) prodrug, tegafur, and two 5-FU modulators, 5-chloro-2,4-dihydroxypyridine (CDHP) and potassium oxonate. CDHP selectively antagonizes the rate-limiting enzyme dihydropyrimidine dehydrogenase in the 5-FU degradation pathway and enhances antitumor effects by increasing blood 5-FU levels. Potassium oxonate also selectively antagonizes orotate phosphoribosyltransferase in the gastrointestinal tract after oral administration and inhibits the formation of 5-fluoronucleotides from 5-FU. In a previous phase II study, monotherapy with S-1 produced a significant response in previously treated non-small cell lung cancer [6]. Because docetaxel and S-1 have different mechanisms of action and toxicity profiles, it may be feasible and efficient to combine these drugs for the treatment of advanced non-small cell lung cancer. Previously, Yoshida et al. reported the feasibility and usefulness of this combination chemotherapy in a clinical trial for advanced gastric cancer [7].

To improve the response rate in previously-treated patients with advanced non-small cell lung cancer, we conducted a phase I/II clinical study of docetaxel plus S-1. In this regimen, docetaxel was administered on day 1 while S-1 was administered on days 1 to 14, according to the potential schedule dependency previously reported by Kano et al. [8]. The primary objectives were to determine the maximum-tolerated dose (MTD) and the recommended dose for this regimen in a phase I study and confirm its efficacy and safety in the phase II study.

2. Experimental Section

2.1. *Eligibility*

Patients were enrolled in this study if they met the following eligibility criteria: cytologically or histologically confirmed diagnosis of incurable, previously treated non-small cell lung cancer; no previous use of docetaxel or uracil plus tegafur (UFT); age between 20–75 years; performance status of ≤1 on the Eastern Cooperative Oncology Group (ECOG) scale; an estimated life expectancy of >12 weeks; adequate bone marrow function (leukocyte count ≥4000/μL, platelet count ≥100,000/μL, and hemoglobin level ≥9.5 g/dL); adequate hepatic function (bilirubin level ≤1.5 mg/dL and a serum ratio of aspartate amino transferase to alanine amino transferase (AST/ALT) ≤2.5 × UNL); adequate renal function (serum creatinine ≤1.5 mg/dL); a measurable lesion according to the Response Evaluation Criteria in Solid Tumors (RECIST) guidelines version 1.0; and provision of written informed consent. The exclusion criteria were: active infection, massive ascites or pleural effusion, symptomatic brain metastasis, uncontrollable diabetes mellitus, or severe comorbidity such as heart disease or renal disease, interstitial pneumonia, watery diarrhea, active concomitant malignancy, pregnancy or lactation, or other medical problems that could prevent compliance with the protocol. The following conditions were necessary: an interval of at least 4 weeks after the end of final therapy and recovery from the previous treatment.

2.2. *Treatment and Dose Escalation Schedules in the Phase I Study*

On day 1 of each cycle, docetaxel (Sanofi-aventis K.K., Tokyo, Japan) diluted with 500 mL of normal saline was administered as a 90-min infusion. S-1 (Taiho Pharmaceutical Company, Tokyo, Japan) was orally administered twice daily on days 1–14. The dose of S-1 was determined according to the patient's body surface area as follows: <1.25 m^2, 40 mg; 1.25–1.50 m^2, 50 mg; and >1.5 m^2, 60 mg. Combination chemotherapy was repeated every 3 weeks until progressive disease (PD) occurred.

In the phase I study, the starting dose of docetaxel was 45 mg/m^2 (level 1). Docetaxel dose escalation was performed as follows: in the patient cohorts containing at least 3 patients at each dose level, if none of the patients treated at a given dose level experienced dose limiting toxicity (DLT) as defined below, patients were entered at the next dose level (50 mg/m^2 at level 2, 60 mg/m^2 at level 3, and 70 mg/m^2 at level 4). If 1 or 2 of the 3 patients in the cohort experienced DLT, 3 additional patients were entered at the same level. MTD was then fixed and dose escalation was discontinued if all 3 patients in the 3-patient cohorts or ≥3 patients in the 6-patient cohorts experienced DLT. Adverse events were assessed in the first two cycles of the phase I study.

In the phase II study, the recommended dose of docetaxel determined in phase I was used in combination with S-1 in the same manner. The treatment regimen was repeated every 21 days until PD, patient withdrawal, or the occurrence of a serious adverse event. Granulocyte colony-stimulating factor (G-CSF) could be administered when either fever ≥38 °C with grade 3 or 4 neutropenia occurred. DLT was defined as: grade 4 neutropenia lasting for ≥4 days, grade 3 febrile neutropenia lasting ≥72 h, grade 3 thrombocytopenia, ≥grade 3 nonhematologic toxicity (besides nausea, vomiting, fatigue, and alopecia), ≥grade 2 interstitial pneumonia, or interruption of the S-1 medication for ≥7 days. If a patient experienced DLT, the docetaxel dose was reduced by one level in the subsequent cycle. To receive a subsequent cycle of chemotherapy, patients had to have leukocyte counts ≥3000/mm^3, neutrophil counts ≥1500/mm^3, platelets ≥100,000/mm^3, serum creatinine <1.5 mg/dL, and reduction in any treatment-related nonhematologic toxicity to <grade 1 (besides alopecia and neuropathy).

2.3. *Toxicity and Response Evaluation*

Toxicity was evaluated according to the Common Terminology Criteria for Adverse Events, version 3.0. Patients' symptoms and general condition were observed periodically. Physical examinations, complete blood counts with differential counts, serum chemistry, and urine tests were carried out at least once per week during the DLT-evaluation period. Tumor response was evaluated according to RECIST version 1.0 every month until the final tumor response was determined. Progression-free survival (PFS) was defined as the time from the date of registration to the date of the first documentation of PD or death. Patients with PFS were censored at the last date when survival was verified. Overall survival (OS) was defined as the time from the date of registration to the date of death. Surviving patients were censored at the last confirmation date of survival. This phase I/II study was conducted in accordance with the Declaration of Helsinki and approved by the Institutional Review Board at each participating hospital. The study was monitored by an independent data and safety monitoring committee.

2.4. *Statistical Considerations*

The primary end point of the phase II study was the rate of response to combination chemotherapy. The study was powered to detect a significant improvement of 18% relative to the 5% estimated from previous studies [1,3]. Assuming a one-sided a = 0.05% and 80% power, sample size was calculated to be 39 patients, with 6 patients at the recommended dose level in the phase I study. PFS and OS were assessed by the Kaplan-Meier method and log-rank test.

3. Results

3.1. Phase I Study

In total, 12 patients were enrolled in the phase I study. None of the three patients in the cohort at level 1 developed DLT. When the docetaxel dose was elevated to level 2, one patient experienced DLT, a grade 3 nonhematologic toxicity. The patient had phenytoin intoxication, which might be due to impairment of the P450 metabolic pathway by S-1. Because the remaining three patients in the cohort at level 2 had no DLT, their docetaxel dose was elevated. At level 3, two patients had DLT, prolonged grade 3 myelosuppression, and grade 3 interstitial pneumonia. The safety committee emphasized the risk of interstitial pneumonia and recommended the termination of the phase I study at level 3. As a result, the MTD and recommended docetaxel dose were 60 mg/m^2 and 50 mg/m^2, respectively.

3.2. Patient Characteristics in Phase II Study

A total of 39 patients (31 men, 8 women; median patient age, 64 years; age range, 46 to 75 years) were enrolled in the phase II study. Patient characteristics are shown in Table 1. The Eastern Cooperative Oncology Group (ECOG) performance status was 0 for 18 patients and 1 for 21 patients. Histologically, there were 24 patients with adenocarcinoma, 11 with squamous cell carcinoma, and 4 with no specified histology. Twenty-nine and 10 patients were at the clinical stages of IV and IIIb, respectively. A total of 120 cycles of therapy were administered. Treatment delay or interruption in the administration of S-1 occurred in 27 cycles (23%). The median number of cycles administered per patient was 3 (range, 1–9). The relative dose intensities were 97.7% for docetaxel and 85.7% for S-1.

Table 1. Characteristics of patients in the phase II study.

Characteristics	N = 39
Age, years	
Median (range)	64 (46–75)
Sex	
Men	31
Women	8
ECOG PS	
0	18
1	21
Stage	
IIIb	10
IV	29
Histology	
Adenocarcinoma	24
Squamous cell carcinoma	11
Not specified	4

ECOG PS: Eastern Cooperative Oncology Group performance status.

3.3. Toxicity

All 39 patients were included in the safety assessment. As shown in Table 2, myelosuppression was the principal toxic effect observed. However, the degree of myelosuppression was generally mild. Grade 3 or 4 leukocytopenia, neutropenia, thrombocytopenia, and anemia occurred in 17 (44%), 26 (67%), 0 (0%), and 0 (0%) patients, respectively. Nonhematologic toxicity was also generally mild and less frequent. Grade 3 or 4 toxicity primarily included loss of appetite (7.7%), fever (5.1%), and interstitial pneumonia (5.1%).

Table 2. Toxicities in the phase II study.

Toxicity	Grade 3	Grade 4	Grade 3 + 4
Hematologic			
Leukocytopenia	15 (38.5%)	2 (5.1%)	17 (43.6%)
Neutropenia	14 (35.9%)	12 (30.8%)	26 (66.7%)
Anemia	0 (0%)	0 (0%)	0 (0%)
Thrombocytopenia	0 (0%)	0 (0%)	0 (0%)
Nonhematologic			
Loss of appetite	3 (7.7%)	0 (0%)	3 (7.7%)
Fever	2 (5.1%)	0 (0%)	2 (5.1%)
Pneumonitis	1 (2.6%)	1 (2.6%)	2 (5.1%)
Stomatitis	1 (2.6%)	0 (0%)	1 (2.6%)
Diarrhea	1 (2.6%)	0 (0%)	1 (2.6%)
Hypercalcemia	1 (2.6%)	0 (0%)	1 (2.6%)
Elevation of γGTP	1 (2.6%)	0 (0%)	1 (2.6%)

3.4. *Efficacy*

Tumor response was evaluated in 39 patients. The median follow-up period was 8 months (range, 1–39 months). The following results were found for treatment response: complete response (CR), 0; partial response (PR), 3; stable disease (SD), 24; PD, 5; and not evaluable (NE), 7. The overall response rate was 3/39 or 7.7% (95% confidence interval (CI), 1.6 –20.9%, $p = 0.31$), a value that was not significantly higher than the threshold response rate statistically estimated from previous studies. The rate of disease control, CR + PR + SD, was 27/39 or 69%. Median PFS and OS were 18.0 weeks (95% CI, 11.3–22.9 weeks) and 53.0 weeks (95% CI, 40.9–134.6 weeks), respectively. The survival curves are shown in Figures 1 and 2.

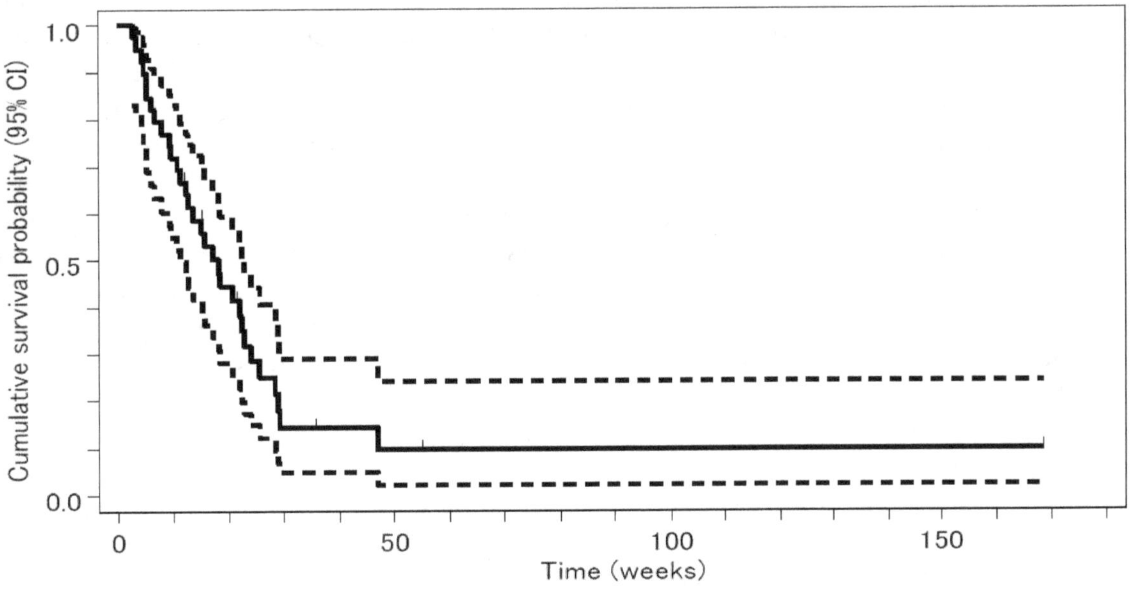

Figure 1. Progression-free survival (PFS) analyzed by the Kaplan-Meyer method is presented as a solid line. Median PFS was 18.0 weeks (95% confidence interval (CI), 11.3–22.9 weeks). The 95% CI is presented as two dashed lines.

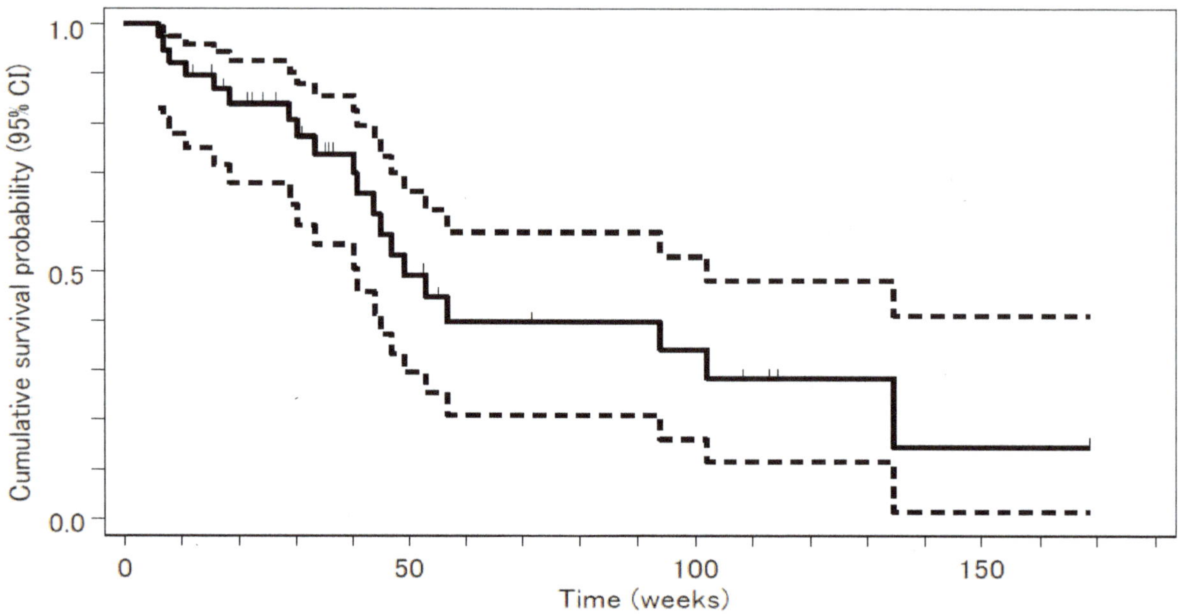

Figure 2. Overall survival (OS) analyzed by the Kaplan-Meyer method is presented as a solid line. Median OS was 53.0 weeks (95% confidence interval (CI), 40.9–134.6 weeks). The 95% CI is presented as two dashed lines.

4. Discussion

In the present study, response rate did not meet the 18% criterion needed to establish a significant improvement relative to the previously reported rate (i.e., the primary endpoint for the efficacy in the phase II study). However, combination chemotherapy was well tolerated and resulted in encouraging survival data.

Based on large-scale randomized controlled trials that compared 75 mg/m^2 docetaxel to optimal supportive care or other anticancer drugs, docetaxel monotherapy is considered to be a standard treatment for advanced non-small cell lung cancer in second-line settings [1,3]. Furthermore, S-1 was confirmed to be effective for previously treated advanced non-small cell lung cancer. Evidence for the efficacy of combination chemotherapy with docetaxel and S-1 has mainly been derived from studies on advanced gastric cancer. S-1 is one of the preferred agents for the treatment of gastric cancer. In fact, docetaxel displayed synergism with S-1 in vitro, improving the response rates in several phase II trials for advanced gastric cancer [7,9–11]. Wada et al. reported the decrease in expression of thymidylate synthase (TS) and dihydropyrimidine dehydrogenase (DPD) and an increase in expression of orotate phosphoribosyl transferase (OPRT) after co-treatment with docetaxel plus FU compared to 5-FU alone in gastric cancer cell lines [9]. DPD catalyzes the metabolic inactivation of 5-FU, while OPRT directly converts 5-FU to 5-fluorouridine-5′-monophosphate (FUMP), an active metabolite that displays anticancer effects. These changes in enzymes that metabolize 5-FU might clarify the enhanced effect of S-1 combined with docetaxel. As reported by Hasegawa et al., a similar synergistic effect is observed in castration-resistant prostate cancer [12]. Interestingly, in the xenograft model, S-1 with low-dose docetaxel could enhance the antitumor effect of S-1.

Several clinical trials have been conducted using docetaxel and S-1 for chemotherapy-naive or previously treated non-small cell lung cancer [9,13–17]. In fact, a triweekly schedule was employed with 40 mg/m^2 as the starting docetaxel dose. Previously, Oki et al. reported the usefulness of biweekly administration of docetaxel [16]. Table 3 contains a summary of results from these clinical studies. Other studies used a fixed docetaxel dose of 40 mg/m^2 + S-1 80 mg/m^2. The relatively low efficacy in these studies was perhaps due to the low fixed dose of chemotherapeutic agents. Therefore, we employed docetaxel dose escalation in the phase I part of the study, and confirmed that 50 mg/m^2 of docetaxel was effective. Moreover, S-1 dosage was determined depending on body surface area (BSA) in each patient in this study, because the fixed dose of S-1 may be too toxic for patients with smaller BSA or ineffective for the patients with larger BSA. Although the response rate in the current study was relatively low compared to that in other studies, the disease control rate was better than those of other studies (69% in this study, 68.9% in Atagi et al., 61% in Segawa et al., 84% in Yanagihara et al., and 49% in Oki et al.) and favorable PFS and OS were obtained. In addition, the PFS was longer than that reported in a previous phase III study [18] where treatment efficacy was compared between docetaxel and gefitinib for previously treated patients with non-small cell lung cancer in Japan; the PFS in the arm treated with docetaxel was 2.0 months. For toxicity, we found that ≥grade 3 myelosuppression was more frequent in our study and may be due to the higher docetaxel dose employed relative to other studies. Nonetheless, nonhematologic toxicity was demonstrated to be mild, and 50 mg/m^2 docetaxel plus S-1 was generally well tolerated.

Table 3. Summary of the results from previous trials of docetaxel plus S-1.

	Author			
	Atagi et al. [12]	**Yanagihara et al. [14]**	**Segawa et al. [13]**	**Oki et al. [15]**
N	29	28	31	49
Docetaxel	40 mg/m^2, day 1 every 3 weeks	40 mg/m^2, day 1 every 3 weeks	40 mg/m^2, day 1 every 3 weeks	35 mg/m^2, day 1, 15 every 4 weeks
S-1	80 mg/m^2, days 1–14	80 mg/m^2, days 1–14	80 mg/m^2, days 1–15	80 mg/m^2, days 1–14
ORR	24.1%	18.4%	16.1%	16.3%
PFS (mo)	3.9	4.4	3.4	3
OS (mo)	11.8	16.1	8.7	9

ORR: overall response rate; OS: overall survival; PFS: progression-free survival.

Takeda et al. reported that in advanced non-small cell lung cancer, the expression of TS and DPD are associated with the response to S-1 and carboplatin [19]. At a low level, their expression was found to be associated with a better response and a longer survival in patients treated with S-1 and carboplatin. Altogether, the expression levels of TS and DPD may be predictive markers for the response to regimens containing S-1. Histologically, squamous cell carcinoma and high-grade carcinoma display higher expression levels for the TS protein and mRNA in non-small cell lung cancer [20,21]. Therefore, a selected patient population with lower expression levels of TS may be most suitable for treatment regimens containing TS-inhibiting agents such as the combination of docetaxel and S-1. We have a plan to conduct a study considering this in the future.

Author Contributions: Conceptualization, K.T. and Y.N.; methodology, K.T.; software, S.T.; validation, S.T., K.T., and J.U.; formal analysis, S.T.; investigation, M.F., T.I., R.M., N.E., S.S., K.M., H.W., and T.Y.; data curation, S.T.; writing—original draft preparation, K.T.; writing—review and editing, J.U.; supervision, Y.N.; funding acquisition, Y.N.

Acknowledgments: We thank the staff at the Clinical Research Support Center Kyushu for their secretarial assistance and for preparing the manuscript.

References

1. Shepherd, F.A.; Dancey, J.; Ramlau, R.; Mattson, K.; Gralla, R.; O'Rourke, M.; Levitan, N.; Gressot, L.; Vincent, M.; Burkes, R.; et al. Prospective randomized trial of docetaxel versus best supportive care in patients with non-small cell lung cancer previously treated with platinum-based chemotherapy. *J. Clin. Oncol.* **2000**, *18*, 2095–2103. [CrossRef] [PubMed]
2. Ringel, I.; Horwitz, S.B. Studies with RP 56976 (taxotere): A semisynthetic analogue of taxol. *J. Natl. Cancer Inst.* **1991**, *83*, 288–291. [CrossRef]

3. Fossella, F.V.; DeVore, R.; Kerr, R.N.; Crawford, J.; Natale, R.R.; Dunphy, F.; Kalman, L.; Miller, V.; Lee, J.S.; Moore, M.; et al. Randomized phase III trial of docetaxel versus vinorelbine or ifosfamide in patients with advanced non-small cell lung cancer previously treated with platinum-containing chemotherapy regimens. *J. Clin. Oncol.* **2000**, *18*, 2354–2362. [CrossRef] [PubMed]
4. Kubota, K.; Watanabe, K.; Kunitoh, H.; Noda, K.; Ichinose, Y.; Katakami, N.; Sugiura, T.; Kawahara, M.; Yokoyama, A.; Yokota, S.; et al. Phase III randomized trial of docetaxel plus cisplatin versus vindesine plus cisplatin in patients with stage IV non-small cell lung cancer: The Japanese Taxotere Lung Cancer Study Group. *J. Clin. Oncol.* **2004**, *22*, 254–261. [CrossRef] [PubMed]
5. Fossella, F.V.; Rigas, J. The use of docetaxel (Taxotere) in patients with advanced non-small cell lung cancer previously treated with platinum-containing chemothepy regimens. *Semin. Oncol.* **1999**, *26*, 9–12. [PubMed]
6. Kawahara, M.; Furuse, K.; Segawa, Y.; Yoshimori, K.; Matsui, K.; Kudoh, S.; Hasegawa, K.; Niitani, H.; S-1 Cooperative Study Group (Lung Cancer Working Group). Phase II study of S-1, a novel oral fluorouracil, in advanced non-small-cell lung cancer. *Br. J. Cancer* **2001**, *85*, 939–943. [CrossRef] [PubMed]
7. Yoshida, K.; Ninomiya, N.; Takakura, N.; Hirabayashi, N.; Takiyama, W.; Sato, Y.; Todo, S.; Terashima, M.; Gotoh, M.; Sakamoto, J.; et al. Phase II study of docetaxel and S-1 combination therapy for advanced or recurrent gastric cancer. *Clin. Cancer Res.* **2006**, *12*, 3402–3407. [CrossRef]
8. Kano, Y.; Akutsu, M.; Tsunoda, S.; Ando, J.; Matsui, J.; Suzuki, K.; Ikeda, T.; Inoue, Y.; Adachi, K. Schedule-dependent interaction between paclitaxel and 5-fluorouracil in human carcinoma cell lines in vitro. *Br. J. Cancer* **1996**, *74*, 704–710. [CrossRef]
9. Wada, Y.; Yoshida, K.; Suzuki, T.; Mizuiri, H.; Konishi, K.; Ukon, K.; Tanabe, K.; Sakata, Y.; Fukushima, M. Synergistic effects of docetaxel and S-1 by modulating the expression of metabolic enzymes of 5-fluorouracil in human gastric cancer cell lines. *Int. J. Cancer* **2006**, *119*, 783–791. [CrossRef]
10. Yamaguchi, K.; Shimamura, T.; Hyodo, I.; Koizumi, W.; Doi, T.; Narahara, H.; Komatsu, Y.; Kato, T.; Saitoh, S.; Akiya, T.; et al. Phase I/II study of docetaxel and S-1 in patients with advanced gastric cancer. *Br. J. Cancer* **2006**, *94*, 1803–1808. [CrossRef]
11. Park, S.R.; Kim, H.K.; Kim, C.G.; Choi, I.J.; Lee, J.S.; Lee, J.H.; Ryu, K.W.; Kim, Y.W.; Bae, J.M.; Kim, N.K. Phase I/II study of S-1 combined with weekly docetaxel in patients with metastatic gastric carcinoma. *Br. J. Cancer* **2008**, *98*, 1305–1311. [CrossRef] [PubMed]
12. Hasegawa, M.; Miyajima, A.; Kosaka, T.; Yasumizu, Y.; Tanaka, N.; Maeda, T.; Shirotake, S.; Ide, H.; Kikuchi, E.; Oya, M. Low-dose docetaxel enhances the sensitivity of S-1 in a xenograft model of human castration resistant prostate cancer. *Int. J. Cancer* **2012**, *130*, 431–442. [CrossRef] [PubMed]
13. Atagi, S.; Kawahara, M.; Kusunoki, Y.; Takada, M.; Kawaguchi, T.; Okishio, K.; Kubo, A.; Uehira, K.; Yumine, K.; Tomizawa, Y.; et al. Phase I/II study of docetaxel and S-1 in patients with previously treated non-small cell lung cancer. *J. Thorac. Oncol.* **2008**, *3*, 1012–1017. [CrossRef] [PubMed]
14. Segawa, Y.; Kiura, K.; Hotta, K.; Takigawa, N.; Tabata, M.; Matsuo, K.; Yoshioka, H.; Hayashi, H.; Kawai, H.; Aoe, K.; et al. A randomized phase II study of a combination of docetaxel and S-1 versus docetaxel monotherapy in patients with non-small cell lung cancer previously treated with platinum-based chemotherapy. *J. Thorac. Oncol.* **2010**, *5*, 1430–1434. [CrossRef] [PubMed]
15. Yanagihara, K.; Yoshimura, K.; Niimi, M.; Yasuda, H.; Sasaki, T.; Nishimura, T.; Ishiguro, H.; Matsumoto, S.; Kitano, T.; Kanai, M.; et al. Phase II study of S-1 and docetaxel for previously treated patients with locally advanced or metastatic non-small cell lung cancer. *Cancer Chemother. Pharmacol.* **2010**, *66*, 913–918. [CrossRef]
16. Oki, Y.; Hirose, T.; Yamaoka, T.; Kusumoto, S.; Shirai, T.; Sugiyama, T.; Okuda, K.; Nakashima, M.; Murata, Y.; Ohmori, T.; et al. Phase II study of S-1, a novel oral fluoropyrimidine, and biweekly administration of docetaxel for previously treated advanced non-small-cell lung cancer. *Cancer Chemother. Pharmacol.* **2011**, *67*, 791–797. [CrossRef]
17. Takiguchi, Y.; Tada, Y.; Gemma, A.; Kudoh, S.; Hino, M.; Yoshimori, K.; Yoshimura, A.; Nagao, K.; Niitani, H. Phase I/II study of docetaxel and S-1, an oral fluorinated pyrimidine, for untreated advanced non-small cell lung cancer. *Lung Cancer* **2010**, *68*, 409–414. [CrossRef]
18. Maruyama, R.; Nishiwaki, Y.; Tamura, T.; Yamamoto, N.; Tsuboi, M.; Nakagawa, K.; Shinkai, T.; Negoro, S.; Imamura, F.; Eguchi, K.; et al. Phase III study, V-15-32, of gefitinib versus docetaxel in previously treated Japanese patients with non-small cell lung cancer. *J. Clin. Oncol.* **2008**, *26*, 4244–4252. [CrossRef]

19. Takeda, M.; Okamoto, I.; Hirabayashi, N.; Kitano, M.; Nakagawa, K. Thymidiylate synthase and dihydropyrimidine dehydrogenase expression levels are associated with response to S-1 plus carboplatin in advanced non-small cell lung cancer. *Lung Cancer* **2011**, *73*, 103–109. [CrossRef]
20. Ceppi, P.; Volante, M.; Saviozzi, S.; Rapa, I.; Novello, S.; Cambieri, A.; Lacono, M.L.; Cappia, S.; Papotti, M.; Scagliotti, G.V. Squamous cell carcinoma of the lung compared with other histotypes shows higher messenger RNA and protein levels for thymidylate synthase. *Cancer* **2006**, *107*, 1589–1596. [CrossRef]
21. Chen, C.Y.; Chang, Y.L.; Shih, J.Y.; Lin, J.W.; Chen, K.Y.; Yang, C.H.; Yu, C.J.; Yang, P.C. Thymidylate synthase and dihydrofolate reductase expression in non-small cell lung carcinoma: The association with treatment efficacy of pemetrexed. *Lung Cancer* **2011**, *74*, 132–138. [CrossRef] [PubMed]

18

RAD51B^{me} Levels as a Potential Predictive Biomarker for PD-1 Blockade Response in Non-Small Cell Lung Cancer

Inês Maria Guerreiro [1,*,†], Daniela Barros-Silva [2,†], Paula Lopes [2,3], Mariana Cantante [2,3], Ana Luísa Cunha [2,3], João Lobo [2,3,4], Luís Antunes [5], Ana Rodrigues [1], Marta Soares [1], Rui Henrique [2,3,4] and Carmen Jerónimo [2,4,*]

1 Department of Medical Oncology, Portuguese Oncology Institute of Porto (IPO-Porto), R. Dr. António Bernardino de Almeida, 4200-072 Porto, Portugal; rodriguesana@me.com (A.R.); martasoares71@gmail.com (M.S.)

2 Cancer Biology and Epigenetics Group, IPO Porto Research Center (GEBC CI-IPOP), Portuguese Oncology Institute of Porto (IPO Porto) & Porto Comprehensive Cancer Center (P.CCC), R. Dr. António Bernardino de Almeida, 4200-072 Porto, Portugal; daniela.barros.silva94@gmail.com (D.B.-S.); lopesanapaula.s@gmail.com (P.L.); marianacantantecf@gmail.com (M.C.); analuisa.cunha@ipoporto.min-saude.pt (A.L.C.); jpedro.lobo@ipoporto.min-saude.pt (J.L.); henrique@ipoporto.min-saude.pt (R.H.)

3 Department of Pathology, Portuguese Oncology Institute of Porto (IPOP), R. Dr. António Bernardino de Almeida, 4200-072 Porto, Portugal

4 Department of Pathology and Molecular Immunology, Institute of Biomedical Sciences Abel Salazar, University of Porto (ICBAS-UP), Rua Jorge de Viterbo Ferreira, 228, 4050-313 Porto, Portugal

5 Cancer Epidemiology Group, IPO Porto Research Center (CI-IPOP), Portuguese Oncology Institute of Porto (IPO-Porto), R. Dr. António Bernardino de Almeida, 4200-072 Porto, Portugal; luis.antunes@ipoporto.min-saude.pt

* Correspondence: ines.m.guerreiro@gmail.com (I.M.G.); carmenjeronimo@ipoporto.min-saude.pt (C.J.)

† Joint first authors.

Abstract: Lung cancer (LC) cells frequently express high levels of programmed death-ligand 1 (PD-L1). Although these levels grossly correlate with the likelihood of response to specific checkpoint inhibitors, the response prediction is rather imperfect, and more accurate predictive biomarkers are mandatory. We examined the methylation profile of *RAD51B* (*RAD51B*^{me}) as a candidate predictive biomarker for anti-PD-1 therapy efficacy in non-small cell lung cancer (NSCLC), correlating with patients' outcome. PD-L1 immunoexpression and *RAD51B*^{me} levels were analysed in NSCLC samples obtained from patients not treated with anti-PD-1 (Untreated Cohort (#1)) and patients treated with PD-1 blockade (Treated Cohort (#2)). Of a total of 127 patients assessed, 58.3% depicted PD-L1 positivity (PD-L1^{+}). *RAD51B*^{me} levels were significantly associated with PD-L1 immunoexpression. Patients with PD-1 blockade clinical benefit disclosed higher *RAD51B*^{me} levels ($p = 0.0390$) and significantly lower risk of disease progression (HR 0.37; 95% CI: 0.15–0.88; $p = 0.025$). Combining *RAD51B*$^{me+}$ with PD-L1^{+} improved the sensitivity of the test to predict immunotherapy response. PD-L1^{+} was also associated with lower risk of death (HR 0.35; 95% CI: 0.15–0.81; $p = 0.014$). Thus, *RAD51B*^{me} levels might be combined with validated predictive biomarker PD-L1 immunostaining to select patients who will most likely experience clinical benefit from PD-1 blockade. The predictive value of *RAD51B*^{me} should be confirmed in prospective studies.

Keywords: *RAD51B* methylation; PD-L1 expression; predictive biomarker; PD-1 blockade

1. Introduction

Lung cancer is the leading cause of cancer death in Europe, with an estimated 470,000 new cases (311,000 in men and 158,200 in women) in 2018 [1]. The estimated mortality in 2018 was 20.1% in both genders, being the most common cause of death from cancer in men (267,000 deaths, 24.8%) and the second most frequent in women (121,000 deaths, 14.2%) [1]. Most patients are diagnosed at advanced stages, with an overall 5-year survival rate of 4–17% depending on the stage and regional differences [2]. The incidence of lung cancer is directly related to tobacco smoking, which is the primary cause of lung cancer, accounting for about 80% to 90% of cases [3]. The risk of lung cancer increases with the extent of smoking measured by the number of packs of cigarettes smoked per day and with the number of years of smoking (pack-years of smoking history) [4].

Since the emergence of personalised targeted therapies, pathology plays a critical role because histologic and genetic features of lung cancer are important determinants of molecular testing and treatment decisions [5–7]. Lung cancer can be classified in non-small cell lung cancer (NSCLC) and small-cell lung cancer [5]. NSCLC is the most frequent class of lung cancer, representing 80% of all cases [4] and includes non-squamous carcinoma and squamous cell carcinoma as major types [5]. Non-squamous carcinoma includes adenocarcinoma, which is the most common subtype of lung cancer [4]. When clear adenocarcinoma, squamous or neuroendocrine morphology or staining pattern is not present, NSCLC is generally classified as not otherwise specified (NOS) [5].

Several predictive biomarkers indicative of therapeutic efficacy have emerged in lung cancer [6]. Immunotherapy, mainly immune checkpoint inhibitors, has changed the treatment paradigm of NSCLC. Immune checkpoints are important to control the immune responses in order to protect tissues from damage when the immune system is activated [8]. The expression of immune checkpoint proteins can be dysregulated by cancer cells, enabling immune evasion, a cancer hallmark [8,9]. Programmed cell death protein 1 (PD-1) is an immune checkpoint receptor expressed on the surface of activated T cells, including a large proportion of tumour-infiltrating lymphocytes from many tumours [8,10]. The binding to its ligands, PD-L1 and PD-L2, inhibits the response of cytotoxic T cells, hence the activation of the pathway PD-1/PD-L1 is a mechanism of immune-escape [11]. PD-L1 is commonly upregulated at the tumour cell surface [8] and is generally expressed in 20% to 40% of NSCLC [12]. There is evidence that infiltrating lymphocytes, mutational burden, and the expression of PD-L1 [13,14] are predictive biomarkers for treatment with checkpoint inhibitors. However, prediction of response is rather imperfect and, thus, more accurate predictive biomarkers are mandatory.

Genome instability leading to the accumulation of genomic aberrations is another characteristic of cancer cells [9]. Double-strand DNA breaks (DSB) may lead to mutations, chromosomal translocations, cell senescence and apoptosis [15,16]; hence, repair mechanisms are essential to maintain genome stability. Homologous recombination repair (HRR) is the leading DNA repair mechanism of double-strand DNA breaks (DSB) that uses the homologous region of the sister chromatid as the replicative template in order to reliably repair DSB [16]. *RAD51* protein has an important activity in HRR, promoting the insertion of the broken ends of the DSB into the sister chromatid [17,18]. Its action is dependent on *RAD51*-like proteins: *RAD51B*, *RAD51C*, *RAD51D*, *XRCC2* and *XRCC3* [17–19]. Defects in the HRR pathway entail cell proliferation despite DNA damage, promoting cancer development [20]. HRR pathway deficiencies seem to be associated with higher expression of PD-L1 and linked to an immune-evasive tumour phenotype [16]. Rieke et al. found that HRR genes hypermethylation is inversely correlated with mRNA transcription and associated with PD-L1 expression in head and neck, lung, and cervix squamous cell carcinomas [18]. As such, the methylation status of these genes could represent new predictive biomarkers for immune checkpoint inhibition.

The aim of this study is to investigate the association of immune checkpoint PD-L1 expression and the status of DNA repair gene *RAD51B* promoter methylation ($RAD51B^{me}$) in advanced NSCLC, correlating with patients' outcome. Additionally, the potential of $RAD51B^{me}$ levels as a candidate predictive biomarker for PD-1 blockade response in NSCLC was also assessed.

2. Materials and Methods

2.1. Patient Selection

We retrospectively analysed patients ≥18 years old, diagnosed with advanced NSCLC (adenocarcinoma, squamous cell carcinoma, and non-small cell lung cancer, not otherwise specified), at the Portuguese Oncology Institute of Porto (IPO-Porto) between 2014 and 2019. All tissue samples were obtained at the time of diagnosis. Samples were routinely fixed, and paraffin-embedded for standard pathological examination by haematoxylin and eosin (H&E) and specific immunostaining for tumour classification, grading, and staging, according to World Health Organization (WHO) Classification of Tumours of the Lung, Pleura, Thymus and Heart (4th Edition, Volume 7). Specimens were evaluated by two lung pathology proficient pathologists (ALC and RH). Biopsy samples available at the archive of the Department of Pathology were obtained for the "Untreated" cohort (Cohort #1, patients not exposed to anti-PD-1 blockade) and "Treated" cohort (Cohort #2, patients exposed to anti-PD-1 blockade anytime during the course of the disease) and were included after approval by the ethics committee of IPO-Porto (CES 15R1/2017).

2.2. Clinical and Pathological Data Collection

Relevant clinical and pathological variables were retrospectively collected for patients' characterisation, including pathological diagnosis (adenocarcinoma, squamous cell carcinoma, not otherwise specified), gender (female, male), age, smoking habits (never smoker, smoker, previous smoker), stage of the disease (stages IIIA to IVB were considered as advanced disease) and type of anti-PD-1 treatment (nivolumab, pembrolizumab, according to the current practice at the time).

All patients whose tumours displayed ≥50% PD-L1 expression did pembrolizumab as a first-line treatment [21], patients whose tumours had 1–49% PD-L1 expression did pembrolizumab [22] or nivolumab as second line treatment, and those with negative PD-L1 expression did nivolumab as a second-line treatment after progression of disease on or after standard platinum-based chemotherapy [23,24]. In patients whose tumours presented a driver mutation (epidermal growth factor receptor (*EGFR*) tyrosine kinase mutation, anaplastic lymphoma kinase (*ALK*) gene rearrangement or c-ROS oncogene 1 (*ROS1*) translocations), treatment with anti-PD-1 was done after progression on or after tyrosine kinase inhibitors and platinum-based chemotherapy.

Response to treatment was assessed by using the Response Evaluation Criteria in Solid Tumours (RECIST): complete response (CR)—disappearance of all target lesions, pathological lymph nodes must have reduction in short axis to <10 mm; partial response (PR)—at least a 30% decrease in the sum of diameters of target lesions, taking as reference the baseline sum diameters; progressive disease (PD)—at least a 20% increase in the sum of diameters of target lesions, taking as reference the smallest sum on study which must demonstrate an absolute increase of at least 5 mm; stable disease (SD)—neither sufficient shrinkage to qualify for PR nor sufficient increase to qualify for PD. Clinical benefit was considered if CR, PR or SD were present.

All procedures performed were in accordance with the ethical standards of the institutional and national research committees and with the 1964 Helsinki declaration and its later amendments or comparable ethical standards.

2.3. Assessment of PD-L1 Expression by Immunohistochemistry

PD-L1 (dilution 1:100, clone 22C3, DAKO) immunostaining was performed on a BenchMark Ultra platform (Ventana, Tucson, AZ, USA) using OptiView DAB detection kit (Ventana, Tucson, AZ, USA) and high pH buffer solution (CC1, Ventana, Tucson, AZ, USA for 40 min at 95 °C) was used for antigen retrieval. Appropriate positive controls were used for each antibody and negative controls consisted of omission of primary antibody. PD-L1 expression was assessed by a proficient pathologist (ALC) who determined the tumour proportion score (TPS), according to the European Society for Medical

Oncology (ESMO) guidelines. TPS was considered negative if <1%, positive intermediate if 1–49%, and positive strong if ≥50%.

2.4. Methylation Analysis

DNA and RNA were extracted from all clinical samples and cell lines using an FFPE RNA/DNA Purification Plus Kit (Norgen, Thorold, ON, Canada), according to the manufacturer's instructions. The bisulfide modification was accomplished using an EZ DNA Methylation-Gold™ Kit (Zymo Research, Orange, CA, USA) that integrates DNA denaturation and the bisulfide conversion processes into one-step, according to the recommended protocol. Evaluation of the DNA repair genes' methylation status was done by quantitative methylation-specific PCR (qMSP) assays and was performed using Xpert Fast SYBR (GRiSP, Porto, Portugal), according to the recommended protocol, in 384-well plates using a Roche LightCycler 480 II. Primers addressing the informative CpG sites within the promoter region were designed using Methyl Primer Express v1 and are described in Table 1. *β-actin* (ACTB) was used as an internal reference gene for normalization.

Table 1. Primer sequences for *ß-Actin* and *RAD51B^{me}*.

Gene	Forward (5′–3′)	Reverse (5′–3′)
ß-Actin	TGGTGATGGAGGAGGTTTAGTAAGT	AACCAATAAAACCTACTCCTCCCTTAA
RAD51B^{me}	AGATTTTTAGGGTCGAGAGC	CGCCCGACTAATTTTTTTAT

2.5. Statistical Analysis

Statistical analysis was conducted separately for each cohort.

Categorical variables are presented as counts and proportions and continuous variables are displayed as mean (standard deviation). Median (interquartile range) is used to describe variables with a highly skewed distribution.

Chi-square test was used to test the association between categorical variables; the Mann–Whitney U test was used to compare continuous variables with skewed distribution. A logistic regression analysis was carried out to identify predictors of PD-L1 expression. The variables considered in the logistic regression model were *RAD51B^{me}* (continuous), sex, age, smoking status and histological subtype.

The area under the receiver operating characteristics curve (AUC, 95% CI) was analysed to assess the performance of the *RAD51B* promotor methylation level as a predictive biomarker for PD-1 blockade response. Specificity, sensitivity, positive predictive value (PPV), negative predictive value (NPV), and accuracy were determined for PD-L1, according to positive vs. negative immune scores and for *RAD51B* methylation by applying an empirical cut-off obtained by ROC curve analysis (sensitivity + (1-specificity)). This cut-off value combines the maximum sensitivity and specificity, ensuring the perfect categorization of the samples as positive and negative for the methylation test. For the analysis of combined *RAD51B^{me+}*/PD-L1^{+}, the test was considered positive when at least one of the variables was plotted, as positive in individual analysis. Diagnostic biomarker performance was calculated, taking into consideration that all the patients included were subjected to anti-PD-1 treatment.

Progression-free survival (PFS) and overall survival (OS) were estimated by means of the Kaplan–Meier method for the Treated Cohort (#2). PFS was defined as the length of time from the beginning of anti-PD-1 blockade until disease progression or death from the disease and OS as the length of time from the beginning of anti-PD-1 blockade until death from any cause. The differences between groups were tested using the log-rank test. Hazard ratios (HRs) from multivariable Cox regression were used to quantify the association between clinicopathological features and survival. *RAD51B* promoter methylation level was considered positive if the quantitative value was above the 75th percentile. A *p*-value smaller than 0.05 (two-sided) indicated statistical significance.

All analyses were performed using IBM SPSS Statistics version 26.0 (SPSS, Chicago, IL, USA) and GraphPad Prism 7.01 (GraphPad Software, La Jolla, CA, USA).

3. Results

Between 2014 and 2019, 293 patients fulfilling the inclusion criteria were analysed. The median age was 64 years, 79.9% were male, and most of the patients (70%) presented adenocarcinoma. A biopsy sample was available in 127 (43.3%) patients (n = 64 in Untreated Cohort (#1) and n = 63 in Treated Cohort (#2)). PD-L1 expression was deemed positive in 58.3% cases (n = 31 in Untreated Cohort (#1) and n = 43 in Treated Cohort (#2)). Table 2 depicts patients' characteristics in the Untreated and Treated cohorts.

Table 2. Clinical and pathological data according to the testing cohorts.

Characteristics	Untreated Cohort (#1) n = 64	Treated Cohort (#2) n = 63
Gender, (n, %)		
Male	51 (79.7)	49 (77.8)
Female	13 (20.3)	14 (22.2)
Age (year), median (IQR)	62.5 (29.0–84.0)	62.0 (32.0–77.0)
Histologic subtype (n, %)		
Adenocarcinoma	41 (64.1)	46 (73.0)
Squamous	22 (34.4)	17 (27.0)
NOS	1 (1.6)	-
Smoking habits (n, %)		
Never	16 (25.0)	10 (15.9)
Smoker	20 (31.3)	20 (31.7)
Previous smoker	28 (43.7)	33 (53.4)
PD-L1 immunoexpression (n, %)		
Negative	33 (51.6)	20 (31.7)
Intermediate (1–49%)	18 (28.1)	14 (22.2)
Strong (≥ 50%)	13 (20.3)	29 (46.0)
Anti-PD-1 agent (n, %)		
Pembrolizumab	n.a.	38 (60.3)
Nivolumab		25 (39.7)
PD-1 blockade (n, %)		
Clinical benefit	n.a.	13 (20.6)
Non-clinical benefit		50 (79.4)
End of PD-1 blockade treatment (n, %)		
Not applicable		18 (28.6)
Disease progression	n.a.	39 (61.9)
Toxicity		6 (9.5)
Progression-free survival since PD-1 blockade, months median (IQR)	n.a.	8.1 (5.1–11.1)
Overall survival since PD-1 blockade, months median (IQR)	n.a.	21.3 (13.7–28.9)
RAD51B^{me} levels (normalized to β-actin), median (IQR)	0.54 (0.16–1.34)	1.08 (0.25–2.06)

n.a.—not applicable; IQR – Interquartil Range.

In the Treated Cohort (#2), 18 patients whose tumours showed ≥50% PD-L1 expression were treated with pembrolizumab in first-line; 19 and 3 patients whose tumours had 1–49% PD-L1 expression were treated with pembrolizumab and nivolumab, respectively, in second-line after progression on chemotherapy. Eighteen patients with PD-L1 negative tumours were treated with nivolumab as a second-line treatment. Four patients with adenocarcinoma carried driver mutations (3 had an *EGFR* tyrosine kinase mutation and 1 had an *ALK* gene rearrangement). As such, anti-PD-1 therapy was administered as a third-line treatment, after progression on tyrosine kinase inhibitors (first-line) and chemotherapy (second-line).

Regarding molecular analysis, *RAD51B*^{me} levels were significantly higher in PD-L1 positive vs. negative cases in both cohorts (Untreated Cohort (#1)—$p = 0.0216$; Treated Cohort (#2)—$p < 0.0001$) (Figure 1). Patients presenting higher *RAD51B*^{me} levels showed a higher chance of having a positive PD-L1 immunoexpression (Untreated cohort (#1) OR: 51.68, 95% CI: 1.77–1512.04, $p = 0.022$; Treated cohort (#2) OR: 45.51, 95% CI: 5.29–391.20, $p = 0.001$), adjusting for sex, age, smoking status and histological subtype (detailed information in Table S1). No differences in *RAD51B*^{me} levels were found between squamous cell carcinoma and adenocarcinoma cases in both cohorts (Untreated Cohort (#1)—$p = 0.774$; Treated Cohort (#2)—$p = 0.520$).

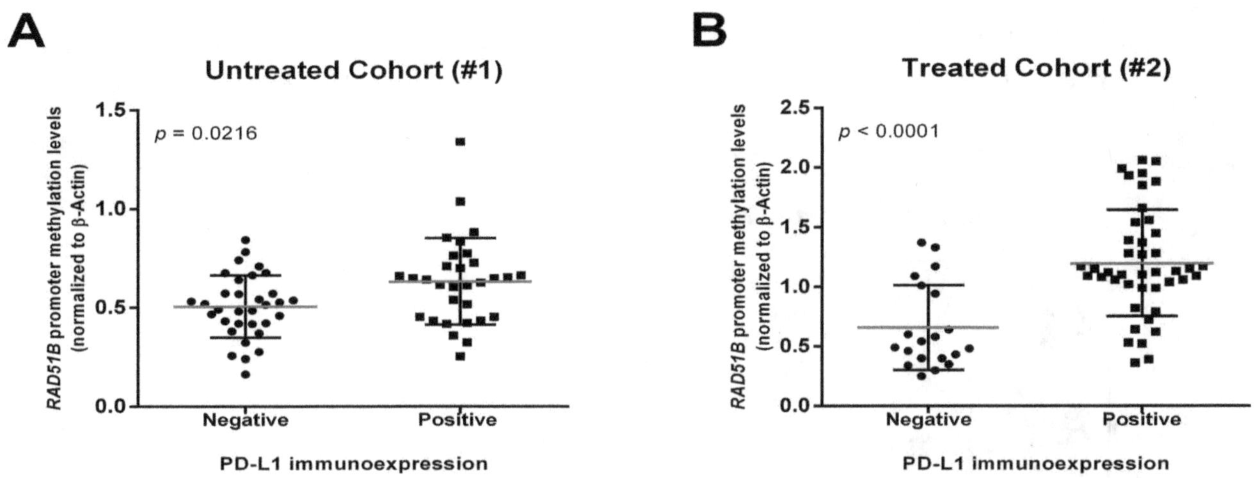

Figure 1. *RAD51B* promoter methylation levels within PD-L1 negative and PD-L1 positive immunoexpression among NSCLC samples. Scatter plot representing *RAD51B* promoter methylation levels distribution obtained by qMSP for (**A**) Untreated Cohort (#1) and (**B**) Treated Cohort (#2) patients, according to negative and positive PD-L1 immunoexpression. Mann–Whitney U-test. Red horizontal line represents the median methylation levels.

RAD51B^{me} levels were significantly higher in patients submitted to immunotherapy, which demonstrated clinical benefit ($p = 0.0390$; Figure 2A). Moreover, patients with positive *RAD51B*^{me} levels (*RAD51B*$^{me+}$ was consider when methylation levels >P75) disclosed clinical benefit independently from PD-L1 expression (Figure 2B). Additionally, *RAD51B*^{me} discriminated between PD-1 blockade clinical benefit and no clinical benefit with 85% specificity and 90% positive predictive value (AUC: 0.758, 95% CI: 0.626–0.889, $p = 0.0015$; Figure 2C and Table 3). Remarkably, combining *RAD51B*$^{me+}$ with PD-L1^{+} improved the sensitivity of the test (68%) to predict immunotherapy response, maintaining high specificity (85%) and increasing positive predictive value (94%).

Table 3. *RAD51B*^{me}, PD-L1 staining and the combination of the two variables performances as predictive biomarkers of PD-1 blockade response in the Treated Cohort (#2).

Predictive Biomarkers of PD-1 Blockade Response			
	***RAD51B*$^{me+}$**	**PD-L1^{+}**	***RAD51B*$^{me+}$/PD-L1^{+}**
Sensitivity	38%	74%	68%
Specificity	85%	54%	85%
Accuracy	48%	70%	71%
PPV	90%	86%	94%
NPV	26%	35%	41%

Abbreviations: PPV: positive predictive value, NPV: negative predictive value.

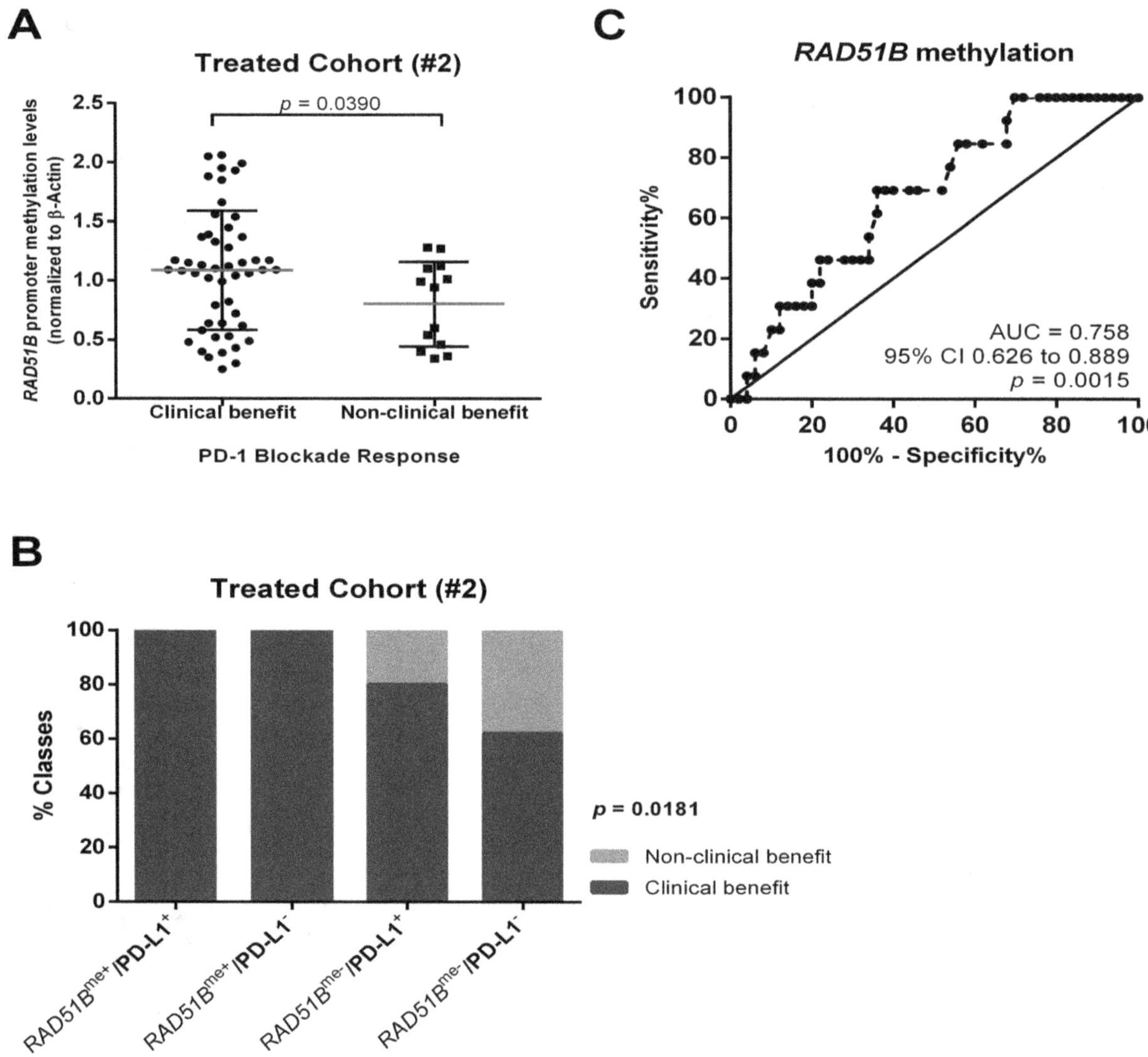

Figure 2. *RAD51B*^{me} levels and PD-L1 positivity associate with PD-1 blockade clinical benefit. (**A**) Scatter plot representing *RAD51B* promoter methylation levels distribution obtained by qMSP in patients with and without clinical benefit from immunotherapy. Mann–Whitney U-test. Red horizontal line represents the median methylation levels; (**B**) Contingency graph displaying the percentage of patients with and without PD-1 blockade clinical benefit, according to *RAD51B* promoter methylation and PD-L1 status. Chi-square test. *RAD51B*^{me} were considered positive when promoter methylation levels >P75; (**C**) Receiver operator characteristic (ROC) curve for discrimination between patients with and without clinical benefit from immunotherapy based on *RAD51B* promoter methylation levels distribution in the Treated Cohort (#2).

The median follow-up time for the Treated Cohort (#2) was 18 months (95% CI: 15.1–20.9). The median PFS was significantly higher in *RAD51B*$^{me+}$ patients ($p = 0.0216$; Figure 3A). Furthermore, patients with *RAD51B*$^{me+}$ disclosed a lower risk of disease progression (HR 0.37; 95% CI: 0.15–0.88; $p = 0.025$) compared with *RAD51B*$^{me-}$. Considering the PD-L1 expression, no significant differences were depicted for PFS ($p = 0.2023$), although PD-L1^{+} patients disclosed a trend for higher PFS (Figure 3B). Nonetheless, PD-L1^{+} associated with a longer OS ($p = 0.0307$) and a lower risk of death (HR 0.35; 95% CI: 0.15–0.81; $p = 0.014$). For *RAD51B*, lower methylation levels tend to associate with shorter OS, despite not being statistically significant. Also, no significant differences were observed for PFS or OS, when combining in panel PD-L1 expression and *RAD51B*^{me} levels.

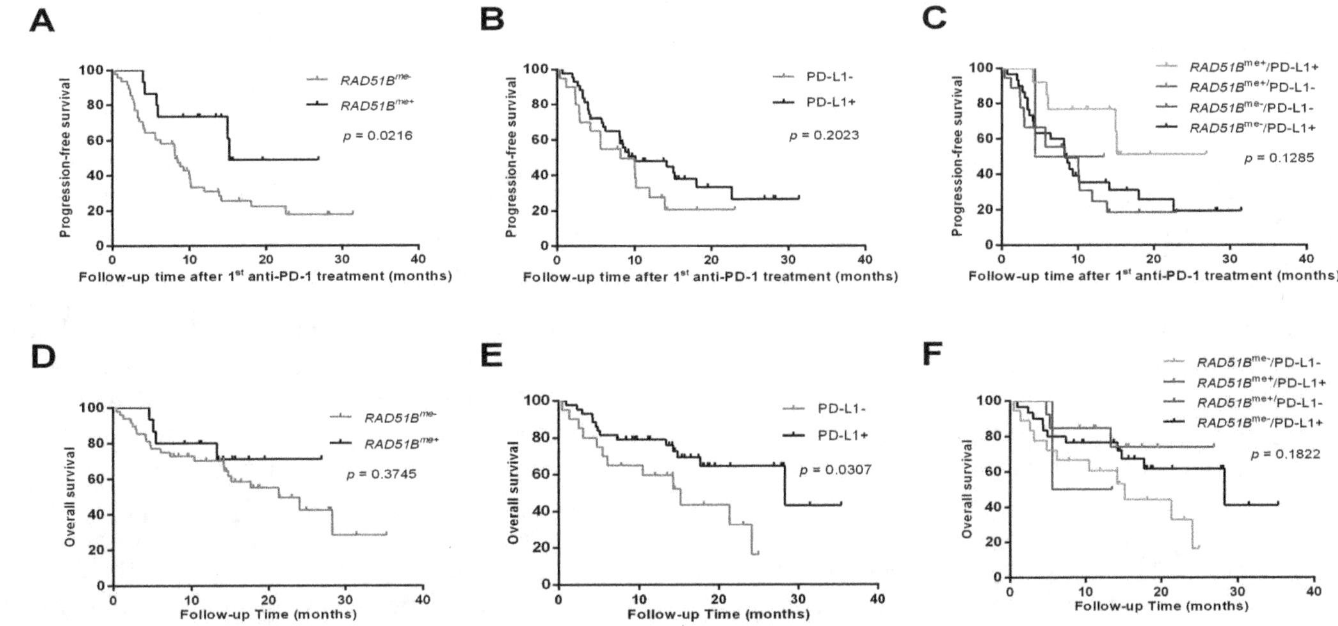

Figure 3. Kaplan–Meier survival curves for progression-free survival (after first anti-PD-1 treatment) of patients according to (**A**) *RAD51B*^{me} status; (**B**) PD-L1 status; and (**C**) combined *RAD51B*^{me} and PD-L1 status. Kaplan–Meier survival curves for patients' overall survival according to (**D**) *RAD51B*^{me} status, (**E**) PD-L1 status, and (**F**) combined *RAD51B*^{me} and PD-L1 status. Log-rank test. *RAD51B*^{me} was considered positive when promoter methylation levels >P75.

4. Discussion

Despite the improvement in lung cancer treatment over the last years, it remains a lethal disease in most cases, mostly due to diagnosis at advanced stages and suboptimal effectiveness of standard therapy. Nonetheless, the emergence of novel therapeutic strategies, including immune-based cancer therapies, has improved the prospects of patients diagnosed at advanced stages of the disease. Indeed, anti-PD-1 treatment for advanced NSCLC has improved the survival of patients [22]. Currently, the most commonly used biomarker to predict this response to anti-PD-1 therapy is PD-L1 immunostaining, although a substantial number of patients with PD-L1 positive immunostaining do not respond [21], highlighting the need for new biomarkers. In NSCLC, similar to other tumours, a higher tumour mutation burden was a strong predictor of immunotherapy efficacy [25–28]. Additionally, defects in the HRR pathway have been associated with higher expression of co-regulatory molecules such as PD-L1, suggesting that deficient homologous recombination, by disabling repair of DNA defects, may lead to neoantigens production with the recruitment of T-cells to the tumour microenvironment. This engages tumour cells to upregulate the expression of PD-L1 as an adaptive resistance mechanism [29]. A recent study demonstrated that DNA methylation profile of NSCLC might also be determinant for the efficacy of anti-PD-1 treatment in stage IV patients [30]. Furthermore, epigenetic alterations in *RAD51B*, specifically DNA promoter methylation, were associated with PD-L1 expression in squamous cell carcinomas [18]. This is a *RAD51* paralog, essential for DSB repair in the homologous recombinant pathway [17]. Thus, we sought to investigate the association of immune checkpoint PD-L1 expression and DNA methylation status of DNA repair gene *RAD51B* in non-small cell lung cancer (NSCLC), correlating with patient outcome.

Overall, the chances of positive PD-L1 expression in advanced NSCLC increased with the level of *RAD51*$^{me+}$. Remarkably, a link between *RAD51B*^{me} and the immune response in NSCLC has been previously suggested [29]. Furthermore, *Rieke et al.* demonstrated that methylation was associated with low mRNA expression levels and with homologous recombination deficiency [18]. Additionally, a significant positive correlation between *RAD51B* methylation status and the inflammatory gene signature, particularly, interferon-gamma (IFN-γ) was disclosed [18]. Interestingly, IFN-γ is an important inducer of PD-L1 expression, which acts via the JAK/STAT1/interferon regulatory factor (IRF) [31] in various types of cancers, including NSCLC. Furthermore, the depletion of *RAD51B* was shown to induce immune response through activation of the STAT3 pathway [32], which activates *CD274* gene/PD-L1 induction [31,33]. Therefore, our results further support the link between homologous repair deficiency by epigenetic regulation and immune checkpoint players, specifically PD-L1. Considering the available literature, assessing the inflammatory profile of these tumours might be useful to determine whether there is a direct effect between DNA repair candidate genes hypermethylation and the expression of immune checkpoint proteins.

Remarkably, $RAD51B^{me+}$ associated with better clinical response to treatment with PD-1 blockade and to a reduction of disease progression by 60%. Conversely, $RAD51B^{me-}$ associated with the absence of clinical benefit, which was even more relevant in negative PD-L1 expression cases. Hence, $RAD51B^{me}$ might constitute a potential biomarker of response to anti-PD-1 therapy. Although $RAD51B^{me}$ depicted lower sensitivity than PD-L1^{+} as a predictive biomarker for treatment with anti-PD-1, it displayed higher specificity.

Although PD-L1 expression has not been described as a strong prognostic factor mostly due to methodological approaches variations, including diverse immunohistochemistry antibodies, dissimilar evaluation for PD-L1 positivity (cut-off % or H-score) and patients' selection [13,34], in our study, both PD-L1^{+} and $RAD51B^{me+}$ associated with better overall survival. Conversely, another research team suggested that *RAD51B* overexpression associates with improved OS in NSCLC patients [35]. Notwithstanding higher promoter methylation levels might entail expression downregulation, several other genetic and epigenetic mechanisms may contribute to this apparent inconsistency. Furthermore, higher *RAD51B* methylation status was depicted in patients with longer progression-free survival after anti-PD-1 treatment, supporting once more the clinical benefit of PD-1 blockade when *RAD51B* promoter is methylated. The shorter overall survival of non-smokers patients may be partially explained by the fact that these patients had a longer median time (higher than 20 months) between diagnosis and the treatment with PD-L1 inhibitors than smokers.

Therefore, PD-L1^{+} and $RAD51B^{me+}$ are promising biomarkers to predict response to PD-1 blockade rather than overall prognostic factors in NSCLC's patients. As such, $RAD51B^{me}$ might represent a new predictive marker potentially assessable in liquid biopsies, allowing for a better selection of patients for anti-PD-1 treatment and eventually for monitoring patients' immunotherapy response throughout the course of the disease. Although our study paves the way for new prospective studies on the *RAD51B* promoter methylation's predictive role in patients with NSCLC treated with anti-PD-1, the retrospective design and small sample size are not neglectable limitations. Nevertheless, all the patients and samples enrolled in the study were analysed using the same criteria both for molecular biology strategies or clinical and pathological data collection. Importantly, other strengths of our research work are the fact that all patients were uniformly treated at the same institution, and all were evaluated by computed tomographic scans at specific timepoints during the course of treatment.

5. Conclusions

Herein, we confirm that higher $RAD51B^{me}$ levels associate with PD-L1 immunoexpression, as well as with immunotherapy's efficacy, in an independent advanced NSCLC patient cohort. Prospective studies, with larger cohorts of patients and extended follow-up periods, are warranted to validate these results and determine whether the methylation profile of this gene might be a predictive tool for selecting patients that will benefit from anti-PD-1 therapy.

Author Contributions: I.M.G. and D.B.-S. collected clinical and pathological data, performed the methylation analysis and the statistical analysis and original draft preparation. P.L. and M.C. did the immunohistochemical staining for PD-L1. A.L.C. and J.L., and R.H. assessed PD-L1 immunoexpression. L.A. contributed to the statistical analysis and interpretation of data. A.R., M.S. and R.H. contributed to the design of the work. C.J. contributed to the conception of the work, review and editing. All authors have read and agreed to the published version of the manuscript.

References

1. Ferlay, J.; Colombet, M.; Soerjomataram, I.; Dyba, T.; Randi, G.; Bettio, M.; Gavin, A.; Visser, O.; Bray, F. Cancer incidence and mortality patterns in Europe: Estimates for 40 countries and 25 major cancers in 2018. *Eur. J. Cancer* **2018**, *103*, 356–387. [CrossRef] [PubMed]
2. Hirsch, F.R.; Scagliotti, G.V.; Mulshine, J.L.; Kwon, R.; Curran, W.J., Jr.; Wu, Y.-L.; Paz-Ares, L. Lung cancer: Current therapies and new targeted treatments. *Lancet* **2017**, *389*, 299–311. [CrossRef]
3. Ettinger, D.S.; Wood, D.E.; Akerley, W.; Bazhenova, L.A.; Borghaei, H.; Camidge, D.R.; Cheney, R.T.; Chirieac, L.R.; D'Amico, T.A.; Dilling, T.J. NCCN guidelines insights: Non–small cell lung cancer, version 4.2016. *J. Natl. Compr. Cancer Netw.* **2016**, *14*, 255–264. [CrossRef] [PubMed]
4. Travis, W.D.; Brambilla, E.; Nicholson, A.G.; Yatabe, Y.; Austin, J.H.; Beasley, M.B.; Chirieac, L.R.; Dacic, S.; Duhig, E.; Flieder, D.B. The 2015 World Health Organization classification of lung tumors: Impact of genetic, clinical and radiologic advances since the 2004 classification. *J. Thorac. Oncol.* **2015**, *10*, 1243–1260. [CrossRef] [PubMed]
5. Mok, T.S. Personalized medicine in lung cancer: What we need to know. *Nat. Rev. Clin. Oncol.* **2011**, *8*, 661–668. [CrossRef]
6. Kerr, K.M.; Bubendorf, L.; Edelman, M.J.; Marchetti, A.; Mok, T.; Novello, S.; O'Byrne, K.; Stahel, R.; Peters, S.; Felip, E. Second ESMO consensus conference on lung cancer: Pathology and molecular biomarkers for non-small-cell lung cancer. *Ann. Oncol.* **2014**, *25*, 1681–1690. [CrossRef]
7. Pardoll, D.M. The blockade of immune checkpoints in cancer immunotherapy. *Nat. Rev. Cancer* **2012**, *12*, 252–264. [CrossRef]
8. Hanahan, D.; Weinberg, R.A. Hallmarks of cancer: The next generation. *Cell* **2011**, *144*, 646–674. [CrossRef]
9. Garon, E.B.; Rizvi, N.A.; Hui, R.; Leighl, N.; Balmanoukian, A.S.; Eder, J.P.; Patnaik, A.; Aggarwal, C.; Gubens, M.; Horn, L. Pembrolizumab for the treatment of non–small-cell lung cancer. *N. Engl. J. Med.* **2015**, *372*, 2018–2028. [CrossRef]
10. Petrelli, F.; Maltese, M.; Tomasello, G.; Conti, B.; Borgonovo, K.; Cabiddu, M.; Ghilardi, M.; Ghidini, M.; Passalacqua, R.; Barni, S. Clinical and Molecular Predictors of PD-L1 Expression in Non–Small-Cell Lung Cancer: Systematic Review and Meta-analysis. *Clin. Lung Cancer* **2018**, *19*, 315–322. [CrossRef]
11. Syn, N.L.; Teng, M.W.; Mok, T.S.; Soo, R.A. De-novo and acquired resistance to immune checkpoint targeting. *Lancet Oncol.* **2017**, *18*, e731–e741. [CrossRef]
12. Shi, Y. Regulatory mechanisms of PD-L1 expression in cancer cells. *Cancer Immunol. Immunother.* **2018**, *67*, 1–9. [CrossRef] [PubMed]
13. Wang, A.; Wang, H.; Liu, Y.; Zhao, M.; Zhang, H.; Lu, Z.; Fang, Y.; Chen, X.; Liu, G. The prognostic value of PD-L1 expression for non-small cell lung cancer patients: A meta-analysis. *Eur. J. Surg. Oncol. (EJSO)* **2015**, *41*, 450–456. [CrossRef] [PubMed]
14. Iarovaia, O.V.; Rubtsov, M.; Ioudinkova, E.; Tsfasman, T.; Razin, S.V.; Vassetzky, Y.S. Dynamics of double strand breaks and chromosomal translocations. *Mol. Cancer* **2014**, *13*, 249. [CrossRef] [PubMed]
15. O'Kane, G.M.; Connor, A.A.; Gallinger, S. Characterization, detection, and treatment approaches for homologous recombination deficiency in cancer. *Trends Mol. Med.* **2017**, *23*, 1121–1137. [CrossRef] [PubMed]
16. Rodrigue, A.; Lafrance, M.; Gauthier, M.C.; McDonald, D.; Hendzel, M.; West, S.C.; Jasin, M.; Masson, J.Y. Interplay between human DNA repair proteins at a unique double-strand break in vivo. *EMBO J.* **2006**, *25*, 222–231. [CrossRef] [PubMed]
17. Gachechiladze, M.; Škarda, J.; Soltermann, A.; Joerger, M. RAD51 as a potential surrogate marker for DNA repair capacity in solid malignancies. *Int. J. Cancer* **2017**, *141*, 1286–1294. [CrossRef]
18. Rieke, D.T.; Ochsenreither, S.; Klinghammer, K.; Seiwert, T.Y.; Klauschen, F.; Tinhofer, I.; Keilholz, U. Methylation of RAD51B, XRCC3 and other homologous recombination genes is associated with expression of immune checkpoints and an inflammatory signature in squamous cell carcinoma of the head and neck, lung and cervix. *Oncotarget* **2016**, *7*, 75379–75393. [CrossRef]

19. Thacker, J. The RAD51 gene family, genetic instability and cancer. *Cancer Lett.* **2005**, *219*, 125–135. [CrossRef]
20. Suwaki, N.; Klare, K.; Tarsounas, M. RAD51 paralogs: Roles in DNA damage signalling, recombinational repair and tumorigenesis. *Semin. Cell Dev. Biol.* **2011**, *22*, 898–905. [CrossRef]
21. Reck, M.; Rodríguez-Abreu, D.; Robinson, A.G.; Hui, R.; Csőszi, T.; Fülöp, A.; Gottfried, M.; Peled, N.; Tafreshi, A.; Cuffe, S. Pembrolizumab versus chemotherapy for PD-L1–positive non–small-cell lung cancer. *N. Engl. J. Med.* **2016**, *375*, 1823–1833. [CrossRef] [PubMed]
22. Herbst, R.S.; Baas, P.; Kim, D.-W.; Felip, E.; Pérez-Gracia, J.L.; Han, J.-Y.; Molina, J.; Kim, J.-H.; Arvis, C.D.; Ahn, M.-J. Pembrolizumab versus docetaxel for previously treated, PD-L1-positive, advanced non-small-cell lung cancer (KEYNOTE-010): A randomised controlled trial. *Lancet* **2016**, *387*, 1540–1550. [CrossRef]
23. Brahmer, J.; Reckamp, K.L.; Baas, P.; Crinò, L.; Eberhardt, W.E.; Poddubskaya, E.; Antonia, S.; Pluzanski, A.; Vokes, E.E.; Holgado, E. Nivolumab versus docetaxel in advanced squamous-cell non–small-cell lung cancer. *N. Engl. J. Med.* **2015**, *373*, 123–135. [CrossRef] [PubMed]
24. Borghaei, H.; Paz-Ares, L.; Horn, L.; Spigel, D.R.; Steins, M.; Ready, N.E.; Chow, L.Q.; Vokes, E.E.; Felip, E.; Holgado, E. Nivolumab versus docetaxel in advanced nonsquamous non–small-cell lung cancer. *N. Engl. J. Med.* **2015**, *373*, 1627–1639. [CrossRef] [PubMed]
25. Hellmann, M.D.; Ciuleanu, T.-E.; Pluzanski, A.; Lee, J.S.; Otterson, G.A.; Audigier-Valette, C.; Minenza, E.; Linardou, H.; Burgers, S.; Salman, P. Nivolumab plus ipilimumab in lung cancer with a high tumor mutational burden. *N. Engl. J. Med.* **2018**, *378*, 2093–2104. [CrossRef] [PubMed]
26. Rizvi, N.A.; Hellmann, M.D.; Snyder, A.; Kvistborg, P.; Makarov, V.; Havel, J.J.; Lee, W.; Yuan, J.; Wong, P.; Ho, T.S. Mutational landscape determines sensitivity to PD-1 blockade in non–small cell lung cancer. *Science* **2015**, *348*, 124–128. [CrossRef]
27. Rizvi, H.; Sanchez-Vega, F.; La, K.; Chatila, W.; Jonsson, P.; Halpenny, D.; Plodkowski, A.; Long, N.; Sauter, J.L.; Rekhtman, N. Molecular determinants of response to anti–programmed cell death (PD)-1 and anti–programmed death-ligand 1 (PD-L1) blockade in patients with non–small-cell lung cancer profiled with targeted next-generation sequencing. *J. Clin. Oncol.* **2018**, *36*, 633–641. [CrossRef]
28. Topalian, S.L.; Drake, C.G.; Pardoll, D.M. Immune checkpoint blockade: A common denominator approach to cancer therapy. *Cancer Cell* **2015**, *27*, 450–461. [CrossRef]
29. Bhattacharya, S.; Srinivasan, K.; Abdisalaam, S.; Su, F.; Raj, P.; Dozmorov, I.; Mishra, R.; Wakeland, E.K.; Ghose, S.; Mukherjee, S. RAD51 interconnects between DNA replication, DNA repair and immunity. *Nucleic Acids Res.* **2017**, *45*, 4590–4605. [CrossRef]
30. Duruisseaux, M.; Martínez-Cardús, A.; Calleja-Cervantes, M.E.; Moran, S.; de Moura, M.C.; Davalos, V.; Piñeyro, D.; Sanchez-Cespedes, M.; Girard, N.; Brevet, M. Epigenetic prediction of response to anti-PD-1 treatment in non-small-cell lung cancer: A multicentre, retrospective analysis. *Lancet Respir. Med.* **2018**, *6*, 771–781. [CrossRef]
31. Abdel-Rahman, O. Correlation between PD-L1 expression and outcome of NSCLC patients treated with anti-PD-1/PD-L1 agents: A meta-analysis. *Crit. Rev. Oncol. Hematol.* **2016**, *101*, 75–85. [CrossRef] [PubMed]
32. Marzec, M.; Zhang, Q.; Goradia, A.; Raghunath, P.N.; Liu, X.; Paessler, M.; Wang, H.Y.; Wysocka, M.; Cheng, M.; Ruggeri, B.A. Oncogenic kinase NPM/ALK induces through STAT3 expression of immunosuppressive protein CD274 (PD-L1, B7-H1). *Proc. Natl. Acad. Sci. USA* **2008**, *105*, 20852–20857. [CrossRef] [PubMed]
33. Akbay, E.A.; Koyama, S.; Carretero, J.; Altabef, A.; Tchaicha, J.H.; Christensen, C.L.; Mikse, O.R.; Cherniack, A.D.; Beauchamp, E.M.; Pugh, T.J. Activation of the PD-1 pathway contributes to immune escape in EGFR-driven lung tumors. *Cancer Discov.* **2013**, *3*, 1355–1363. [CrossRef] [PubMed]
34. Zhou, Z.-J.; Zhan, P.; Song, Y. PD-L1 over-expression and survival in patients with non-small cell lung cancer: A meta-analysis. *Transl. Lung Cancer Res.* **2015**, *4*, 203–208. [CrossRef] [PubMed]
35. Wu, M.; Sheng, Z.; Jiang, L.; Liu, Z.; Bi, Y.; Shen, Y. Overexpression of RAD51B predicts a preferable prognosis for non-small cell lung cancer patients. *Oncotarget* **2017**, *8*, 91471–97480. [CrossRef] [PubMed]

19

Prognostic Significance of Glucose Metabolism as GLUT1 in Patients with Pulmonary Pleomorphic Carcinoma

Hisao Imai [1], Kyoichi Kaira [2,3,*], Hideki Endoh [4], Kazuyoshi Imaizumi [5], Yasuhiro Goto [5], Mitsuhiro Kamiyoshihara [6], Takayuki Kosaka [7], Toshiki Yajima [2,8], Yoichi Ohtaki [8], Takashi Osaki [9], Yoshihito Kogure [10], Shigebumi Tanaka [11], Atsushi Fujita [12], Tetsunari Oyama [13], Koichi Minato [1], Takayuki Asao [14] and Ken Shirabe [2,8]

1 Division of Respiratory Medicine, Gunma Prefectural Cancer Center, Ota 373-8550, Japan; m06701014@gunma-u.ac.jp (H.I.); kminato@gunma-cc.jp (K.M.)
2 Department of Innovative Immune-Oncology Therapeutics, Gunma University Graduate School of Medicine, Maebashi 371-8511, Japan; yajimatos@yahoo.co.jp (T.Y.); kshirabe@gunma-u.ac.jp (K.S.)
3 Department of Respiratory Medicine, Comprehensive Cancer Center, International Medical Center, Saitama University Hospital, Hidaka 350-1298, Japan
4 Department of Thoracic Surgery, Saku Central Hospital Advanced Care Center, Saku 385-0051, Japan; hidend0509@yahoo.co.jp
5 Department of Respiratory Medicine, Fujita Health University, Toyoake 470-1192, Japan; jeanluc@fujita-hu.ac.jp (K.I.); gotoyasu510@gmail.com (Y.G.)
6 Department of General Thoracic Surgery, Japanese Red Cross Maebashi Hospital, Maebashi 371-0811, Japan; micha2005jp@yahoo.co.jp
7 Division of Thoracic Surgery, Takasaki General Medical Center, Takasaki 370-0829, Japan; tkosaka133@gmail.com
8 Department of General Surgical Science, Gunma University Graduate School of Medicine, Maebashi 371-8511, Japan; yohtakiadvanced@gmail.com
9 Department of Respiratory Medicine, Shibukawa Medical Center, Shibukawa 377-0280, Japan; tosaki@xb4.so-net.ne.jp
10 Department of Respiratory Medicine, Nagoya Medical Center, Nagoya 460-0001, Japan; yo-kogure@umin.ac.jp
11 Department of Respiratory Surgery, Isesaki Municipal Hospital, Isesaki 372-0817, Japan; tanakasigebumi@yahoo.co.jp
12 Division of Thoracic Surgery, Gunma Prefectural Cancer Center, Ota 373-8550, Japan; afujita@gunma-cc.jp
13 Department of Diagnostic Pathology, Gunma University Graduate School of Medicine, Maebashi 371-8511, Japan; oyama@gunma-u.ac.jp
14 Big Data Center for Integrative Analysis, Gunma University Initiative for Advance Research, Maebashi 371-8511, Japan; asao@gunma-u.ac.jp
* Correspondence: kkaira1970@yahoo.co.jp

Abstract: Glucose metabolism is necessary for tumor progression, metastasis, and survival in various human cancers. Glucose transporter 1 (GLUT1), in particular, plays an important role in the mechanism of ^{18}F-FDG (2-[^{18}F]-fluoro-2-deoxy-d-glucose) within tumor cells. However, little is known about the clinicopathological significance of GLUT1 in patients with pulmonary pleomorphic carcinoma (PPC). Adenocarcinoma, squamous cell carcinoma, adenosquamous cell carcinoma, poorly differentiated carcinoma, large cell carcinoma, and others were identified as epithelial components, and spindle-cell type, giant-cell type, and both spindle- and giant-cell types were identified as sarcomatous components. This study was performed to determine the prognostic impact of GLUT1 expression in PPC. Patients with surgically resected PPC (n = 104) were evaluated by immunohistochemistry analysis to detect GLUT1 expression and determine the Ki-67 labeling index using specimens of the resected tumors. GLUT1 was highly expressed in 48% (50/104) of all patients, 42% (20/48) of the patients with an adenocarcinoma component, and 53% (30/56) of the patients with a nonadenocarcinoma component. High expression of GLUT1 was significantly associated with advanced stage, vascular invasion, pleural invasion, and tumor cell proliferation as determined by Ki-67 labeling. GLUT1 expression and tumor cell proliferation were significantly correlated according to the Ki-67 labeling in all patients (Spearman's rank; r = 0.25, $p < 0.01$). In multivariate analysis, GLUT1 was identified as a significant independent marker for predicting a poor prognosis. GLUT1 is an independent prognostic factor for predicting the poor prognosis of patients with surgically resected PPC.

Keywords: pulmonary pleomorphic carcinoma; prognostic factor; glucose transporter 1

1. Introduction

Pulmonary pleomorphic carcinoma (PPC) is a rare disease with an incidence of 0.1%–0.4% among all lung cancers and shows a poor prognosis because of its resistance to systemic chemotherapy [1]. PPC includes carcinomatous and sarcomatoid components and is classified as a subtype of sarcomatoid carcinoma of the lung by the World Health Organization histologic classification of lung neoplasms [2,3]. Because of its rarity and low treatment efficacy, most patients with PPC exhibit recurrence even after complete surgical resection; moreover, there are no standard treatments for patients with advanced and inoperable PPC. The development of appropriate treatments and identification of predictive biomarkers are critical for improving the prognosis of patients with complex histologies, such as PPC.

Glucose metabolism is associated with tumor progression and metastases, and is used in molecular imaging, such as 2-[^{18}F]-fluoro-2-deoxy-d-glucose (^{18}F-FDG) positron emission tomography (PET), to detect cancers [4]. Although there are several types of glucose transporters (GLUTs), glucose transporter 1 (GLUT1) and GLUT3 are strongly expressed on the membrane of tumor cells, and a meta-analysis demonstrated GLUT1 to be a prognostic marker for predicting worse outcomes in patients with lung cancer [4]. ^{18}F-FDG accumulates in tumor cells via GLUT1, a process closely associated with poor prognosis and tumor progression in patients with lung cancer [5]. We previously showed that ^{18}F-FDG uptake in PPC is closely related to the presence of GLUT1 and angiogenesis, and that the accumulation of ^{18}F-FDG and the expression level of GLUT1 were significantly higher in patients with PPC than those with other nonsmall cell lung cancer (NSCLC) [6]. This indicates that tumor glucose metabolism involving GLUT1 plays a crucial role in the carcinogenesis of PPC. ^{18}F-FDG-PET can be used to detect primary and metastatic lesions for disease staging in patients with PPC. From a pathological perspective, studies are needed to determine how the expression of GLUT1 in cancer-specific glucose metabolism reflects the survival and metastasis of patients with PPC. However, little is known about the clinicopathological relevance of GLUT1 expression in patients with PPC.

In this clinicopathological study, we examined the prognostic role of GLUT1 expression in patients with surgically resected PPC.

2. Experimental Section

2.1. Patients

Between August 2001 and October 2015, 104 patients with histologically confirmed PPC who underwent surgical resection at multiple institutions were enrolled in this study. Pleomorphic carcinoma was diagnosed according to the 2015 World Health Organization Classification of Tumours [2]. Diagnoses were confirmed by light microscopy and immunohistochemistry. PPC was defined as NSCLC containing at least 10% sarcomatoid components. This study included 104 surgically resected primary tumors in accordance with institutional guidelines and the Declaration of Helsinki. The institutional review boards of all participating institutions approved this study. Mortality and recurrence were determined using medical records. The tumor samples were collected in our previous study [7–9].

2.2. *Immunohistochemical Staining*

GLUT1 expression was assessed by immunohistochemical staining using a rabbit anti-GLUT1 polyclonal antibody (Abcam, Cambridge, UK; 1:200 dilution). The reaction was visualized using the Histofine Simple Stain MAX-PO (Multi) Kit (Nichirei, Tokyo, Japan), according to the manufacturer's instructions. The detailed protocol for immunostaining has been published elsewhere [4]. Negative controls were incubated without primary antibody, and no staining was observed. GLUT1 expression was considered positive only if distinct cytoplasmic and plasma membrane staining was present. GLUT1 expression was scored as follows: 1, ≤10% of tumor area stained; 2, 11%–25% stained; 3, 26%–50% stained; 4, 51%–75% stained; and 5, ≥76% stained. Tumors in which the stained tumor cells were scored ≥4 were considered as "high-expression" tumors.

Immunohistochemical staining for Ki-67 was performed as described previously [4] using a murine monoclonal antibody against Ki-67 (Dako, Glostrup, Denmark; 1:40 dilution). Highly cellular areas of the immunostained sections were assessed for Ki-67. All epithelial cells with nuclear staining of any intensity were defined as high-expression epithelial cells. Approximately 1000 nuclei were counted on each slide. Proliferative activity was assessed as the percentage of Ki-67-stained nuclei (Ki-67 labeling index) in the sample. The median Ki-67 labeling index value was evaluated, and tumor cells with greater than median Ki-67 labeling index value were defined as high-expression tumor cells. All sections were assessed by light microscopy in a blinded manner by at least two investigators. In case of discrepancies, both investigators evaluated the slides simultaneously until reaching a final consensus. Neither of the investigators had knowledge of the patient outcomes.

2.3. *Statistical Analysis*

Statistical analyses were performed using Student's t- and χ^2-tests for continuous and categorical variables, respectively. Correlations were analyzed using nonparametric Spearman's rank tests. The Kaplan–Meier method was used to estimate survival as a function of time, and survival differences were analyzed by log-rank tests. Overall survival (OS) was defined as the time from tumor resection to death from any cause. Disease-free survival (DFS) was defined as the time between tumor resection and the first episode of disease progression or death. Univariate and multivariate survival analyses were performed using Cox proportional hazards models and a logistic regression model for radical surgery. $p < 0.05$ was considered to indicate statistical significance. All statistical analyses were performed using GraphPad Prism version 7 (GraphPad Software, San Diego, CA, USA) and JMP Pro version 14.0 (SAS Institute, Inc., Cary, NC, USA).

3. Results

3.1. *Patient Demographics and Immunohistochemistry*

GLUT1 expression was assessed in 104 patients (79 males, 25 females; median age 69 years, range 35–88 years) and correlated with patient's clinical information. All patients were diagnosed using resected primary tumors. Histologic analysis revealed that 29 patients with PPC harbored a combination of carcinomatous and sarcomatous components. In the remaining 75 primary tumors, carcinomatous components were identified in 48 patients with adenocarcinoma, 13 with squamous cell carcinoma, 8 with adenosquamous cell carcinoma, 2 with poorly differentiated carcinoma, and 4 with Pe. Of the sarcomatous components, 69 patients exhibited spindle-cell type, 10 giant-cell type, and 25 both spindle- and giant-cell types. Each percentage of epithelial and sarcomatous components is shown in Supplementary Figure S1. The day of surgery was considered the starting day for measuring postoperative survival. The median follow-up period was 476 days (range, 30–4519 days).

Patient demographics data according to GLUT1 expression are listed in Table 1. Immunohistochemical analyses were performed for 104 primary sites with PPC. GLUT1 was stained on the cell membranes of tumor specimens, and there was no evidence of normal tissue without red blood cells. Figure 1 shows the representative images of GLUT1 expression in patients with PPC. Figure 2 shows the distribution of GLUT1 expression according to a scoring system. The frequencies of scores 1, 2, 3 4, and 5 for GLUT1 were 11%, 3%, 25%, 32%, and 19%, respectively. The percentage of samples showing high GLUT1 expression was 48% (50/104). High expression of GLUT1 was found to be significantly associated with advanced stage, vascular invasion, pleural invasion, and tumor cell proliferation, as determined by the Ki-67 index. There was a significant correlation between GLUT1 expression and tumor cell proliferation according to the Ki-67 labeling index in all patients (Spearman's rank; $r = 0.25$, $p < 0.01$).

Table 1. Patient demographics according to GLUT1 expression.

Variables	**GLUT1 Expression in All Patients**			
	Total (n = 104)	**High (n = 50)**	**Low (n = 54)**	***p*-Value**
		Age		
<69 years/≥69 years	54/50	30/20	24/30	0.12
		Gender		
Male/Female	79/25	35/15	44/10	0.25
		Smoking		
Yes/No	84/20	40/10	44/10	>0.99
		T factor		
T1-2/T3-4	65/39	25/25	40/14	0.11
		N factor		
Absent/Present	72/32	33/17	39/15	0.53
		Stage		
I-II/III-IV	69/35	28/22	41/13	0.03*
		Lymphatic permeation		
Absent/Present	41/63	17/33	24/30	0.31
		Vascular invasion		
Absent/Present	31/73	9/41	22/32	0.02*
		Pleural invasion		
Absent/Present	48/56	17/33	31/13	<0.01*
		Adjuvant chemotherapy		
Absent/Present	77/27	35/15	42/12	0.38
		Ki-67 labeling index		
High/Low	50/54	31/19	19/35	<0.01*
		*** <0.05**		

* $p < 0.05$ was considered statistically significant. t-test score was for continuous variables, and χ^2 test for categorical variables.

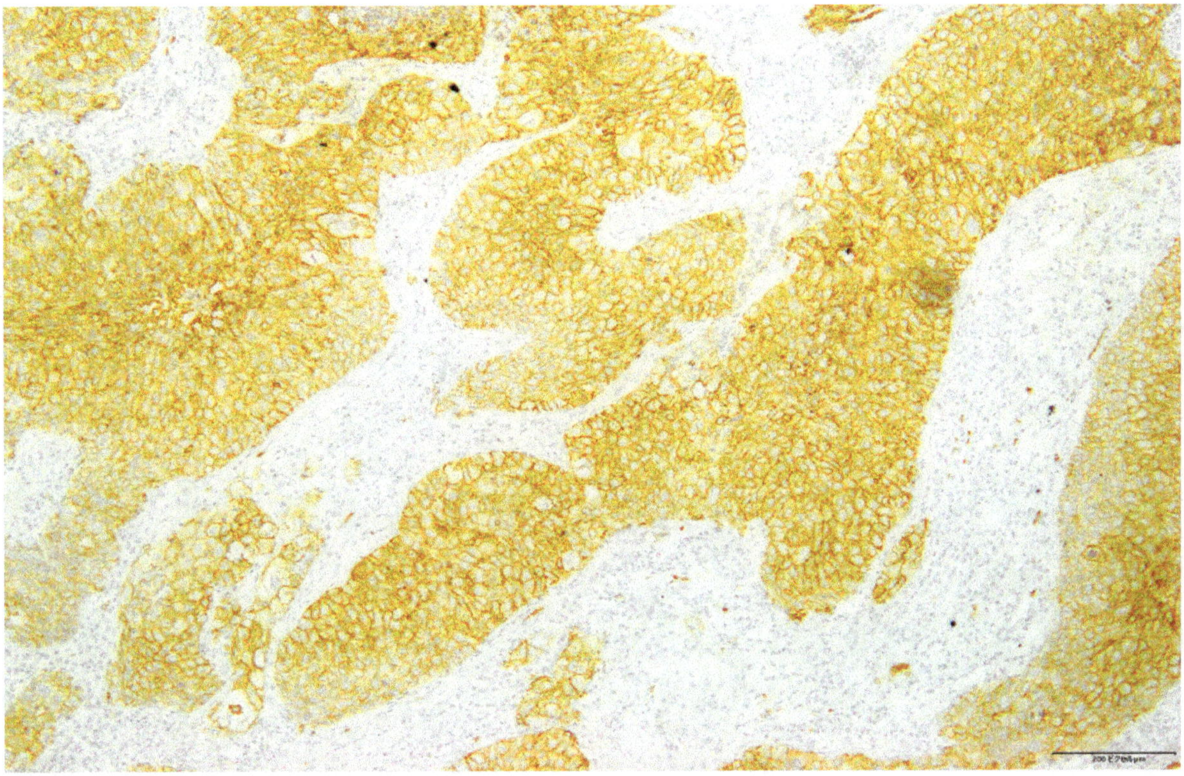

A

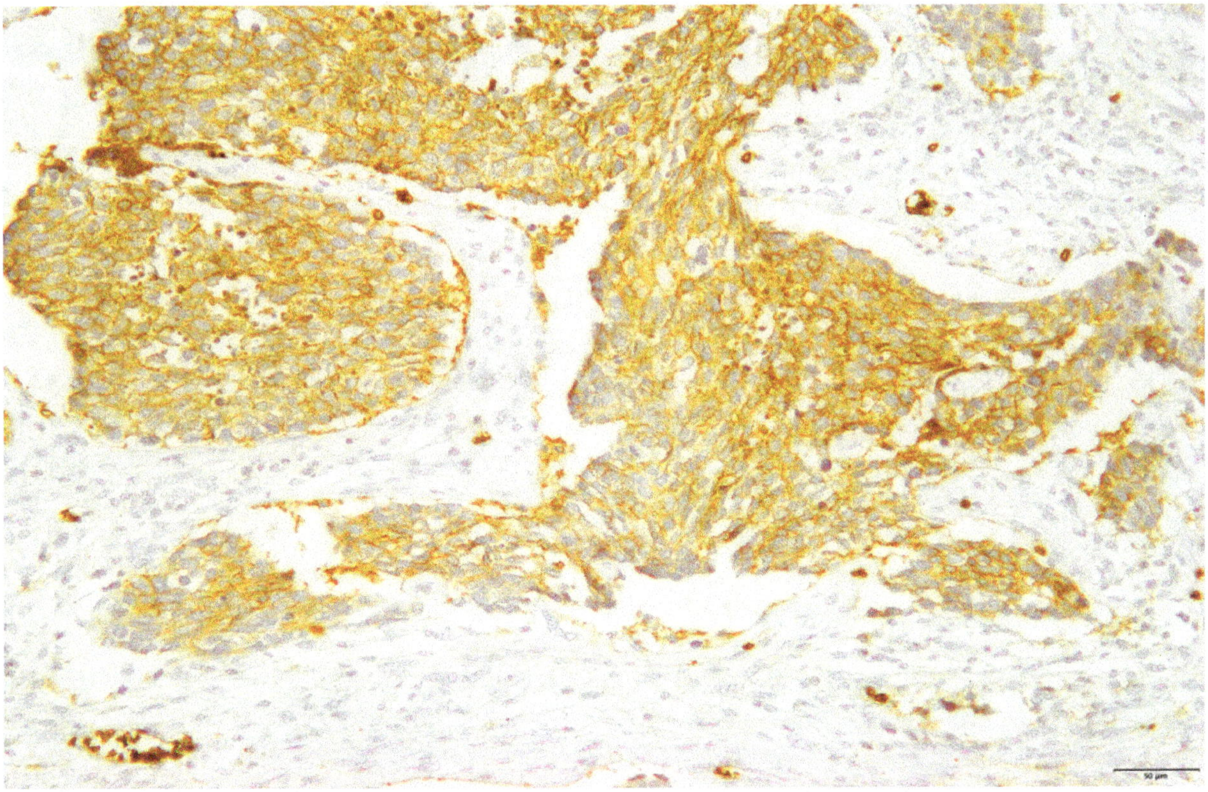

B

Figure 1. *Cont.*

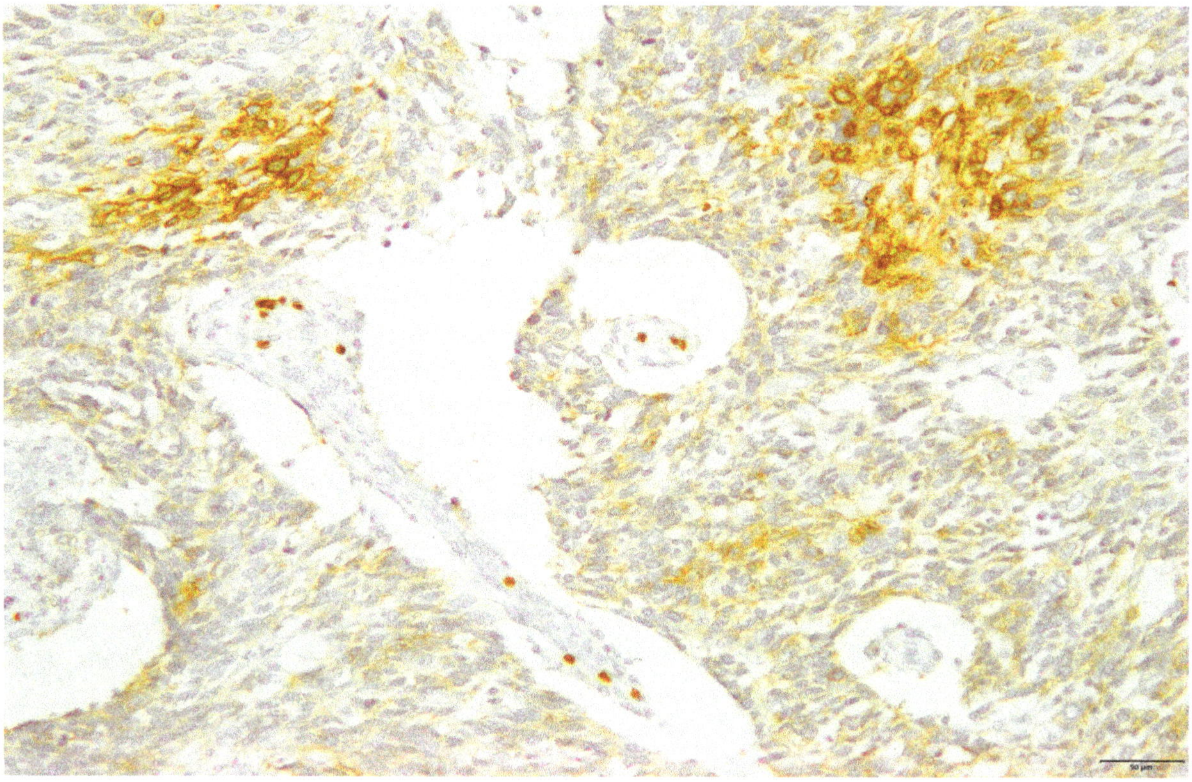

C

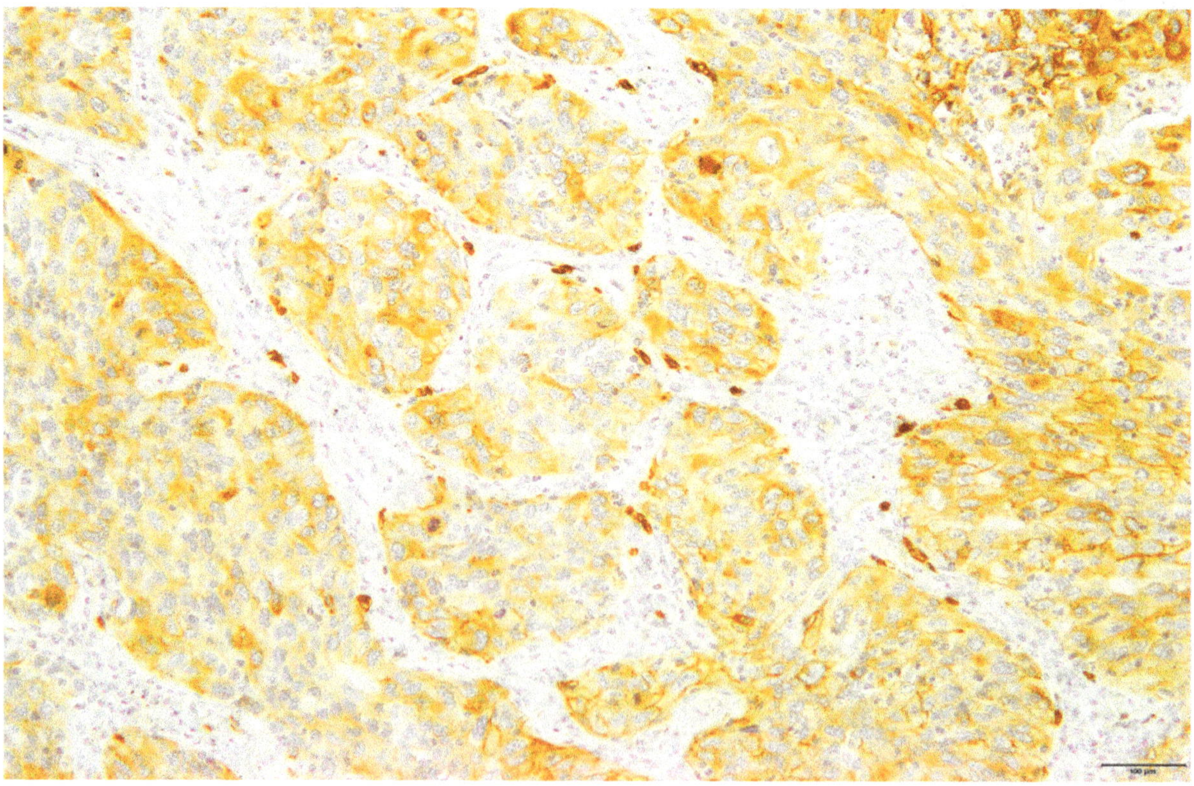

D

Figure 1. *Cont.*

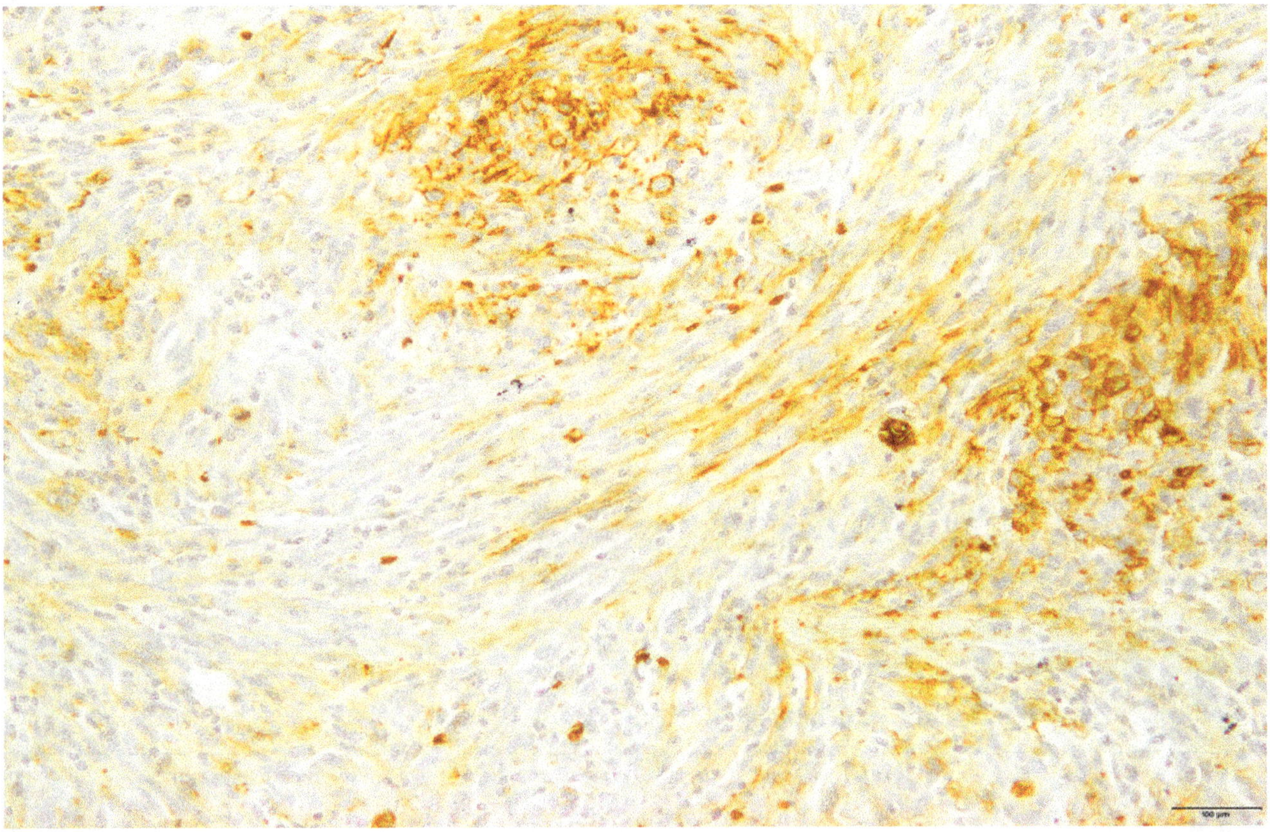

E

Figure 1. An 88-year-old male with PPC including a component of squamous cell carcinoma (**A**) GLUT1 was stained on the membrane of tumor cells, showing a score of 4. A 78-year-old female with PPC including components of squamous cell carcinoma and spindle cells: GLUT1 was stained throughout the squamous cell carcinomas (**B**) and partial lesions of spindle cells (**C**). A 77-year-old male with PPC including components of adenosquamous cell carcinoma and giant cells: GLUT1 was stained throughout the epithelial cells (**D**) and sarcomatous cells (**E**).

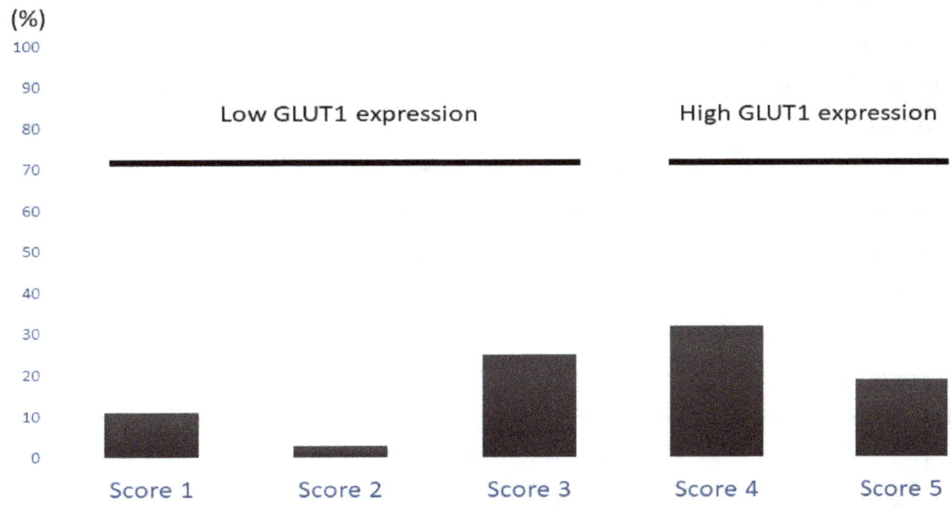

Figure 2. Distribution of GLUT1 expression according to scoring system. The frequencies of scores 1, 2, 3 4, and 5 for GLUT1 were 11%, 3%, 25%, 32%, and 19%, respectively.

Next, epithelial histological types such as adenocarcinoma (AC) and non-AC were assessed. No significant difference in the frequency of high GLUT1 expression was observed between patients with AC (20/48) and non-AC (30/56) ($p = 0.24$).

3.2. Univariate and Multivariate Survival Analysis

The median DFS and OS of all patients were 449 and 991 days, respectively. In the analysis according to the epithelial histology, the median DFS and OS of patients with AC and non-AC components were 522 and 1038 days and 336 and 507 days, respectively. In total, 60 patients died, and recurrence after initial surgery was observed in 59 patients. The above survival information has been previously described [7–9]. The results of the survival analysis are listed in Table 2. The Kaplan-Meier survival curve of all patients with high or low GLUT1 expression is shown in Figure 3. According to the univariate analysis, disease stage and GLUT1 were identified as significant factors for predicting worse OS after surgery and disease stage; pleural invasion and GLUT1 displayed a close association with poor DFS. The different variables with a cut-off of $p < 0.05$ were screened based on the results of the univariate log-rank test. In all patients, the disease stage and GLUT1 were confirmed as independent prognostic factors related to worse OS and DFS by multivariate analysis. Next, we analyzed the prognostic significance of GLUT1 expression according to the epithelial histological types of PPC (AC and non-AC component). Figure 3 shows the Kaplan-Meier survival curve of patients with AC and non-AC components. In univariate analysis, patients with a non-AC component with high GLUT1 expression showed a significantly worse OS and DFS than low GLUT1 expression compared to those with an AC component.

Table 2. Univariate and multivariate survival analysis in all patients.

Variables	Overall survival (OS) in Total Patients				
	Univariate Analysis		Multivariate Analysis		
	1-Year Rate (%)	*p*-Value	HR	95% CI	*p*-Value
Age (<69/≥69)	48/73	0.41			
Gender (female/male)	60/58	0.66			
p-stage (I-II/III-IV)	75/29	<0.01*	1.53	1.21–2.12	<0.01*
Ly (present/absent)	52/71	0.21			
v (present/absent)	59/61	0.23			
Pl (present/absent)	53/66	0.07			
Adjuvant CTx (present/absent)	66/57	0.18			
GLUT1 expression (high/low)	43/75	<0.01*	1.72	1.29–2.34	<0.01*
Ki-67 labeling index (high/low)	60/61	0.77			
	Disease-Free Survival (DFS) in Total Patients				
Age (<69/≥69)	41/69	0.12			
Gender (female/male)	58/46	0.17			
p-stage (I-II/III-IV)	67/31	<0.01*	1.58	1.19–2.09	<0.01*
ly (present/absent)	47/68	0.04			
v (present/absent)	56/62	0.08			
pl (present/absent)	43/71	<0.01*	1.15	0.57–1.02	0.07
Adjuvant CTx (present/absent)	57/52	0.97			
GLUT1 expression (high/low)	36/72	<0.01*	1.44	1.08–1.95	0.01*
Ki-67 labeling index (high/low)	51/59	0.64			

CI = confidence interval; *$p < 0.05$ is considered statistically significant, calculated with continuous variable; ly, lymphatic permeation; v, vascular invasion; pl, pleural invasion; GLUT1, glucose transporter 1; and HR, hazard ratio.

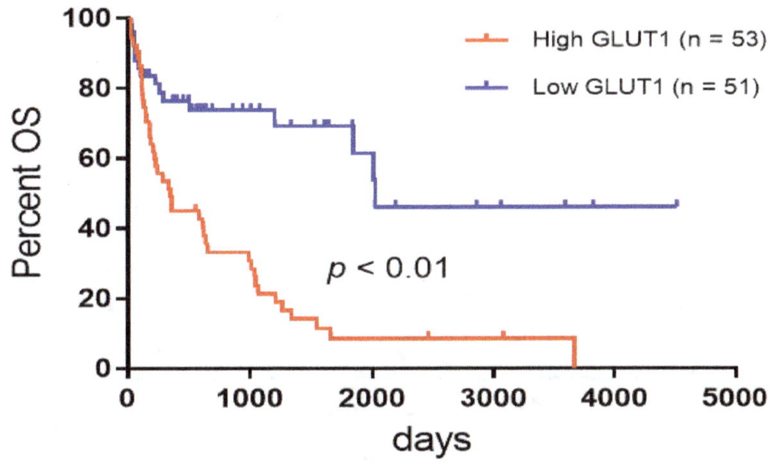

A

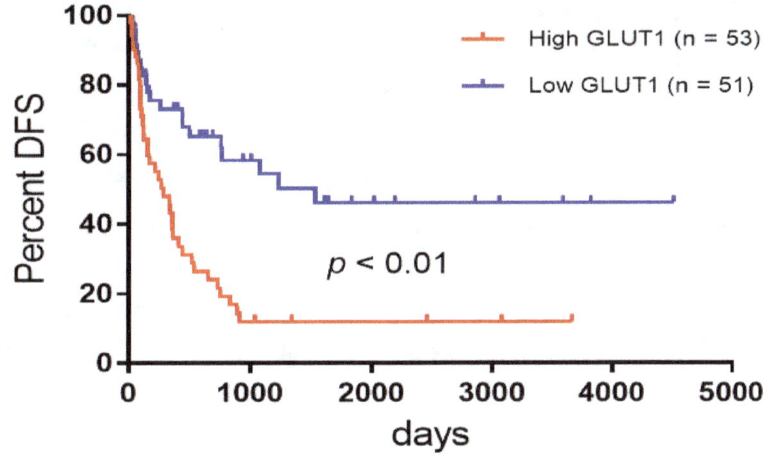

B

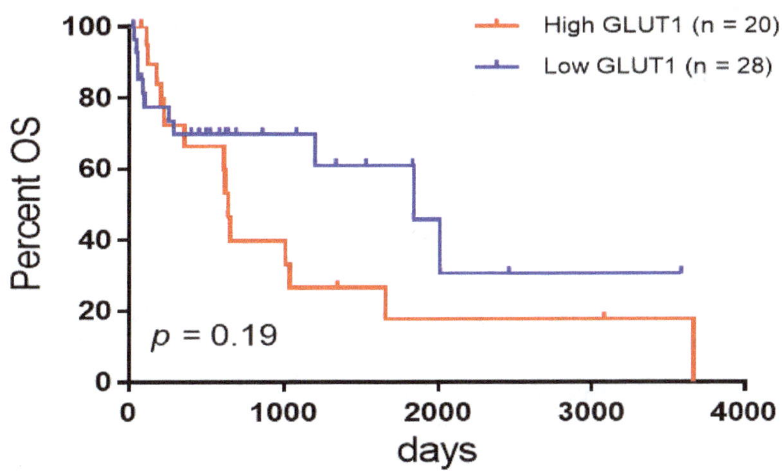

C

Figure 3. *Cont.*

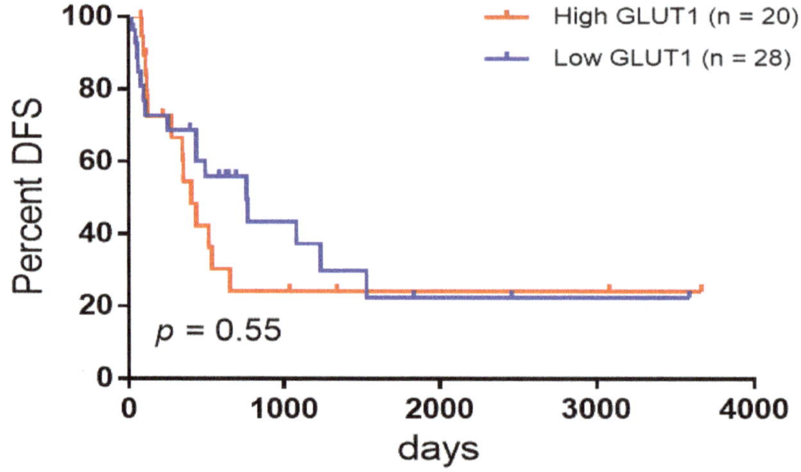

D

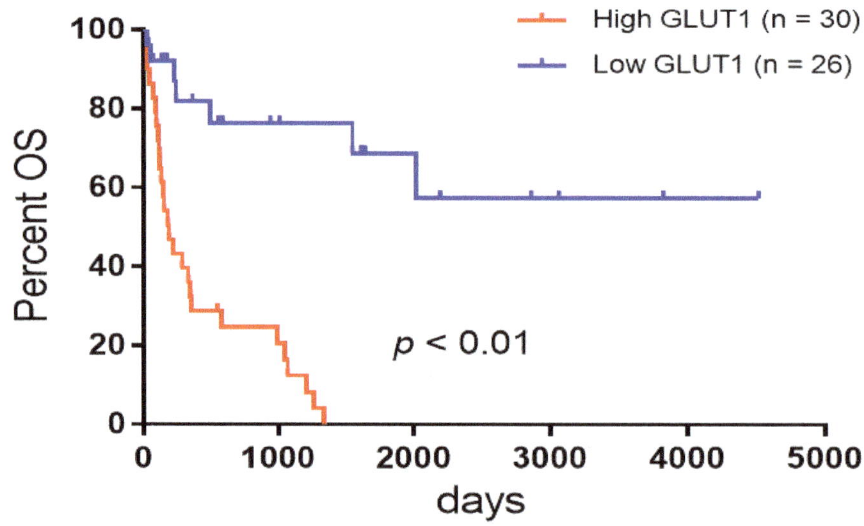

E

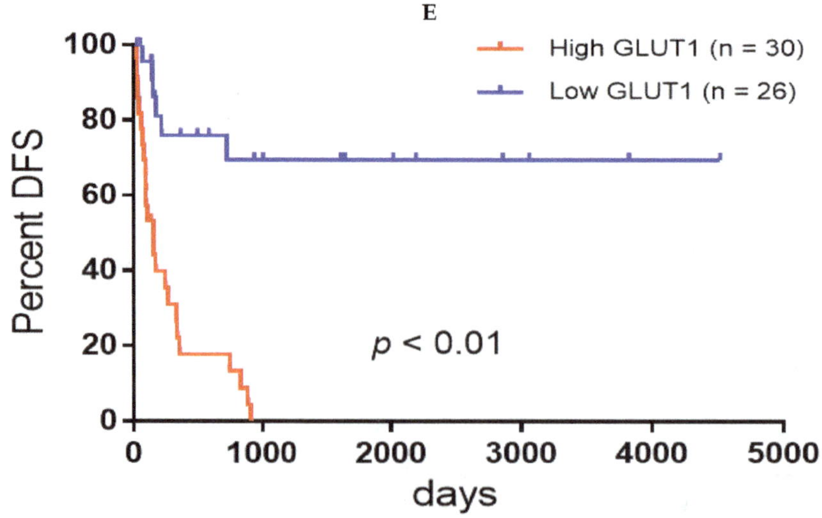

F

Figure 3. Kaplan-Meier survival curves for all patients (**A**,**B**), those with adenocarcinoma (**C**,**D**), and those with nonadenocarcinoma (**E**,**F**). Patients with high GLUT1 expression exhibited a significantly worse OS (A) and DFS (B) than those with low GLUT1 expression. No significant difference in the OS (C) and DFS (D) was observed between patients with adenocarcinoma with high and low GLUT1 expression, whereas the OS (E) and DFS (F) in patients with nonadenocarcinoma were significantly lower in those with high GLUT1 expression than in those low GLUT1 expression.

Figure 4 shows the forest plot of the one-year OS and DFS rates according to GLUT1 expression for each variable. Patients with high GLUT1 expression exhibited a worse OS and DFS than those with low GLUT1 expression for different variables except for stages III and IV.

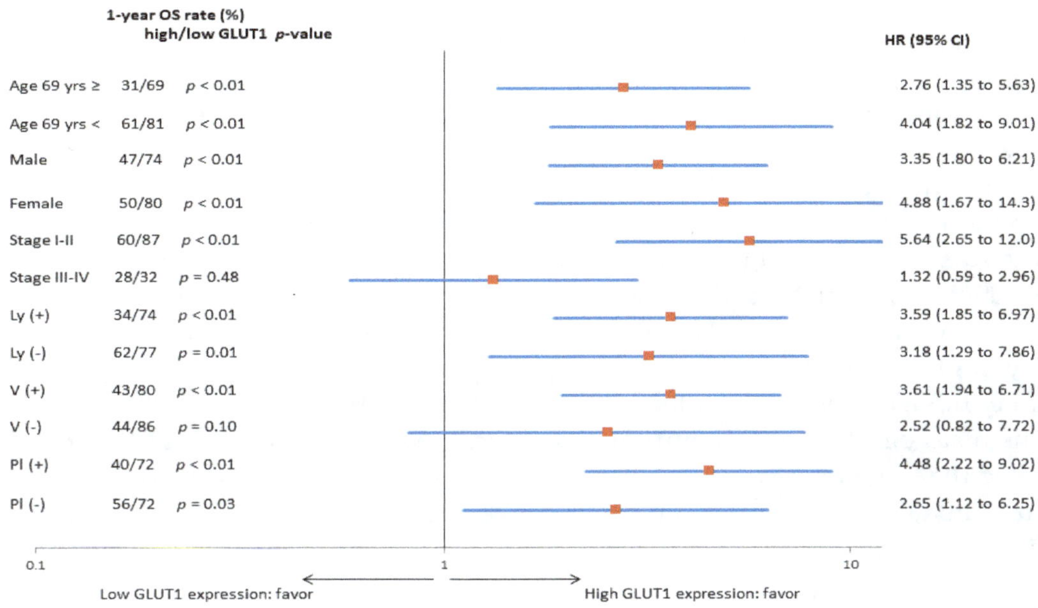

A

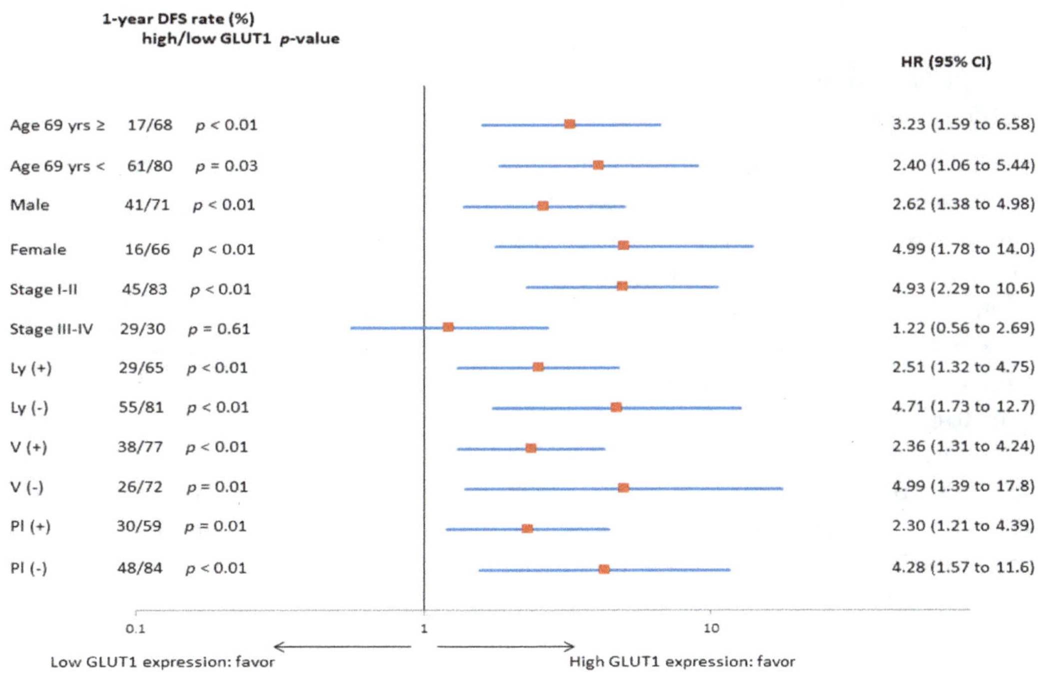

B

Figure 4. (**A**) Forest plot of one-year OS rate according to GLUT1 expression for each variable. (**B**) Forest plot of one-year DFS rate according to GLUT1 expression for each variable.

4. Discussion

We examined the prognostic significance of GLUT1 expression in patients with surgically resected PPC. We found that overexpression of GLUT1 is an independent factor for predicting poor outcomes and is useful as a prognostic marker in patients with a non-AC component. In the patients with non-AC, OS and DFS showed the highest difference between low-GLUT1 and high-GLUT1 compared with all patients and subgroup patients with AC component. The value of GLUT1 as a prognostic marker differed according to the epithelial histology of PPC.

A previous meta-analysis of 1423 patients with lung cancer revealed a relationship between GLUT1 expression and clinicopathological parameters [5]. This study described that positive expression of GLUT1 was significantly associated with squamous cell carcinoma, poorly differentiated tumors, lymph node metastases, large tumor size, and advanced tumor stage. In the present study, no significant difference in the frequency of high GLUT1 expression was observed between patients with non-AC and AC components. In our analysis according to epithelial histology, however, high expression of GLUT1 was identified as a significant factor for predicting worse outcomes in patients with a non-AC component compared to those with an AC component. A previous study reported that the accumulation of FDG was closely linked to poor prognosis in patients with AC, indicating the prognostic role of glucose metabolism as a significant prognostic predictor [10]. Although the limited sample size may have biased our results, our study suggests that the role of GLUT1 as a prognostic predictor in the histology of the AC component differs between patients with PPC and NSCLC. Here, we demonstrated that high expression of GLUT1 was strongly correlated with advanced stage, vascular invasion, pleural invasion, and tumor cell proliferation. These findings correspond to those of a study on NSCLC [5].

Recently, we reported the prognostic significance of amino acid transporter 1 (LAT1) expression in patients with surgically resected NSCLC [7]. LAT1 was highly expressed in patients with PPC, and there was a close relationship between high LAT1 expression and a worse prognosis. In the analysis according to histological type, the expression of LAT1 was significantly lower in patients with an AC component than in those without an AC component; however, the role of LAT1 as a predictive marker related to poor prognosis did not differ between patients with AC and non-AC. This contradicts the findings of the current study.

There were several limitations to our study. First, the sample size was small because PPC is a rare entity, which may have biased the results. However, compared to previous studies, this was a large-scale investigation using tumor samples collected from multiple institutions. As it is difficult to definitively diagnose PPC using biopsy samples, we collected tumor samples from patients with surgically resected PPC. Second, the expression of GLUT1 has been shown to be closely associated with tumor progression, metastases, and survival of PPC; however, it remains unknown whether GLUT1 expression is correlated with the uptake of ^{18}F-FDG within PPC tumor cells. Although a previous exploratory study indicated a close relationship between GLUT1 expression and ^{18}F-FDG accumulation in patients with PPC, it is necessary to validate this correlation using different cohorts with more than 100 tumor samples. Finally, GLUT1 is found to be a targeting molecule for PPC; however, inhibition of glucose metabolism may be harmful to normal cells rather than cancer cells. Therefore, it may be difficult to administer inhibitors of GLUT1 as a treatment for PPC with a non-AC component in clinical practice. Further studies are needed to develop a selective inhibitor of GLUT1 to diminish the tumor growth and metastases of PPC.

5. Conclusions

GLUT1 is an independent predictor of poor prognosis in patients with surgically resected PPC, particularly in those with an AC component. Although GLUT1 is widely expressed in human cancers, tumor glucose metabolism was identified as an essential factor related to tumor cell proliferation, survival, and pathogenesis. Additional studies are needed to determine the therapeutic potential of GLUT1 inhibitors in patients with advanced PPC.

Author Contributions: Conceptualization, H.I. and K.K.; methodology, K.K.; software, K.K.; validation, H.I.; formal analysis, K.K.; investigation, H.I. and K.K.; resources, H.E., K.I., Y.G., M.K., T.K., T.Y., Y.O., T.O. (Takashi Osaki), Y.K., S.T., and A.F.; data curation, H.I.; writing—original draft preparation, H.I., K.K., H.E., K.I., Y.G., M.K., T.K., T.Y., Y.O., T.O. (Takashi Osaki), Y.K., S.T., and A.F.; writing—review and editing, H.I., K.K., H.E., K.I., Y.G., M.K., T.K., T.Y., Y.O., T.O. (Takashi Osaki), Y.K., S.T., A.F., and T.O. (Tetsunari Oyama); visualization, T.O. (Tetsunari Oyama); supervision, T.A. and K.S.; project administration, K.K.; funding acquisition, K.M. All authors have read and agreed to the published version of the manuscript.

Acknowledgments: We thank Kimihiro Shimizu and Akira Mogi with Gunma University Hospital, Osamu Kawashima with Shibukawa Medical Center, Masayuki Sugano with Takasaki Medical Center, Ryohei Yamamoto with Saku Central Hospital Advanced Care Center, and Yukio Seki with Nagoya Medical Center for the collection of materials and patient treatment information. We would also like to thank Editage (www.editage.jp) for English language editing.

References

1. Chang, Y.L.; Lee, Y.C.; Shih, J.Y.; Wu, C.T. Pulmonary pleomorphic (spindle) cell carcinoma: Peculiar clinicopathologic manifestations different from ordinary non-small cell carcinoma. *Lung Cancer* **2001**, *34*, 91–97. [CrossRef]
2. Kerr, K.M.; Pelosi, G.; Austin, J.H.M. Pleomorphic, spindle cell, and giant cell carcinoma. In *WHO Classification of Tumours of the Lung, Pleura, Thymus and Heart*; Travis, W.D., Brambilla, E., Burke, A.P., Marx, A., Nicholson, A.G., Eds.; IARC Press: Lyon, France, 2015; Volume 7, pp. 88–90.
3. Fishback, N.F.; Travis, W.D.; Moran, C.A.; Guinee, D.G., Jr.; McCarthy, W.F.; Koss, M.N. Pleomorphic (spindle/giant cell) carcinoma of the lung. A clinicopathologic correlation of 78 cases. *Cancer* **1994**, *73*, 2936–2945. [CrossRef]
4. Kaira, K.; Endo, M.; Abe, M.; Nakagawa, K.; Ohde, Y.; Okumura, T.; Takahashi, T.; Murakami, H.; Tsuya, A.; Nakamura, Y.; et al. Biologic correlation of 2-[18F]-fluoro-2-deoxy-D-glucose uptake on positron emission tomography in thymic epithelial tumors. *J. Clin. Oncol.* **2010**, *28*, 3746–3753. [CrossRef] [PubMed]
5. Zhang, B.; Xie, Z.; Li, B. The clinicopathologic impacts and prognostic significance of GLUT1 expression in patients with lung cancer: A meta-analysis. *Gene* **2019**, *689*, 76–83. [CrossRef] [PubMed]
6. Kaira, K.; Endo, M.; Abe, M.; Nakagawa, K.; Ohde, Y.; Okumura, T.; Takahashi, T.; Murakami, H.; Tsuya, A.; Nakamura, Y.; et al. Biologic correlates of ^{18}F-FDG uptake on PET in pulmonary pleomorphic carcinoma. *Lung Cancer* **2011**, *71*, 144–150. [CrossRef] [PubMed]
7. Kaira, K.; Kawashima, O.; Endoh, H.; Imaizumi, K.; Goto, Y.; Kamiyoshihara, M.; Sugano, M.; Yamamoto, R.; Osaki, T.; Tanaka, S.; et al. Expression of amino acid transporter (LAT1 and 4F2hc) in pulmonary pleomorphic carcinoma. *Hum. Pathol.* **2019**, *84*, 142–149. [CrossRef] [PubMed]
8. Kaira, K.; Kamiyoshihara, M.; Kawashima, O.; Endoh, H.; Imaizumi, K.; Sugano, M.; Tanaka, S.; Fujita, A.; Kogure, Y.; Shimizu, A.; et al. Prognostic impact of β2 adrenergic receptor expression in surgically resected pulmonary pleomorphic carcinoma. *Anticancer Res.* **2019**, *39*, 395–403. [CrossRef] [PubMed]
9. Imai, H.; Shimizu, K.; Kawashima, O.; Endoh, H.; Imaizumi, K.; Goto, Y.; Kamiyoshihara, M.; Sugano, M.; Yamamoto, R.; Tanaka, S.; et al. Clinical significance of various drug-sensitivity markers in patients with surgically resected pulmonary pleomorphic carcinoma. *Cancers* **2019**, *11*, 1636. [CrossRef]
10. Kaira, K.; Shimizu, K.; Kitahara, S.; Yajima, T.; Atsumi, J.; Kosaka, T.; Ohtaki, Y.; Higuchi, T.; Oyama, T.; Asao, T.; et al. 2-Deoxy-2-[fluorine-18] fluoro-d-glucose uptake on positron emission tomography is associated with programmed death ligand-1 expression in patients with pulmonary adenocarcinoma. *Eur. J. Cancer* **2018**, *101*, 181–190. [CrossRef] [PubMed]

20

Comparative Efficacy of Targeted Therapies in Patients with Non-Small Cell Lung Cancer

Tung Hoang [1], Seung-Kwon Myung [1,2,3,*], Thu Thi Pham [4,5], Jeongseon Kim [1] and Woong Ju [6,7]

1 Department of Cancer Biomedical Science, National Cancer Center Graduate School of Cancer Science and Policy, Goyang 10408, Korea; 75256@ncc.re.kr (T.H.); jskim@ncc.re.kr (J.K.)
2 Division of Cancer Epidemiology and Management, National Cancer Center Research Institute, Goyang 10408, Korea
3 Department of Family Medicine and Center for Cancer Prevention and Detection, National Cancer Center Hospital, Goyang 10408, Korea
4 Health Data Science Program, Institute of Public Health, Charité Universitätsmedizin Berlin, 10117 Berlin, Germany; thuphamhup@gmail.com
5 Molecular Epidemiology Research Group, Max Delbrück Center for Molecular Medicine (MDC), 13125 Berlin, Germany
6 Department of Obstetrics and Gynecology, Ewha Womans University College of Medicine, Seoul 07804, Korea; goodmorning@ewha.ac.kr
7 Medical Research Institute, Ewha Womans University College of Medicine, Seoul 07804, Korea
* Correspondence: msk@ncc.re.kr

Abstract: This study aims to investigate the efficacy of targeted therapies in the treatment of non-small cell lung cancer (NSCLC) by using a network meta-analysis of clinical trials. PubMed, EMBASE, Cochrane Library, and Clinicaltrials.gov were searched by using keywords related to the topic on 19 September 2018. Two investigators independently selected relevant trials by pre-determined criteria. A pooled response ratio (RR) for overall response rate (ORR) and a hazard ratio (HR) for progression-free survival (PFS) were calculated based on both the Bayesian and frequentist approaches. A total of 128 clinical trials with 39,501 participants were included in the final analysis of 14 therapeutic groups. Compared with chemotherapy, both ORR and PFS were significantly improved for afatinib, alectinib, and crizotinib, while only PFS was significantly improved for cabozantinib, ceritinib, gefitinib, and osimertinib. Consistency was observed between the direct and indirect comparisons based on the Bayesian approach statistically and the frequentist approach visually. Cabozantinib and alectinib showed the highest probability for the first-line treatment ranking in ORR (62.5%) and PFS (87.5%), respectively. The current network meta-analysis showed the comprehensive evidence-based comparative efficacy of different types of targeted therapies, which would help clinicians use targeted therapies in clinical practice.

Keywords: non-small cell lung cancer; targeted therapy; network meta-analysis

1. Introduction

Lung cancer is the most common cancer and the leading cause of cancer death worldwide, with approximately 2.1 million new cases (11.6% of the total new cases) and 1.76 million deaths (18.4% of the total deaths) [1,2]. Of the two major types of lung cancer, non-small cell lung cancer (NSCLC) accounts for about 85% to 90% of all lung cancers, which typically has a slower rate and double time than small cell lung cancer [3,4].

Among several treatment options for NSCLC treatment recommended by the latest updated National Comprehensive Cancer Network (NCCN) guideline, targeted cancer therapy with various pathways is one of the new generations of cancer treatments [5]. Some cell surface receptors such as epidermal growth factor receptor (EGFR), anaplastic lymphoma kinase (ALK), and receptor of silencing 1 (ROS1) are overactive in the pathology of NSCLC [6,7]. Also, B-Raf proto-oncogene (BRAF), kirsten rat sarcoma 2 viral oncogene homolog (KRAS) and a kinase upstream of mitogen-activated protein kinase (MEK) have generated recent interest [8]. Other inhibitors of human epidermal growth factor receptor 2 (HER2), 'rearranged during transfection' proto-oncogene (RET), and tyrosine-protein kinase Met (MET) have also been approved for the treatment of NSCLC [9–11]. Although the efficacy of targeted therapies has been evaluated through large-scale randomized controlled trials and has already been approved by the Food and Drug Administration (FDA), their comparative efficacy has not been investigated.

Therefore, we performed a network meta-analysis (NMA) of clinical trials to compare and rank targeted therapies for the treatment of patients with NSCLC.

2. Materials and Methods

2.1. Search Strategy and Keywords

Eligible studies were identified by searching PubMed, EMBASE, Cochrane library, and Clinicaltrials.gov databases from their inception until September 19, 2018, limiting to human subjects and a clinical trial. The keywords for literature search were as follows: 'ado-trastuzumab', 'afatinib', 'alectinib', 'bevacizumab', 'brigatinib', 'cabozantinib', 'ceritinib', 'cetuximab', 'crizotinib', 'dabrafenib', 'erlotinib', 'gefitinib', 'osimertinib', 'ramucirumab', 'trametinib', 'vandetanib', and 'vemurafenib' for intervention factors; 'non-small cell lung cancer' for an outcome factor; and 'clinical trial' and 'randomized controlled trial' for type of study. The bibliographies of relevant articles were also reviewed to identify additional studies related to this topic. The literature search was restricted to studies published in English.

2.2. Selection of Relevant Studies

We included head-to-head or controlled trials that: compared the efficacy of FDA-approved targeted drugs with chemotherapy or placebos in the treatment of NSCLC; reported the outcomes on overall response rates (ORRs) and/or hazard ratios (HRs) for progression-free survival (PFS).

Two investigators (Hoang and Myung) independently selected relevant trials searched from the databases. The following variables were extracted from all the included studies: study name (first author, published year, and specific trial title, if possible), period and country, regimen of the intervention and the comparison, number of participants, and main outcomes.

2.3. Data Analysis

The pooled response ratio (RR) for ORRs based on an arm-based approach, HR for PFS based on a contrast-based approach, and their 95% confidence intervals (95% CIs) were calculated for estimating the differences between treatment groups.

We measured inconsistency, which implies statistical disagreement between direct and indirect comparisons [12,13]. The generalized linear model was applied for the Bayesian NMA [14]. Binomial likelihood and logit link function were applied for arm-based data of ORR, while normal likelihood and identity link function were used for contrast-based data of natural logarithm HR in the Bayesian approach [14]. Also, Bayesian model assumptions in the Bayesian analysis were assessed by the convergence diagnostics of the Markov chain Monte Carlo [14].

Based on the ranking probabilities of each therapy in different treatment lines, we calculated the surface under the cumulative ranking line (SUCRA) value and performed k-means clustering analysis to group the similar treatments [15,16].

For the statistical analysis of this NMA, we used different packages including pcnetmeta, gemtc, and netmeta in the R statistical environment [17–19]. Results from both the Bayesian approach (pcnetmeta and gemtc packages) and the frequentist approach (netmeta package) and were presented.

Finally, we calculated a decremental hazard-response ratio (DHRR) to obtain a decreased amount of HR per a unit of RR (compared to a dummy group) as in the following formula:

$$\mathrm{DHRR} = -\frac{\mathrm{HR} - \mathrm{HR_o}}{\mathrm{RR} - \mathrm{RR_o}}$$

where $\mathrm{HR_o}$ and $\mathrm{RR_o}$ are a baseline hazard ratio and a response ratio of chemotherapy vs. a dummy group, respectively.

3. Results

3.1. Selection of Relevant Studies

Figure S1 shows the flow diagram for selection of relevant studies. We identified 7279 articles from four different databases (PubMed, EMBASE, Cochrane Library, and Clinicaltrials.gov) using the keywords and hand-search from relevant bibliographies. After excluding 845 duplicated records and 5815 irrelevant studies, the full text of the remaining 619 articles were reviewed. Overall, a total of 128 parallel clinical trials were included in the current network meta-analysis.

3.2. Study Characteristics

The general characteristics of the included studies (eReferences in the Supplement) were summarized in Table S1. A total of 39,501 study participants were assigned to receive 14 different treatments including 12 targeted therapies, 1 chemotherapy, and 1 dummy. Sixty-four % of all the studies involved the comparisons between EGFR-targeted drugs and other treatments.

3.3. Network Geometry

Figure 1 shows the network geometry for ORR and PFS to represent graphical comparisons among various treatments. The comparative efficacy between erlotinib vs. chemotherapy/bevacizumab vs. dummy/erlotinib vs. dummy was frequently investigated for ORR, while the comparative efficacy between erlotinib vs. chemotherapy/gefitinib vs. chemotherapy/gefitinib vs. dummy/bevacizumab vs. dummy/erlotinib vs. dummy was done for PFS.

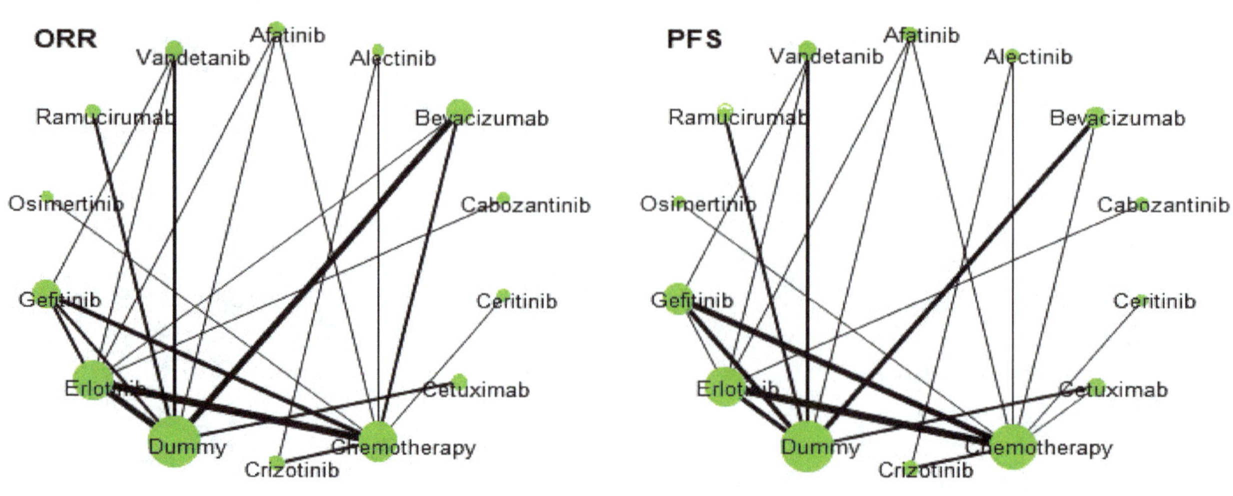

Figure 1. Network geometry of comparisons for overall response rate (ORR) and progression-free survival (PFS).

3.4. Assumption Checking

Figures S2 and S3 show a heat map, which provides visual inconsistency between direct and indirect comparisons in the frequentist approach. There was a big difference between inconsistency before and after the detachment in some treatment comparisons. However, no inconsistency was observed in the Bayesian approach (Figures S4 and S5).

Substantial heterogeneity was detected in both ORR and PFS, with the global $I^2 = 78\%$ for both outcomes as well as for either a pairwise pooled effect or a consistency effect (Table S2).

The width of every line reflects the number of studies. The size of the circles is proportional to the number of study participants. A dummy group is a placebo or a control group without additional treatment.

3.5. Comparative Efficacy

Compared to chemotherapy, afatinib, alectinib, ceritinib, and crizotinib were found to have a higher ORR with RRs ranging between 2.26 (95% CI, 1.34–3.82) for crizotinib and 3.75 (95% CI, 1.80–7.94) for ceritinib (Figure 2). Also, cabozantinib, gefitinib, and osimertinib vs. chemotherapy were found to improve PFS with HRs ranging from 0.17 (95% CI, 0.10–0.29) for alectinib to 0.78 (0.67–0.91) for gefitinib (Figure 3).

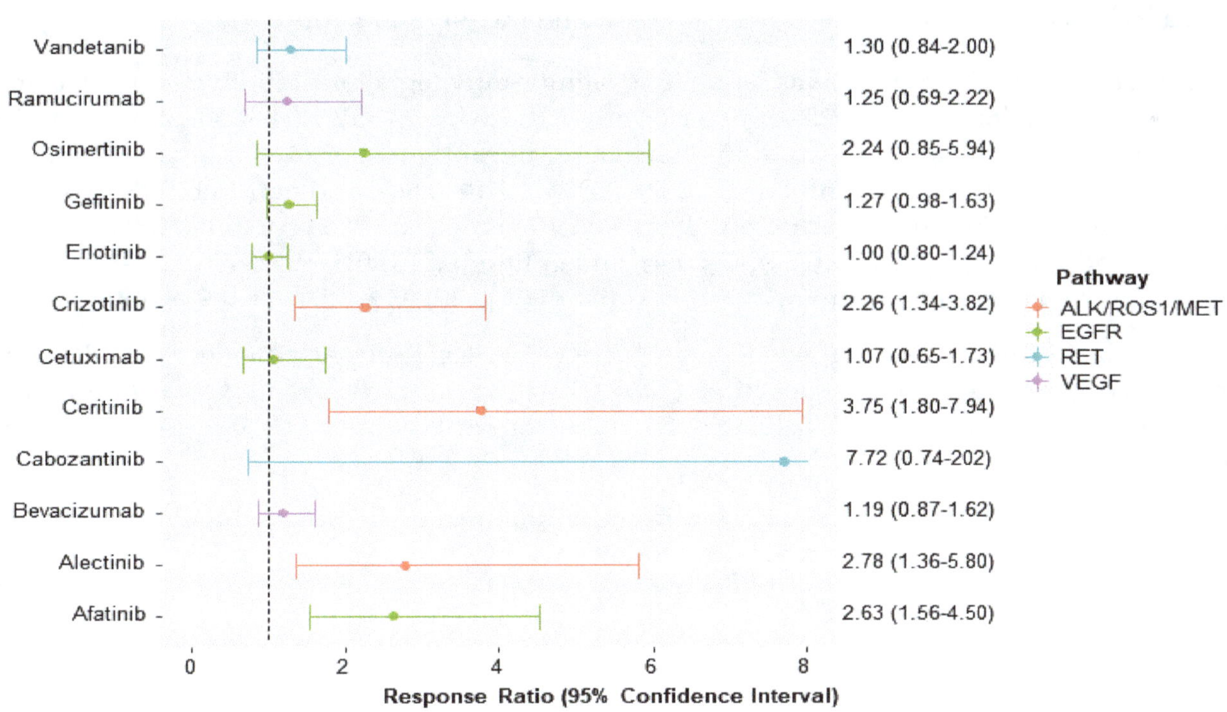

Figure 2. Response ratio for overall response rate of each targeted therapy vs. chemotherapy.

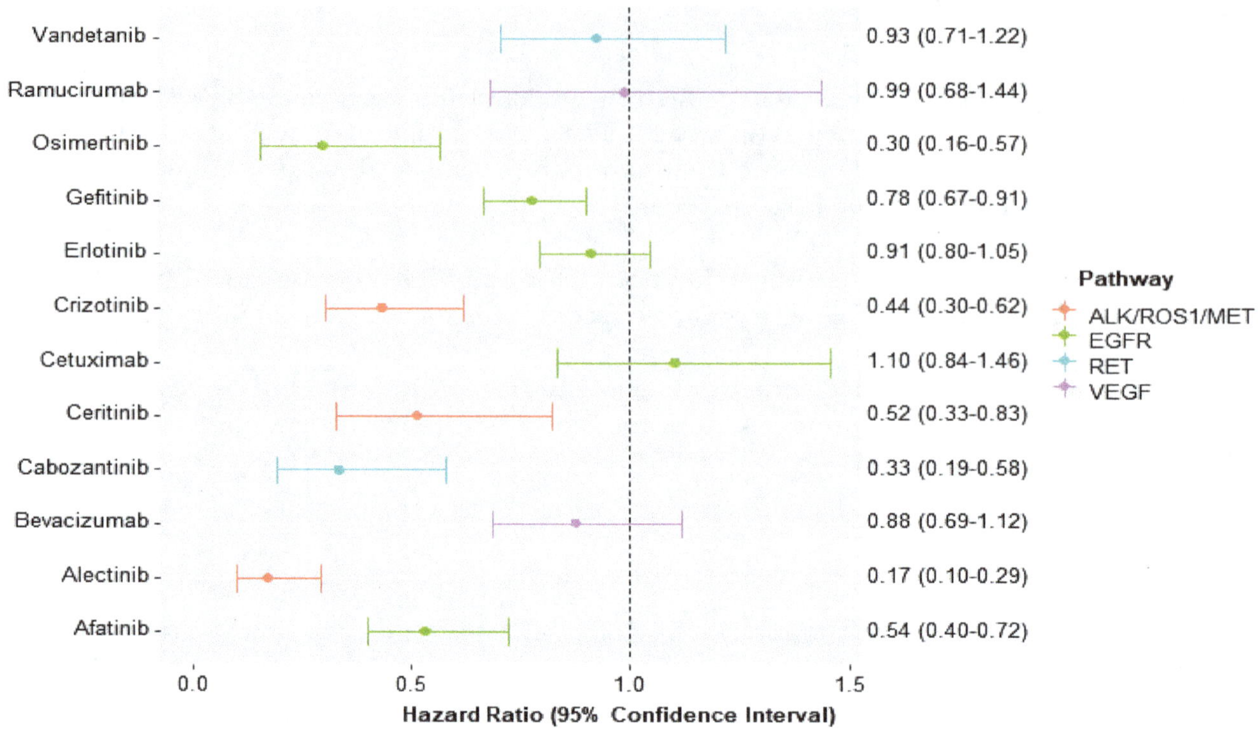

Figure 3. Hazard ratio for progression-free survival of each targeted therapy vs. chemotherapy.

Tables 1 and 2 show the league tables representing the comparative efficacy of targeted therapies for ORR and PFS in the network meta-analysis based on the Bayesian approach.

Among EGFR inhibitors, ORR was found to be significantly higher in afatinib treatment, compared to cetuximab (RR, 2.46; 95% CI, 1.25–4.90), erlotinib (RR, 2.64; 95% CI, 1.54–4.58), and gefitinib (RR, 2.08; 95% CI, 1.18-3.68) (Table 1). Also, afatinib had a significantly longer PFS, compared to cetuximab (HR, 0.49; 95% CI, 0.33–0.71), erlotinib (HR, 0.59; 95% CI 0.44–0.80), and gefitinib (HR, 0.69; 95% CI, 0.50–0.95) (Table 2). Osimertinib was found to improve PFS, compared to cetuximab (HR, 0.27; 95% CI, 0.14–0.55), erlotinib (HR, 0.33; 95% CI, 0.17–0.64), and gefitinib (HR, 0.39; 95% CI, 0.20–0.75) (Table 2). Gefitinib showed a better PFS compared to cetuximab (HR, 0.70; 95% CI, 0.53–0.94) (Table 2).

Regarding ALK/ROS1/MET targeted drugs, there were no significant differences in ORR between each pair of crizotinib, ceritinib, and alectinib (Table 1). However, alectinib showed a superior efficacy compared to either crizotinib (HR, 0.40; 95% CI, 0.25–0.64) or ceritinib (HR, 0.33; 0.17–0.67) for PFS (Table 2).

As for VEGF pathway (bevacizumab and ramucizumab) and RET targeted therapy (cabozantinib and vandetanib), only cabozantinib was found to improve PFS compared to vandetanib (HR, 0.36; 95% CI, 0.20–0.66) (Table 2).

3.6. Sensitivity Analysis

Findings of the direct pairwise meta-analysis and the relative effect estimates for ORR and PFS using the frequentist approach are presented in Tables S3–S5. The findings were similar to those by using the Bayesian approach (Tables 1 and 2).

Table 1. Comparative efficacy of targeted therapies for overall response rate in the network meta-analysis based on the Bayesian approach.

Afat	0.95 (0.38–2.31)	*2.22 (1.25–3.98)*	0.34 (0.01–3.81)	0.71 (0.28–1.73)	*2.46 (1.25–4.90)*	*2.63 (1.56–4.50)*	1.18 (0.55–2.46)	*3.53 (2.06–6.15)*	*2.64 (1.54–4.58)*	*2.08 (1.18–3.68)*	1.18 (0.39–3.51)	2.11 (1.00–4.49)	*2.03 (1.07–3.88)*
1.06 (0.43–2.62)	Alec	*2.34 (1.08–5.22)*	0.36 (0.01–4.26)	0.74 (0.26–2.10)	*2.60 (1.10–6.27)*	*2.78 (1.36–5.80)*	1.24 (0.67–2.27)	*3.74 (1.75–8.22)*	*2.79 (1.32–6.02)*	*2.20 (1.03–4.78)*	1.24 (0.37–4.21)	2.24 (0.90–5.71)	2.15 (0.93–5.03)
0.45 (0.25–0.80)	*0.42 (0.19–0.93)*	Beva	0.15 (0.01–1.63)	*0.31 (0.14–0.70)*	1.11 (0.70–1.78)	1.19 (0.87–1.62)	*0.52 (0.28–0.96)*	*1.59 (1.25–2.05)*	1.19 (0.87–1.63)	0.94 (0.66–1.32)	0.53 (0.19–1.46)	0.95 (0.54–1.69)	0.92 (0.59–1.41)
2.93 (0.26–78.11)	2.79 (0.23–76.6)	6.49 (0.62–170)	Cabo	2.08 (0.17–57.3)	7.21 (0.67–193)	7.72 (0.74–202)	3.45 (0.30–92.0)	10.36 (0.99–272)	7.74 (0.75–201)	6.09 (0.58–162)	3.45 (0.27–104)	6.20 (0.56–166)	5.95 (0.56–157)
1.43 (0.58–3.57)	1.35 (0.48–3.78)	*3.16 (1.43–7.12)*	0.49 (0.02–5.78)	Ceri	*3.51 (1.45–8.60)*	*3.75 (1.80–7.94)*	1.66 (0.68–4.13)	*5.04 (2.30–11.2)*	*3.76 (1.74–8.25)*	*2.96 (1.36–6.54)*	1.68 (0.50–5.65)	*3.02 (1.18–7.83)*	*2.89 (1.23–6.89)*
0.41 (0.20–0.80)	*0.38 (0.16–0.91)*	0.90 (0.56–1.44)	0.14 (0.01–1.49)	*0.28 (0.12–0.69)*	Cetu	1.07 (0.65–1.73)	0.47 (0.23–0.96)	1.44 (0.96–2.14)	1.07 (0.67–1.72)	0.84 (0.51–1.38)	0.48 (0.16–1.41)	0.86 (0.45–1.65)	0.82 (0.48–1.41)
0.38 (0.22–0.64)	*0.36 (0.17–0.74)*	0.84 (0.62–1.15)	0.13 (0.00–1.35)	*0.27 (0.13–0.56)*	0.93 (0.58–1.53)	Chem	*0.44 (0.26–0.75)*	*1.34 (1.03–1.77)*	1.00 (0.80–1.25)	0.79 (0.61–1.02)	0.45 (0.17–1.17)	0.80 (0.45–1.45)	0.77 (0.50–1.19)
0.86 (0.41–1.82)	0.81 (0.44–1.49)	*1.90 (1.04–3.51)*	0.29 (0.01–3.28)	0.60 (0.24–1.48)	*2.11 (1.04–4.34)*	*2.26 (1.34–3.82)*	Criz	*3.03 (1.69–5.50)*	*2.26 (1.29–4.03)*	1.78 (0.99–3.20)	1.01 (0.34–3.03)	1.81 (0.84–3.99)	1.74 (0.89–3.45)
0.28 (0.16–0.49)	*0.26 (0.12–0.57)*	*0.63 (0.49–0.80)*	0.10 (0.00–1.01)	*0.20 (0.09–0.43)*	0.70 (0.47–1.04)	*0.75 (0.57–0.98)*	*0.33 (0.18–0.59)*	Dum	*0.75 (0.58–0.96)*	*0.59 (0.44–0.78)*	*0.33 (0.12–0.91)*	0.60 (0.36–1.00)	*0.57 (0.40–0.82)*
0.38 (0.22–0.65)	*0.36 (0.17–0.76)*	0.84 (0.61–1.15)	0.13 (0.00–1.33)	*0.26 (0.12–0.57)*	0.93 (0.58–1.50)	1.00 (0.80–1.24)	*0.44 (0.25–0.78)*	*1.34 (1.05–1.72)*	Erlo	0.79 (0.59–1.04)	0.45 (0.16–1.19)	0.80 (0.46–1.42)	0.77 (0.51–1.16)
0.48 (0.27–0.85)	*0.45 (0.21–0.98)*	1.07 (0.76–1.51)	0.16 (0.01–1.72)	*0.34 (0.15–0.74)*	1.19 (0.73–1.94)	1.27 (0.98–1.63)	0.56 (0.31–1.01)	*1.70 (1.28–2.27)*	1.27 (0.96–1.68)	Gefi	0.57 (0.21–1.53)	1.02 (0.57–1.83)	0.98 (0.63–1.51)
0.85 (0.29–2.56)	0.80 (0.24–2.70)	1.88 (0.68–5.22)	0.29 (0.01–3.75)	0.59 (0.18–2.01)	2.09 (0.71–6.26)	2.24 (0.85–5.94)	0.99 (0.33–2.97)	*3.01 (1.10–8.30)*	2.24 (0.84–6.07)	1.77 (0.65–4.84)	Osim	1.80 (0.59–5.63)	1.73 (0.60–5.02)
0.47 (0.22–1.00)	0.44 (0.18–1.12)	1.05 (0.59–1.85)	0.16 (0.01–1.79)	*0.33 (0.13–0.84)*	1.16 (0.61–2.23)	1.25 (0.69–2.22)	0.55 (0.25–1.19)	*1.67 (1.00–2.78)*	1.25 (0.71–2.20)	0.98 (0.55–1.76)	0.56 (0.18–1.70)	Ramu	0.96 (0.51–1.79)
0.49 (0.26–0.94)	0.46 (0.20–1.07)	1.09 (0.71–1.69)	0.17 (0.01–1.77)	*0.34 (0.15–0.81)*	1.21 (0.71–2.09)	1.30 (0.84–2.00)	0.57 (0.29–1.13)	*1.74 (1.22–2.51)*	1.30 (0.86–1.97)	1.02 (0.66–1.59)	0.58 (0.20–1.67)	1.04 (0.56–1.96)	Vand

Drugs are reported in alphabetical order. Data in the right-upper triangle are RRs (95% confidence interval, CI) in the row-defining treatment compared with the column-defining treatment. RRs higher than 1 favor the row-defining treatment (the first drug in alphabetical order). RRs for the opposite comparison of ORR are in the left-lower triangle. Each comparison is shown twice in the table, once with drug A vs. drug B and once with drug B vs. drug A. Significant results are in italic and underscored. RR, response ratio; CI, confidence interval; ORR: overall response rate; Afat, afatinib; Alec, alectinib; Beva, bevacizumab; Cabo, cabozantinib; Ceri, ceritinib; Cetu, cetuximab; Chem, chemotherapy; Criz, crizotinib; Dum, dummy; Erlo, erlotinib; Gefi, gefitinib; Osim, osimertinib; Ramu, ramucirumab; Vand, vandetanib.

Table 2. Comparative efficacy of targeted therapies for progression-free survival in the network meta-analysis based on the Bayesian approach.

Afat	*3.10 (1.69–5.65)*	*0.61 (0.43–0.87)*	1.61 (0.87–2.98)	1.03 (0.60–1.79)	*0.49 (0.33–0.71)*	*0.54 (0.40–0.72)*	1.23 (0.78–1.96)	*0.43 (0.32–0.58)*	*0.59 (0.44–0.80)*	*0.69 (0.50–0.95)*	1.79 (0.88–3.63)	*0.54 (0.35–0.84)*	*0.58 (0.40–0.84)*
0.32 (0.18–0.59)	Alec	*0.20 (0.11–0.35)*	0.52 (0.24–1.11)	*0.33 (0.17–0.67)*	*0.16 (0.09–0.28)*	*0.17 (0.10–0.29)*	*0.40 (0.25–0.64)*	*0.14 (0.08–0.24)*	*0.19 (0.11–0.33)*	*0.22 (0.13–0.38)*	0.58 (0.25–1.33)	*0.17 (0.09–0.33)*	*0.19 (0.10–0.33)*
1.64 (1.15–2.33)	*5.08 (2.87–9.04)*	Beva	*2.63 (1.46–4.76)*	*1.69 (1.01–2.86)*	0.80 (0.59–1.08)	0.88 (0.69–1.12)	*2.02 (1.32–3.10)*	*0.71 (0.58–0.86)*	0.96 (0.76–1.23)	1.13 (0.88–1.45)	*2.93 (1.47–5.82)*	0.89 (0.60–1.30)	0.95 (0.70–1.28)
0.62 (0.34–1.15)	1.93 (0.90–4.12)	*0.38 (0.21–0.69)*	Cabo	0.64 (0.31–1.32)	*0.30 (0.16–0.55)*	*0.33 (0.19–0.58)*	0.77 (0.40–1.49)	*0.27 (0.15–0.47)*	*0.37 (0.21–0.63)*	*0.43 (0.24–0.76)*	1.11 (0.48–2.60)	*0.34 (0.18–0.65)*	*0.36 (0.20–0.66)*
0.97 (0.56–1.67)	*3.00 (1.50–6.02)*	*0.59 (0.35–0.99)*	1.55 (0.76–3.20)	Ceri	*0.47 (0.27–0.81)*	*0.52 (0.33–0.83)*	1.19 (0.67–2.14)	*0.42 (0.26–0.68)*	*0.57 (0.35–0.92)*	0.67 (0.41–1.09)	1.73 (0.78–3.85)	*0.52 (0.29–0.95)*	*0.56 (0.33–0.96)*
2.05 (1.41–2.99)	*6.37 (3.54–11.5)*	1.26 (0.92–1.71)	*3.30 (1.80–6.07)*	*2.12 (1.24–3.64)*	Cetu	1.10 (0.84–1.46)	*2.54 (1.62–3.98)*	0.89 (0.70–1.13)	1.21 (0.91–1.59)	*1.42 (1.06–1.89)*	*3.68 (1.83–7.39)*	1.11 (0.74–1.67)	1.19 (0.85–1.66)
1.86 (1.38–2.51)	*5.77 (3.42–9.73)*	1.14 (0.89–1.44)	*2.99 (1.72–5.21)*	*1.92 (1.21–3.06)*	0.91 (0.69–1.20)	Chem	*2.30 (1.61–3.29)*	*0.81 (0.68–0.95)*	1.09 (0.96–1.25)	*1.29 (1.10–1.50)*	*3.33 (1.75–6.34)*	1.01 (0.70–1.46)	1.08 (0.82–1.41)
0.81 (0.51–1.29)	*2.51 (1.57–4.00)*	*0.50 (0.32–0.76)*	1.30 (0.67–2.52)	0.84 (0.47–1.50)	*0.39 (0.25–0.62)*	*0.44 (0.30–0.62)*	Criz	*0.35 (0.24–0.52)*	*0.48 (0.33–0.70)*	*0.56 (0.38–0.83)*	1.45 (0.69–3.04)	*0.44 (0.26–0.73)*	*0.47 (0.30–0.73)*
2.30 (1.71–3.11)	*7.15 (4.14–12.4)*	*1.41 (1.16–1.71)*	*3.71 (2.12–6.49)*	*2.38 (1.46–3.91)*	1.12 (0.88–1.43)	*1.24 (1.05–1.46)*	*2.85 (1.92–4.22)*	Dum	*1.36 (1.16–1.59)*	*1.59 (1.34–1.89)*	*4.13 (2.12–8.02)*	1.25 (0.90–1.73)	*1.33 (1.05–1.68)*
1.70 (1.26–2.30)	*5.27 (3.07–9.07)*	1.04 (0.82–1.32)	*2.73 (1.60–4.68)*	*1.76 (1.09–2.85)*	0.83 (0.63–1.09)	0.91 (0.80–1.05)	*2.10 (1.44–3.07)*	*0.74 (0.63–0.86)*	Erlo	1.17 (0.98–1.40)	*3.05 (1.57–5.88)*	0.92 (0.64–1.33)	0.98 (0.76–1.28)
1.45 (1.05–1.99)	*4.49 (2.62–7.75)*	0.88 (0.69–1.13)	*2.33 (1.32–4.10)*	1.50 (0.92–2.44)	*0.70 (0.53–0.94)*	*0.78 (0.67–0.91)*	*1.79 (1.21–2.63)*	*0.63 (0.53–0.74)*	0.85 (0.71–1.02)	Gefi	*2.59 (1.33–5.03)*	0.78 (0.54–1.14)	0.84 (0.64–1.10)
0.56 (0.28–1.14)	1.73 (0.75–3.97)	*0.34 (0.17–0.68)*	0.90 (0.38–2.10)	0.58 (0.26–1.28)	*0.27 (0.14–0.55)*	*0.30 (0.16–0.57)*	0.69 (0.33–1.44)	*0.24 (0.12–0.47)*	*0.33 (0.17–0.64)*	*0.39 (0.20–0.75)*	Osim	*0.30 (0.14–0.64)*	*0.32 (0.16–0.65)*
1.84 (1.18–2.89)	*5.72 (3.02–10.9)*	1.13 (0.77–1.66)	*2.97 (1.55–5.68)*	*1.91 (1.06–3.47)*	0.90 (0.60–1.36)	0.99 (0.68–1.44)	*2.28 (1.37–3.82)*	0.80 (0.58–1.12)	1.09 (0.75–1.56)	1.27 (0.88–1.85)	*3.31 (1.56–6.94)*	Ramu	1.07 (0.71–1.61)
1.73 (1.19–2.50)	*5.36 (2.99–9.67)*	1.06 (0.78–1.43)	*2.78 (1.53–5.06)*	*1.79 (1.04–3.06)*	0.84 (0.60–1.17)	0.93 (0.71–1.22)	*2.13 (1.36–3.33)*	*0.75 (0.59–0.95)*	1.02 (0.78–1.32)	1.19 (0.91–1.57)	*3.10 (1.54–6.23)*	0.94 (0.62–1.40)	Vand

Drugs are reported in alphabetical order. Data in the right-upper triangle are HRs (95% CI) in the row-defining treatment compared with the column-defining treatment. HRs lower than 1 favour the row-defining treatment (the first drug in alphabetical order). HRs for the opposite comparison of PFS are in the left-lower triangle. Each comparison is shown twice in the table, once with drug A vs. drug B and once with drug B vs. drug A. Significant results are in italic and underscored. HR, hazard ratio; CI, confidence interval; PFS: progression-free survival. Afat, afatinib; Alec, alectinib;. Beva, bevacizumab; Cabo, cabozantinib; Ceri, ceritinib; Cetu, cetuximab; Chem, chemotherapy;. Criz, crizotinib; Dum, dummy; Erlo, erlotinib; Gefi, gefitinib; Osim, osimertinib; Ramu, ramucirumab; Vand, vandetanib.

3.7. Treatment Ranking

The Gelman plot for checking Bayesian model assumption shows a low chain reduction over time for both ORR and PFS outcomes, and the chains seem roughly converged after maximum 10,000 iterations in chain (Figures S6 and S7). Also, cabozantinib and alectinib were found to become the first-line therapies with the highest treatment ranking probabilities of 62.5% for ORR and 87.5% for PFS, respectively (Tables S6 and S7 and Figure S8). In the k-means clustering analysis of SUCRA, ceritinib, alectinib, crizotinib, osimertinib, cabozantinib, and afatinib showed the more efficacy compared with the remaining treatment (Figure S9).

Figure S10 reports the two-dimensional graphs about RR for ORR and HR for PFS in the comparison with dummy group. DHRR indicated the decrease of HR obtained per 1 unit increase of RR for osimertinib (0.34), alectinib (0.28), bevacizumab (0.38), and vandetanib (0.14), which are higher than that for other drugs relating to EGFR, ALK/ROS1/MET, VEGF, and RET pathways.

4. Discussion

4.1. Summary of Findings

In the current comprehensive network meta-analysis, compared to chemotherapy, most of the targeted drugs including afatinib, alectinib, cabozantinib, ceritinib, crizotinib, gefitinib, and osimertinib showed a significantly higher efficacy in ORR and PFS. Among EGFR inhibitors, afatinib was found to improve both ORR and PFS, vs. cetuximab, erlotinib, or gefitinib treatment. Furthermore, alectinib and cabozantinib also showed the lower risk of disease progression, compared to other drugs in the ALK/ROS1/MET and RET pathways.

There was no inconsistency between direct and indirect comparisons in most treatments based on the Bayesian approach. The findings of the NMA based on both the frequentist and Bayesian approach were similar in pooled effect sizes as well as a significant direction. Also, Bayesian assumptions were ensured by convergence diagnostics.

4.2. Comparison with Previous Studies

Previous reports related to EGFR inhibitors showed consistent findings with the current study. A recent meta-analysis of 90 retrospective or prospective cohort studies and clinical trials showed the comparable effect of gefitinib vs. erlotinib [20]. The RR (95% CI) for ORR and HR (95% CI) for PFS were 1.05 (1.00–1.11) and 1.00 (0.95–1.04), respectively [20]. Another network meta-analysis of 11 clinical trials also showed the similar PFS between gefitinib and erlotinib [21]. However, unlike our findings, the third-generation EGFR inhibitor osimertinib was found to have a longer PFS (HR 0.71, 95% CI 0.54–0.95), and the significant difference between the second-generation EGFR inhibitor afatinib and standard of care (either gefitinib or erlotinib) was not observed (HR 0.96, 95% CI, 0.86–1.17) [21].

In a large medical chart review of 1471 participants with ALK-positive NSCLC among a total of 27,375 recorded subjects from seven countries, crizotinib showed a significant improvement in complete response (odds ratio (OR) = 2.65, 95% CI = 1.69–4.15) and reduction of recurrence/progression (odds ratio = 0.38, 95% CI = 0.24–0.59) compared to controls [22]. Also, a recent network meta-analysis of ALK inhibitors showed consistent findings among treatments in both ORR and PFS outcomes [23]. In Fan et al.'s study, a remarkable improvement in ORR was shown: the ORs (95%CI) for crizotinib, ceritinib, and alextinib were 11.69 (4.29–36.56), 7.85 (3.44–19.27), and 6.04 (3.33–11.71), compared to chemotherapy, respectively [23]. The superior efficacy of alectinib in PFS might be associated with the resistance to crizotinib among ALK-positive NSCLC patients, which reduces therapeutic response to crizotinib [24,25]. Although ceritinib is also a second-generation ALK inhibitor, our study showed that there is no signicant difference in the efficacy between ceritinib and crizotinib. Similarly, the recent meta-analyses of pooled estimates reported that crizotinib might have higher ORR [66% (58–74%) vs. 52% (38–66%)] and longer PFS [9.27 months (8.28–10.26) vs. 5.92 months (4.36–7.48)] than ceritinib, although no statistical test was performed [26]. It remains unclear why ceritinib did not show a superior efficacy unlike alectinib.

4.3. *Strengths and Limitations*

To the best of our knowledge, this is the first network meta-analysis which summarized the direct and indirect evidence on the comparative efficacy of targeted therapies in the treatment of NSCLC. Also, this compiled a large dataset, and the method was valid by checking several assumptions. In addition, this network meta-analysis included clinical trials only, which had a higher level of evidence than observational studies and allowed us to obtain the precise estimates.

Despite the strengths, there are several limitations in the current study. The efficacy of targeted therapies was evaluated through ORR and PFS surrogates only. We did not perform subgroup analyses by different treatment lines and patients of different mutations as well. Also, the potential heterogeneity was observed with approximately 78% for both ORR and PFS outcomes. Finally, among 34,969 subjects included for the analysis of ORR outcome, the small number of patients received cabozatinib (38 subjects, Table S1). Also, a big difference in ORRs between the two arms (10.5% for cabozatinib vs. 2.6% erlotinib) might lead to the large error margins for the comparative effect of cabozantinib and other treatments (Figure 2 and Table 1).

5. Conclusions

In summary, the current study showed the comprehensive evidence-based comparative efficacy of different types of targeted therapies, which would help clinicians use targeted therapies in clinical practice. Cabozantinib and alectinib showed the highest probability for the first-line treatment ranking in ORR and PFS, respectively.

Supplementary Materials:
Figure S1: Flow diagram for selection of relevant studies, Figure S2: Inconsistency-detecting heat map between direct and indirect comparisons for overall response rate in the frequentist approach, Figure S3: Inconsistency-detecting heat map between direct and indirect comparisons for progression-free survival in the frequentist approach, Figure S4: Node-splitting analysis of inconsistency for the comparison of overall response rate in the Bayesian approach, Figure S5: Node-splitting analysis of inconsistency for the comparison of progression-free survival in the Bayesian approach, Figure S6: Convergence diagnostics for the comparison of overall response rate, Figure S7: Convergence diagnostics for the comparison of progression-free survival, Figure S8: Treatment ranking plots according to overall response rate and progression-free survival, Figure S9: Cluster ranking plot based on SUCRA values of the overall response rate and progression free-survival of treatments, Figure S10: Two-dimensional graphs for response ratio and hazard ratio compared to dummy group, Table S1: General characteristics of the studies included in the final analysis, Table S2: Test for heterogeneity, Table S3: Direct pairwise comparative efficacy in the frequentist approach, Table S4: Comparative efficacy of targeted therapies for overall response rate in the network meta-analysis based on the frequentist approach, Table S5: Comparative efficacy of targeted therapies for progression-free survival in the network meta-analysis based on the frequentist approach, Table S6: Treatment ranking probability based on overall response rate, Table S7: Treatment ranking probability based on progression-free survival, eReferences: List of studies included in the network meta-analysis.

Author Contributions: Conceptualization, S.-K.M. and T.H.; methodology, S.-K.M. and T.H.; formal analysis, T.H.; investigation, T.H. and S.-K.M.; data curation, T.H. and S.-K.M.; writing—original draft preparation, T.H.; writing—review and editing, S.-K.M., T.T.P., T.H., J.K., and W.J. All authors have read and agreed to the published version of the manuscript.

References

1. Bray, F.; Ferlay, J.; Soerjomataram, I.; Siegel, R.L.; Torre, L.A.; Jemal, A. Global cancer statistics 2018: GLOBOCAN estimates of incidence and mortality worldwide for 36 cancers in 185 countries. *CA Cancer J. Clin.* **2018**, *68*, 394–424. [CrossRef] [PubMed]
2. International Agency for Research on Cancer: GLOBOCAN. Fact Sheet by Cancer Type: Lung Cancer. Available online: http://gco.iarc.fr/today/fact-sheets-cancers (accessed on 4 July 2019).

3. Dai, L.; Lin, Z.; Cao, Y.; Chen, Y.; Xu, Z.; Qin, Z. Targeting EIF4F complex in non-small cell lung cancer cells. *Oncotarget* **2017**, *8*, 55731–55735. [CrossRef] [PubMed]
4. Zappa, C.; Mousa, S.A. Non-small cell lung cancer: Current treatment and future advances. *Transl. Lung Cancer Res.* **2016**, *5*, 288–300. [CrossRef] [PubMed]
5. National Comprehensive Cancer Network (NCCN). Non-Small Cell Lung Cancer. *Clinical Practice Guidelines in Oncology (Version 1.2018)*. Available online: https://www.nccn.org (accessed on 4 July 2019).
6. Prabhu, V.V.; Devaraj, N. Epidermal growth factor receptor tyrosine kinase: A potential target in treatment of non-small-cell lung carcinoma. *J. Environ. Pathol. Toxicol. Oncol.* **2017**, *36*, 151–158. [CrossRef] [PubMed]
7. Toschi, L.; Rossi, S.; Finocchiaro, G.; Santoro, A. Non-small cell lung cancer treatment (r)evolution: Ten years of advances and more to come. *Ecancermedicalscience* **2017**, *11*, 787. [CrossRef] [PubMed]
8. Brustugun, O.T.; Khattak, A.M.; Tromborg, A.K.; Beigi, M.; Beiske, K.; Lund-Iversen, M.; Helland, A. BRAF-mutations in non-small cell lung cancer. *Lung Cancer* **2014**, *84*, 36–38. [CrossRef] [PubMed]
9. Gainor, J.F.; Shaw, A.T. Novel targets in non-small cell lung cancer: ROS1 and RET fusions. *Oncologist* **2013**, *18*, 865–875. [CrossRef] [PubMed]
10. Gelsomino, F.; Facchinetti, F.; Haspinger, E.R.; Garassino, M.C.; Trusolino, L.; De Braud, F.; Tiseo, M. Targeting the MET gene for the treatment of non-small-cell lung cancer. *Crit. Rev. Oncol. Hematol.* **2014**, *89*, 284–299. [CrossRef] [PubMed]
11. Mar, N.; Vredenburgh, J.J.; Wasser, J.S. Targeting HER2 in the treatment of non-small cell lung cancer. *Lung Cancer* **2015**, *87*, 220–225. [CrossRef] [PubMed]
12. Rouse, B.; Chaimani, A.; Li, T. Network meta-analysis: An introduction for clinicians. *Intern. Emerg. Med.* **2017**, *12*, 103–111. [CrossRef] [PubMed]
13. Shim, S.; Yoon, B.H.; Shin, I.S.; Bae, J.M. Network meta-analysis: Application and practice using Stata. *Epidemiol. Health* **2017**, *39*, e2017047. [CrossRef] [PubMed]
14. Neupane, B.; Richer, D.; Bonner, A.J.; Kibret, T.; Beyene, J. Network meta-analysis using R: A review of currently available automated packages. *PLoS ONE* **2014**, *9*, e115065. [CrossRef] [PubMed]
15. Kassambara, A.; Fabian, M. Factoextra: Extract and Visualize the Results of Multivariate Data Analyses. Available online: http://www.sthda.com/english/rpkgs/factoextra (accessed on 12 December 2019).
16. Salanti, G.; Ades, A.E.; Ioannidis, J.P. Graphical methods and numerical summaries for presenting results from multiple-treatment meta-analysis: An overview and tutorial. *J. Clin. Epidemiol.* **2011**, *64*, 163–171. [CrossRef] [PubMed]
17. Lin, L.; Zhang, J.; Chu, H. Pcnetmeta: Methods for Patient-Centered Network Meta-Analysis. Available online: https://cran.r-project.org/web/packages/pcnetmeta/pcnetmeta.pdf (accessed on 9 November 2019).
18. Rucker, G.; Schwarzer, G.; Krahn, U.; Konig, J. Netmeta: Network Meta-Analysis Using Frequentist Methods. Available online: https://cran.r-project.org/web/packages/netmeta/netmeta.pdf (accessed on 9 November 2019).
19. Van Valkenhoef, G.; Kuiper, J. Gemtc: Network Meta-Analysis Using Bayesian Methods. Available online: https://cran.r-project.org/web/packages/gemtc/gemtc.pdf (accessed on 9 November 2019).
20. Yang, Z.; Hackshaw, A.; Feng, Q.; Fu, X.; Zhang, Y.; Mao, C.; Tang, J. Comparison of gefitinib, erlotinib and afatinib in non-small cell lung cancer: A meta-analysis. *Int. J. Cancer* **2017**, *140*, 2805–2819. [CrossRef] [PubMed]
21. Lin, J.Z.; Ma, S.K.; Wu, S.X.; Yu, S.H.; Li, X.Y. A network meta-analysis of nonsmall-cell lung cancer patients with an activating EGFR mutation: Should osimertinib be the first-line treatment? *Medicine* **2018**, *97*, e11569. [CrossRef] [PubMed]
22. DiBonaventura, M.; Higginbottom, K.; Meyers, A.; Morimoto, Y.; Ilacqua, J. Comparative effectiveness of crizotinib among ALK+ NSCLC patients across the United States, Western Europe, and Japan. *Value Health* **2016**, *19*, A711. [CrossRef]
23. Fan, J.; Fong, T.; Xia, Z.; Zhang, J.; Luo, P. The efficacy and safety of ALK inhibitors in the treatment of ALK-positive non-small cell lung cancer: A network meta-analysis. *Cancer Med.* **2018**, *7*, 4993–5005. [CrossRef] [PubMed]
24. Dagogo-Jack, I.; Shaw, A.T. Crizotinib resistance: Implications for therapeutic strategies. *Ann. Oncol.* **2016**, *27*, iii42–iii50. [CrossRef] [PubMed]

25. Gainor, J.F.; Dardaei, L.; Yoda, S.; Friboulet, L.; Leshchiner, I.; Katayama, R.; Dagogo-Jack, I.; Gadgeel, S.; Schultz, K.; Singh, M.; et al. Molecular mechanisms of resistance to first- and second-generation ALK inhibitors in ALK-rearranged lung cancer. *Cancer Discov.* **2016**, *6*, 1118–1133. [CrossRef] [PubMed]
26. Hoang, T.; Myung, S.K.; Pham, T.T.; Park, B. Efficacy of Crizotinib, Ceritinib, and Alectinib in ALK-Positive Non-Small Cell Lung Cancer Treatment: A Meta-Analysis of Clinical Trials. *Cancers* **2020**, *12*, 526. [CrossRef] [PubMed]

Permissions

All chapters in this book were first published by MDPI; hereby published with permission under the Creative Commons Attribution License or equivalent. Every chapter published in this book has been scrutinized by our experts. Their significance has been extensively debated. The topics covered herein carry significant findings which will fuel the growth of the discipline. They may even be implemented as practical applications or may be referred to as a beginning point for another development.

The contributors of this book come from diverse backgrounds, making this book a truly international effort. This book will bring forth new frontiers with its revolutionizing research information and detailed analysis of the nascent developments around the world.

We would like to thank all the contributing authors for lending their expertise to make the book truly unique. They have played a crucial role in the development of this book. Without their invaluable contributions this book wouldn't have been possible. They have made vital efforts to compile up to date information on the varied aspects of this subject to make this book a valuable addition to the collection of many professionals and students.

This book was conceptualized with the vision of imparting up-to-date information and advanced data in this field. To ensure the same, a matchless editorial board was set up. Every individual on the board went through rigorous rounds of assessment to prove their worth. After which they invested a large part of their time researching and compiling the most relevant data for our readers.

The editorial board has been involved in producing this book since its inception. They have spent rigorous hours researching and exploring the diverse topics which have resulted in the successful publishing of this book. They have passed on their knowledge of decades through this book. To expedite this challenging task, the publisher supported the team at every step. A small team of assistant editors was also appointed to further simplify the editing procedure and attain best results for the readers.

Apart from the editorial board, the designing team has also invested a significant amount of their time in understanding the subject and creating the most relevant covers. They scrutinized every image to scout for the most suitable representation of the subject and create an appropriate cover for the book.

The publishing team has been an ardent support to the editorial, designing and production team. Their endless efforts to recruit the best for this project, has resulted in the accomplishment of this book. They are a veteran in the field of academics and their pool of knowledge is as vast as their experience in printing. Their expertise and guidance has proved useful at every step. Their uncompromising quality standards have made this book an exceptional effort. Their encouragement from time to time has been an inspiration for everyone.

The publisher and the editorial board hope that this book will prove to be a valuable piece of knowledge for researchers, students, practitioners and scholars across the globe.

List of Contributors

Alice Blondel, Amine Benberghout and Rémy Pedeux
INSERM U1242, Chemistry Oncogenesis Stress and Signaling, CLCC Eugène Marquis, 35033 Rennes, France

Charles Ricordel
INSERM U1242, Chemistry Oncogenesis Stress and Signaling, CLCC Eugène Marquis, 35033 Rennes, France
CHU Rennes, Service de Pneumologie, Université de Rennes 1, 35033 Rennes, France

Federico Nichetti, Francesca Ligorio, Emma Zattarin, Diego Signorelli, Arsela Prelaj, Claudia Proto, Giulia Galli, Giulia Apollonio and Roberto Ferrara
Department of Medical Oncology, Fondazione IRCCS Istituto Nazionale dei Tumori, 20133 Milan, Italy

Marina Chiara Garassino and Giuseppe Lo Russo
Department of Medical Oncology, Fondazione IRCCS Istituto Nazionale dei Tumori, 20133 Milan, Italy
Unit of Thoracic Oncology, Medical Oncology Department 1, Fondazione IRCCS Istituto Nazionale dei Tumori, 20133 Milan, Italy

Antonio Marra
Department of Medical Oncology, Istituto Europeo di Oncologia, 20141 Milan, Italy

Luca Porcu
Department of Oncology, IRCCS Istituto di Ricerche Farmacologiche Mario Negri, 20156 Milan, Italy

Filippo de Braud
Department of Medical Oncology, Fondazione IRCCS Istituto Nazionale dei Tumori, 20133 Milan, Italy
Department of Oncology and Hemato-Oncology, University of Milan, 20122 Milan, Italy

Hwani Ryu
Division of Radiation Biomedical Research, Korea Institute of Radiological & Medical Sciences (KIRAMS), Seoul 01812, Korea
Department of Biology, Korea University, Seoul 02841, Korea

Toshio Oyama
Department of Pathology, Yamanashi Central Hospital, Yamanashi 400-8506, Japan

Hyo Jeong Kim, Jie-Young Song, Sang-Gu Hwang, Jae-Sung Kim and Jiyeon Ahn
Division of Radiation Biomedical Research, Korea Institute of Radiological & Medical Sciences (KIRAMS), Seoul 01812, Korea

Joon Kim
Department of Biology, Korea University, Seoul 02841, Korea

Thi Hong Nhung Bui and Hyun-Kyung Choi
Department of Medicinal Chemistry, Jungwon University, Goesan 28024, Korea

Hiroshi Gyotoku, Hiroyuki Yamaguchi, Hiroshi Ishimoto, Hirokazu Taniguchi, Hiroaki Senju, Katsumi Nakatomi, Noriho Sakamoto, Yasushi Obase and Hiroshi Mukae
Department of Respiratory Medicine, Nagasaki University Graduate School of Biomedical Sciences, Nagasaki University, Nagasaki 852-8523, Japan

Shuntaro Sato
Clinical Research Center, Nagasaki University Hospital, Nagasaki 852-8501, Japan

Tomoyuki Kakugawa
Department of Respiratory Medicine, Nagasaki University Graduate School of Biomedical Sciences, Nagasaki University, Nagasaki 852-8523, Japan
Department of Pulmonology and Gerontology, Yamaguchi University Graduate School of Medicine, Ube 755-0046, Japan

Minoru Fukuda
Department of Respiratory Medicine, Nagasaki University Graduate School of Biomedical Sciences, Nagasaki University, Nagasaki 852-8523, Japan
Clinical Oncology Center, Nagasaki University Hospital, Nagasaki 852-8501, Japan

Hiroshi Soda
Department of Respiratory Medicine, Sasebo City General Hospital, Nagasaki 857-8511, Japan

Kazuto Ashizawa
Clinical Oncology Center, Nagasaki University Hospital, Nagasaki 852-8501, Japan

Rumi Higuchi, Daichi Shikata and Sotaro Otake
Lung Cancer and Respiratory Disease Center, Yamanashi Central Hospital, Yamanashi 400-8506, Japan

Takahiro Nakagomi, Taichiro Goto and Yujiro Yokoyama
Lung Cancer and Respiratory Disease Center, Yamanashi Central Hospital, Yamanashi 400-8506, Japan
Department of Surgery, School of Medicine, Keio University, Tokyo 160-8582, Japan

Yosuke Hirotsu, Kenji Amemiya and Hitoshi Mochizuki
Genome Analysis Center, Yamanashi Central Hospital, Yamanashi 400-8506, Japan

Masao Omata
Genome Analysis Center, Yamanashi Central Hospital, Yamanashi 400-8506, Japan
Department of Gastroenterology, The University of Tokyo Hospital, Tokyo 113-8655, Japan

Inês Maria Guerreiro, Ana Rodrigues and Marta Soares
Department of Medical Oncology, Portuguese Oncology Institute of Porto (IPO-Porto), R. Dr. António Bernardino de Almeida, 4200-072 Porto, Portugal

Daniela Barros-Silva
Cancer Biology and Epigenetics Group, IPO Porto Research Center (GEBC CI-IPOP), Portuguese Oncology Institute of Porto (IPO Porto) & Porto Comprehensive Cancer Center (P.CCC), R. Dr. António Bernardino de Almeida, 4200-072 Porto, Portugal

Paula Lopes, Mariana Cantante and Ana Luísa Cunha
Cancer Biology and Epigenetics Group, IPO Porto Research Center (GEBC CI-IPOP), Portuguese Oncology Institute of Porto (IPO Porto) & Porto Comprehensive Cancer Center (P.CCC), R. Dr. António Bernardino de Almeida, 4200-072 Porto, Portugal
Department of Pathology, Portuguese Oncology Institute of Porto (IPOP), R. Dr. António Bernardino de Almeida, 4200-072 Porto, Portugal

João Lobo and Rui Henrique
Cancer Biology and Epigenetics Group, IPO Porto Research Center (GEBC CI-IPOP), Portuguese Oncology Institute of Porto (IPO Porto) & Porto Comprehensive Cancer Center (P.CCC), R. Dr. António Bernardino de Almeida, 4200-072 Porto, Portugal
Department of Pathology, Portuguese Oncology Institute of Porto (IPOP), R. Dr. António Bernardino de Almeida, 4200-072 Porto, Portugal
Department of Pathology and Molecular Immunology, Institute of Biomedical Sciences Abel Salazar, University of Porto (ICBAS-UP), Rua Jorge de Viterbo Ferreira, 228, 4050-313 Porto, Portugal

Luís Antunes
Cancer Epidemiology Group, IPO Porto Research Center (CI-IPOP), Portuguese Oncology Institute of Porto (IPO-Porto), R. Dr. António Bernardino de Almeida, 4200-072 Porto, Portugal

Carmen Jerónimo
Cancer Biology and Epigenetics Group, IPO Porto Research Center (GEBC CI-IPOP), Portuguese Oncology Institute of Porto (IPO Porto) & Porto Comprehensive Cancer Center (P.CCC), R. Dr. António Bernardino de Almeida, 4200-072 Porto, Portugal
Department of Pathology and Molecular Immunology, Institute of Biomedical Sciences Abel Salazar, University of Porto (ICBAS-UP), Rua Jorge de Viterbo Ferreira, 228, 4050-313 Porto, Portugal

Kosuke Hashimoto, Ou Yamaguchi, Atsuto Mouri, Ayako Shiono, Yu Miura, Yoshitake Murayama, Kunihiko Kobayashi and Hiroshi Kagamu
Department of Respiratory Medicine, Comprehensive Cancer Center, International Medical Center, Saitama Medical University, 1397-1 Yamane, Hidaka-City, Saitama 350-1298, Japan

Ichiei Kuji
Department of Nuclear Medicine, Comprehensive Cancer Center, International Medical Center, Saitama Medical University, 1397-1 Yamane, Hidaka-City, Saitama 350-1298, Japan

Matteo Canale, Elisa Chiadini and Paola Ulivi
Biosciences Laboratory, Istituto Scientifico Romagnolo per lo Studio e la Cura dei Tumori (IRST) IRCCS, 47014 Meldola, Italy

Elisabetta Petracci
Biostatistics and Clinical Trials Unit, Istituto Scientifico Romagnolo per lo Studio e la Cura dei Tumori (IRST) IRCCS, 47014 Meldola, Italy

Angelo Delmonte, Giuseppe Bronte, Alberto Verlicchi, Marco Angelo Burgio and Lucio Crinò
Department of Medical Oncology, Istituto Scientifico Romagnolo per lo Studio e la Cura dei Tumori (IRST) IRCCS, 47014 Meldola, Italy

Vienna Ludovini, Sara Baglivo and Giulio Metro
Department of Medical Oncology, Santa Maria della Misericordia Hospital, 06129 Perugia, Italy

Alessandra Dubini
Department of Pathology, Morgagni-Pierantoni Hospital, 47121 Forlì, Italy

Maximilian Papi
Department of Medical Oncology, Per gli Infermi Hospital, Rimini 47923, Italy

Nicoletta De Luigi
UOS Oncology, Istituto per la Sicurezza Sociale, State Hospital, Cailungo 47893, San Marino, Italy

Rita Chiari
Department of Medical Oncology, Ospedali Riuniti Padova Sud "M. Teresa di Calcutta", ULSS6 Euganea, 35131 Padova, Italy

Lorenza Landi
Department of Medical Oncology, S. Maria delle Croci Hospital, 48121 Ravenna, Italy

Hisao Imai and Koichi Minato
Division of Respiratory Medicine, Gunma Prefectural Cancer Center, Ota 373-8550, Japan

Kyoichi Kaira
Department of Innovative Immune-Oncology Therapeutics, Gunma University Graduate School of Medicine, Maebashi 371-8511, Japan
Department of Respiratory Medicine, Comprehensive Cancer Center, International Medical Center, Saitama University Hospital, Hidaka 350-1298, Japan

Hideki Endoh
Department of Thoracic Surgery, Saku Central Hospital Advanced Care Center, Saku 385-0051, Japan

Kazuyoshi Imaizumi and Yasuhiro Goto
Department of Respiratory Medicine, Fujita Health University, Toyoake 470-1192, Japan

Mitsuhiro Kamiyoshihara
Department of General Thoracic Surgery, Japanese Red Cross Maebashi Hospital, Maebashi 371-0811, Japan

Takayuki Kosaka
Division of Thoracic Surgery, Takasaki General Medical Center, Takasaki 370-0829, Japan

Toshiki Yajima and Ken Shirabe
Department of Innovative Immune-Oncology Therapeutics, Gunma University Graduate School of Medicine, Maebashi 371-8511, Japan
Department of General Surgical Science, Gunma University Graduate School of Medicine, Maebashi 371-8511, Japan

Yoichi Ohtaki
Department of General Surgical Science, Gunma University Graduate School of Medicine, Maebashi 371-8511, Japan

Takashi Osaki
Department of Respiratory Medicine, Shibukawa Medical Center, Shibukawa 377-0280, Japan

Yoshihito Kogure
Department of Respiratory Medicine, Nagoya Medical Center, Nagoya 460-0001, Japan

Shigebumi Tanaka
Department of Respiratory Surgery, Isesaki Municipal Hospital, Isesaki 372-0817, Japan

Atsushi Fujita
Division of Thoracic Surgery, Gunma Prefectural Cancer Center, Ota 373-8550, Japan

Tetsunari Oyama
Department of Diagnostic Pathology, Gunma University Graduate School of Medicine, Maebashi 371-8511, Japan

Takayuki Asao
Big Data Center for Integrative Analysis, Gunma University Initiative for Advance Research, Maebashi 371-8511, Japan

Yuki Katayama, Takayuki Shimamoto, Masahiro Iwasaku, Nobuyo Tamiya, Takako Mouri, Naoko Okura, Yoshie Morimoto and Yoshiko Kaneko
Department of Pulmonary Medicine, Graduate School of Medical Science, Kyoto Prefectural University of Medicine, Kyoto 602-8566, Japan

Junji Uchino and Tadaaki Yamada
Department of Respiratory Medicine, Kyoto Prefectural University of Medicine, Kyoto 6020841, Japan
Department of Pulmonary Medicine, Graduate School of Medical Science, Kyoto Prefectural University of Medicine, Kyoto 602-8566, Japan

Takahiro Yamada
Department of Pulmonary Medicine, Matsushita Memorial Hospital, Moriguchi 570-8540, Japan

Shinsuke Shiotsu
Department of Pulmonary Medicine, Japanese Red Cross Kyoto Daiichi Hospital, Kyoto 605-0981, Japan

Yusuke Chihara
Department of Pulmonary Medicine, Uji-Tokushukai Medical Center, Uji 611-0041, Japan
Department of Pulmonary Medicine, Graduate School of Medical Science, Kyoto Prefectural University of Medicine, Kyoto 602-8566, Japan

Osamu Hiranuma
Department of Pulmonary Medicine, Otsu City Hospital, Otsu 520-0804, Japan
Department of Respiratory Medicine, Otsu City Hospital, Shiga 520-0804, Japan

Mai Asano and Michiaki Fukui
Department of Endocrinology and Metabolism, Graduate School of Medical Science, Kyoto Prefectural University of Medicine, Kyoto 602-8566, Japan

Jorge García-González, Juan Ruiz-Bañobre and Luis León-Mateos
Medical Oncology Department, University Clinical Hospital of Santiago de Compostela and Translational Medical Oncology Group (Oncomet), Health Research Institute of Santiago de Compostela (IDIS), CIBERONC, 15706 Santiago de Compostela, Spain

Francisco J. Afonso-Afonso
Medical Oncology Department, Complexo Hospitalario Universitario de Ferrol, 15405 A Coruña, Spain

Margarita Amenedo-Gancedo
Medical Oncology Department, Centro Oncológico de Galicia, 15009 A Coruña, Spain

María del Carmen Areses-Manrique and José Luis Fírvida Pérez
Medical Oncology Department, Complexo Hospitalario Universitario de Ourense, 32005 Ourense, Spain

Begoña Campos-Balea and Natalia Fernández-Núñez
Medical Oncology Department, Hospital Universitario Lucus Augusti, 27003 Lugo, Spain

Joaquín Casal-Rubio and Martín Lázaro-Quintela
Medical Oncology Department, Complexo Hospitalario Universitario de Vigo, 36213 Vigo, Spain

Diego Pérez Parente, Leonardo Crama and Pedro Ruiz-Gracia
Lung Cancer Medical Department, Roche Farma S.A., 28042 Madrid, Spain

Lucía Santomé-Couto
Medical Oncology Department, Hospital POVISA, 36211 Vigo, Spain

Yujin Kim, Bo Bin Lee, Dongho Kim and Duk-Hwan Kim
Department of Molecular Cell Biology, Sungkyunkwan University School of Medicine, Suwon 440-746, Korea
Department of Molecular Cell Biology, Sungkyunkwan University School of Medicine, Suwon 16419, Korea

Sangwon Um
Department of Internal Medicine, Samsung Medical Center, Sungkyunkwan University School of Medicine, Seoul 135-710, Korea

Eun Yoon Cho and Joungho Han
Department of Pathology, Samsung Medical Center, Sungkyunkwan University School of Medicine, Seoul 135-710, Korea
Department of Pathology, Samsung Medical Center, Sungkyunkwan University School of Medicine, Seoul 06351, Korea

Young Mog Shim
Department of Thoracic and Cardiovascular Surgery, Samsung Medical Center, Sungkyunkwan University, School of Medicine, Seoul 06351, Korea

Akira Nakao and Masaki Fujita
Department of Respiratory Medicine, Faculty of Medicine, Fukuoka University, Fukuoka 814-0180, Japan

Chikara Sakaguchi
Department of Pulmonary Medicine, Rakuwakai Otowa Hospital, Kyoto 607-8062, Japan

Tomoyuki Araya
Department of Respiratory Medicine, National Hospital Organization, Kanazawa Medical Center, Ishikawa 920-8650, Japan

Noriya Hiraoka
Department of Respiratory Medicine, Japanese Red Cross Kyoto Daiichi Hospital, Kyoto 605-0981, Japan

Tamotsu Ishizuka
Third Department of Internal Medicine, Faculty of Medical Sciences, University of Fukui, Fukui 910-1193, Japan

Hidetaka Uramoto
Department of Thoracic Surgery, Kanazawa Medical University, Ishikawa 920-0293, Japan

Hisao Imai
Division of Respiratory Medicine, Gunma Prefectural Cancer Center, Gunma 373-8550, Japan

Takayuki Takeda
Department of Respiratory Medicine, Japanese Red Cross Society Kyoto Daini Hospital, Kyoto 602-8026, Japan
Department of Pulmonary Medicine, Japanese Red Cross Kyoto Daini Hospital, Kyoto 602-8026, Japan

Masayuki Kawasaki
Department of Respiratory Medicine, National Hospital Organization, Omuta National Hospital, Fukuoka 837-0911, Japan

Noboru Hattori
Department of Molecular and Internal Medicine, Graduate School of Biomedical & Health Sciences, Hiroshima University, Hiroshima 734-8553, Japan

Keita Nakatomi
Department of Respiratory Medicine, Kyushu Central Hospital of the Mutual Aid Association of Public School Teachers, Fukuoka 815-8588, Japan

Kiyoaki Uryu
Department of Respiratory Medicine, Yao Tokushukai General Hospital, Osaka 581-0011, Japan

Minoru Fukuda
Second Department of Internal Medicine, Nagasaki University Hospital, Nagasaki 852-8523, Japan

Yasuki Uchida
Department of Respiratory Medicine, Shiga University of Medical Science Hospital, Shiga 520-2192, Japan

Toshihide Yokoyama
Department of Respiratory Medicine, Kurashiki Central Hospital, Okayama 710-8602, Japan

Masaya Akai
Department of Respiratory Medicine, Japanese Red Cross Fukui Hospital, Fukui 918-8501, Japan

Tadashi Mio
Division of Respiratory Medicine, Center for Respiratory Diseases, National Hospital Organization Kyoto Medical Center, Kyoto 612-8555, Japan

Seiji Nagashima
Department of Respiratory Medicine, National Hospital Organization Nagasaki Medical Center, Nagasaki 856-0835, Japan

Helena Linardou
4th Oncology Department, Metropolitan Hospital, 18547 Athens, Greece

Kenichi Yoshimura
Center for Integrated Medical Research, Hiroshima University Hospital, Hiroshima University, Hiroshima 734-8553, Japan

Maria Francesca Alvisi and Eliana Rulli
Laboratory of Methodology for Clinical Research, Department of Oncology, Istituto di Ricerche Farmacologiche Mario Negri IRCCS, 20156 Milan, Italy

Monica Ganzinelli
Unit of Thoracic Oncology, Medical Oncology Department 1, Fondazione IRCCS Istituto Nazionale dei Tumori, 20133 Milan, Italy

Elisa Caiola, Gloriana Ndembe, Massimo Broggini and Mirko Marabese
Laboratory of Molecular Pharmacology, Department of Oncology, Istituto di Ricerche Farmacologiche Mario Negri IRCCS, 20156 Milan, Italy

Fabiana Letizia Cecere
Division of Medical Oncology 1, IRCCS Regina Elena National Cancer Institute, 00144 Rome, Italy

Anna Cecilia Bettini
UO Oncologia Medica, ASST Papa Giovanni XXIII, 24127 Bergamo, Italy

Amanda Psyrri
Section of Oncology, Department of Internal Medicine, Attikon Hospital, National Kapodistrian University of Athens, 12462 Athens, Greece

Michele Milella
Department of Medicine, Section of Medical Oncology, University and Hospital Trust of Verona, 37126 Verona, Italy

Alessandra Fabbri
Department of Pathology and Laboratory Medicine, Fondazione IRCCS Istituto Nazionale dei Tumori, 20133 Milan, Italy

Marcella De Maglie and Pierpaolo Romanelli
Mouse & Animal Pathology Lab, Fondazione Filarete, 20139 Milan, Italy
Department of Veterinary Medicine, University of Milan, 20122 Milan, Italy

Seokjin Haam
Department of Thoracic and Cardiovascular Surgery, Ajou University School of Medicine, Suwon 16499, Korea

Samuel Murray
Biomarker Solutions Ltd., London EC1V 2NX, UK

Koichi Takayama
Research Institute for Diseases of the Chest, Graduate School of Medical Sciences, Kyushu University, Fukuoka 8190395, Japan
Department of Respiratory Medicine, Kyoto Prefectural University of Medicine, Kyoto 6020841, Japan
Department of Pulmonary Medicine, Graduate School of Medical Science, Kyoto Prefectural University of Medicine, Kyoto 602-8566, Japan

Shoji Tokunaga
Medical Information Center, Kyushu University Hospital, Fukuoka 8190395, Japan

Tomotoshi Imanaga
Department of respiratory disease, Nippon Steel Yawata Memorial Hospital, Kitakyushu 8058508, Japan

Ryotaro Morinaga
Department of Medical Oncology, Oita University Faculty of Medicine, Yuhu 8795593, Japan

Noriyuki Ebi
Department of Respiratory Medicine, Iizuka Hospital, Iizuka, 8208505, Japan

Sho Saeki
Department of Respiratory Medicine, Kumamoto University Hospital, Kumamoto 8608556, Japan

Kazuya Matsukizono
Department of Internal Medicine, Kagoshima City Hospital, Kagoshima 8908544, Japan

Hiroshi Wataya
Department of Internal Medicine, Saiseikai Fukuoka General Hospital, Fukuoka 8100001, Japan

Pildu Jeong and Wun-Jae Kim
Department of Urology, College of Medicine, Chungbuk National University, Cheongju 28644, Korea

Young Wha Koh and Jae-Ho Han
Department of Pathology, Ajou University School of Medicine, Suwon 16499, Korea

Dohun Kim
Department of Thoracic and Cardiovascular Surgery, Chungbuk National University Hospital, College of Medicine, Chungbuk National University, Cheongju 28644, Korea

Hyun Woo Lee
Department of Hematology-Oncology, Ajou University School of Medicine, Suwon 16499, Korea

Ok-Jun Lee
Department of Pathology, College of Medicine, Chungbuk National University, Cheongju 28644, Korea

Yoichi Nakanishi
Research Institute for Diseases of the Chest, Graduate School of Medical Sciences, Kyushu University, Fukuoka 8190395, Japan

Chih-Yu Chen, Bing-Ru Wu, Chia-Hung Chen, Wen-Chien Cheng and Chih-Yen Tu
Division of Pulmonary and Critical Care Medicine, Department of Internal Medicine, China Medical University Hospital, Taichung 40447, Taiwan School of Medicine, China Medical University, Taichung 40402, Taiwan

Wei-Chun Chen and Te-Chun Hsia
Division of Pulmonary and Critical Care Medicine, Department of Internal Medicine, China Medical University Hospital, Taichung 40447, Taiwan
Department of Respiratory Therapy, China Medical University, Taichung 40402, Taiwan
Hyperbaric oxygen therapy center, China Medical University Hospital, Taichung 40447, Taiwan

Wei-Chih Liao
Division of Pulmonary and Critical Care Medicine, Department of Internal Medicine, China Medical University Hospital, Taichung 40447, Taiwan
School of Medicine, China Medical University, Taichung 40402, Taiwan
Hyperbaric oxygen therapy center, China Medical University Hospital, Taichung 40447, Taiwan

Chih-Yi Chen
Department of Surgery, Chung Shan Medical University Hospital, Taichung 40201, Taiwan

Tung Hoang and Jeongseon Kim
Department of Cancer Biomedical Science, National Cancer Center Graduate School of Cancer Science and Policy, Goyang 10408, Korea

Seung-Kwon Myung
Department of Cancer Biomedical Science, National Cancer Center Graduate School of Cancer Science and Policy, Goyang 10408, Korea
Division of Cancer Epidemiology and Management, National Cancer Center Research Institute, Goyang 10408, Korea
Department of Family Medicine and Center for Cancer Prevention and Detection, National Cancer Center Hospital, Goyang 10408, Korea

Thu Thi Pham
Health Data Science Program, Institute of Public Health, Charité Universitätsmedizin Berlin, 10117 Berlin, Germany
Molecular Epidemiology Research Group, Max Delbrück Center for Molecular Medicine (MDC), 13125 Berlin, Germany

Woong Ju
Department of Obstetrics and Gynecology, EwhaWomans University College of Medicine, Seoul 07804, Korea
Medical Research Institute, EwhaWomans University College of Medicine, Seoul 07804, Korea

Index

www.ingramcontent.com/pod-product-compliance
Lightning Source LLC
LaVergne TN
LVHW080927210926
848485LV00004B/749